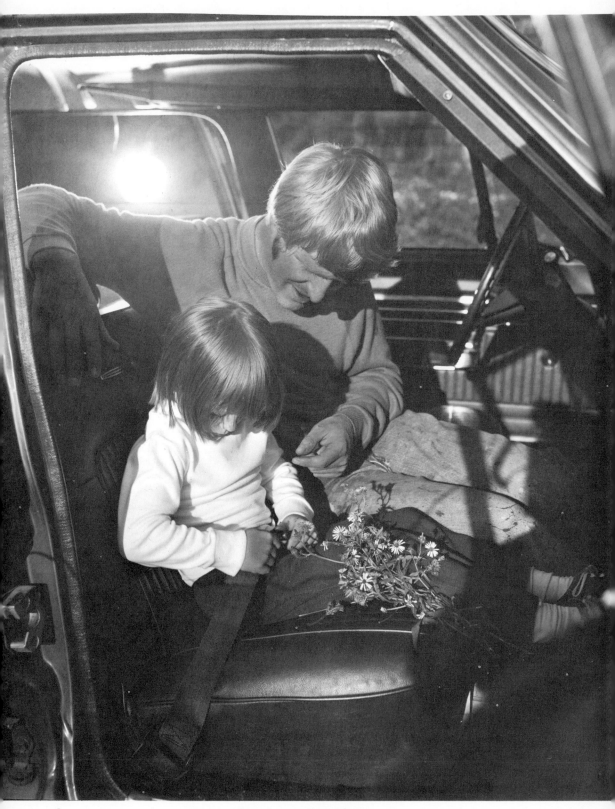

—Buckling up for safety—

HEALTH EDUCATION
IN THE
ELEMENTARY SCHOOL

FOURTH EDITION

CARL E. WILLGOOSE, Ed.D. BOSTON UNIVERSITY

1974 W. B. SAUNDERS COMPANY
PHILADELPHIA • LONDON • TORONTO

W. B. Saunders Company: West Washington Square
Philadelphia, Pa. 19105

12 Dyott Street
London, WC1A 1DB

833 Oxford Street
Toronto 18, Ontario

Health Education in the Elementary School   ISBN 0-7216-9367-9

Last digit is the print number: 9   8   7   6   5   4   3   2   1

PREFACE
TO THE FOURTH EDITION

It was Prometheus the "forethinker," that fire-bearing Titan, who sought a "heroic" civilization in which the unyielding spirit of mankind could be expressed. Hesiod, Aeschylus, and Plato proclaimed the Promethean will in terms of human power, hopes, and the intent of heaven reconciled at last. This may be the ultimate state of health and well-being that emerges in the ideal. It may also mean that the multidimensional nature of health is so all-encompassing that the present security as well as the future of the society itself lies in the education of school children.

No longer will just any education do. As the President's Committee on Health Education has cautioned, it is now imperative to *educate* for healthful living, for it is no longer possible to stem the tide of human illness and despair by improved medical and surgical techniques, more hospitals and social workers, and more sophisticated health care centers. The message calls for prevention. The time is for learning—and at an early age. It is time for a total effort—for teachers and their community of citizens to work together.

There is no person in the American public school system in a better position to make a significant contribution to the health of school children than the classroom teacher in the elementary school. This teacher holds the key for improving child health: with her interest, enthusiasm, and professional understanding, the school health program moves ahead; without her support the health program never really gets started.

In the belief that the potential ability of the classroom teacher is great, this edition sets forth several means to an end. The early chapters are concerned with the general topic of school health and the health status of the child. They stress the detection and referral role of the teacher and the unique opportunity to function efficiently with the school health service personnel and other health-related groups in the community. Then follows a discussion of the school environment and its bearing on general behavior and learning. No attempt has been made in these early chapters to be complete in dealing with school health services and healthful school environment. These are major areas of study in themselves. They are briefly presented here so that the elementary school teacher can see the relationship they have to total school health and their connection with health instruction in and about the classroom.

The major part of the book is specifically concerned with health instruction and the movement away from health teaching as a "do-gooder" activity to a carefully organized and programmed part of the total school curriculum. It is designed to furnish the elementary school teacher with a quantity of orderly and practical information to be of help in planning, carrying out and evaluating health teaching. The concern is for inner-city children as well as those from rural and suburban areas. The direction throughout the text is toward a broad program of essential health topics, taught in a warm and effective style, that will not only transmit ideas but also clarify student values and affect student behavioral patterns.

A great many sources of information have been used, and the research and curriculum materials of several individuals and organizations have been employed to make this edition a thoroughly up-to-date text. Materials which appear on p. 124 of this publication were used by permission of, and copyrighted in 1970 by, Minnesota Mining and Manufacturing Company.

Carl E. Willgoose

CONTENTS

9

10

11

1 THE NATURE AND SCOPE OF HEALTH EDUCATION

"Not even an army with banners flying is as powerful as an idea whose hour has come."

—Carlyle

When the President's Committee on Health Education became operational in early 1972 it was acknowledged with some degree of concern that because of the major health problems in the country the health care of the citizenry could no longer be assured through purely medical approaches. More specifically it was made clear that continued biomedical advances and improved health services to the population will continue to fall short of meeting individual and community needs. Simply stated, there are too many people and too many health problems. Consequently, the Committee recommended that from then on the health education of the public must be a prime consideration for health maintenance.

Educating for health is hardly a new idea, but it is, as Carlyle so fittingly put it, "... an idea whose hour has come."

ROADMAP FOR SURVIVAL

In any age the capacity or wherewithal *to do* has been the *sine qua non*, the indispensable quality in man. With this level of wellness it is possible to strive and struggle through life seeking not only to survive, but to achieve a certain happiness. This is accomplished "not by acquiescing with what is but by struggling for something else, not by accepting but by doing, not by receiving but by

giving, not by rest but by activity."[1] Any stable happiness, therefore, is related to the ability of the organism to be active. Weak muscles, poor hearing or vision, diseased tissues, or an emotional disturbance weaken the organism and curtail its ability to be active and survive.

Fortunately, there is more to a life in a lifetime than mere survival, because survival is not an end in itself. To his credit John Garcia asks "Survival for what?" In answer he suggests a rational purpose relative to man's ability to predict and control the total environment.[2] He quickly points out that to do this in the years ahead one must set as a personal goal the ultimate expansion of *awareness*. The deliberate choice to expand awareness is an end in itself—and happiness the prime effect.

The significance of the Garcia message is that it points in a direction that a nation of people will have to go if they are to go anywhere at all. The heightened awareness of the human organism that Garcia speaks of will be advanced when there is a desire to improve health status toward a maximum level. However, it is only when individuals are sensitive to

[1]Lawton, Shailer U., and Frederick R. Rogers. *Educational Paths to Virtue—I.* Newton, Mass.: Pleides Co., 1937, p. 47.

[2]Garcia, John David. *The Moral Society: A Rational Alternative to Death.* New York: Julian, 1971.

1

the preciousness of life and the potentialities of a fully awakened human being that they will consider high-level wellness worthy of serious attention. After all, it is pretty obvious that the half sick body will make accomplishments and partly adjust to almost any kind of punishment and deprivation, and still survive at a subclinical level. Yet, when real awareness takes hold even the skeptic speaks out. When one experiences illness which interferes with his immediate ambitions he is apt to express himself somewhat the way Schopenhauer did after getting out of a sickbed:

"The greatest of follies is to neglect one's health for other virtues in life."

THE FULL VIEW OF HEALTH

It is literally impossible to expect to achieve a state of high-level wellness if children and adults continue to take the narrow view and think of health simply as a condition in which there is no immediate ache, strain, or infection. It is for this very reason that the World Health Organization of the United Nations defines health in a comprehensive way as "a state of complete physical, mental and social well-being, and not merely the absence of disease and infirmity."[3]

The real meaning of the WHO definition is to be found in the direction it gives to life and living. Implied is that man's health potential is on a continuum, with near death at one end and optimal health at the other. It is frequently a fluctuating state. Hoyman classifies man's health status into five levels.[4]

The observation that a state of health has far-reaching consequences was clearly illustrated by Julian Huxley, when he said that "... the highest and most sacred duty of man is seen as the proper utilization of the untapped resources of

[3]Constitution of the World Health Organization, *Chronicles of the World Health Organization, 1*:29–43; Geneva: World Health Organization, 1947, p. 3.

[4]Hoyman, Howard S. "Our Modern Concept of Health," *Journal of School Health, 32*:253–264, September 1962.

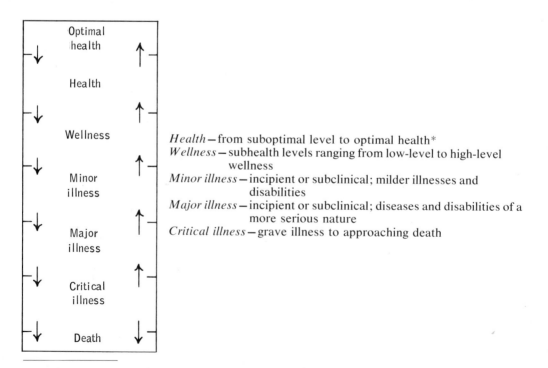

Health—from suboptimal level to optimal health*
Wellness—subhealth levels ranging from low-level to high-level wellness
Minor illness—incipient or subclinical; milder illnesses and disabilities
Major illness—incipient or subclinical; diseases and disabilities of a more serious nature
Critical illness—grave illness to approaching death

*The level at which an individual's living approaches his full desirable potentialities (e.g., Dr. Albert Schweitzer, Grandma Moses, Konrad Adenauer).

human beings."[5] Involved here is the whole of man's capacity for expression. It is multidimensional—anthropological, biological, psychological, economic, and even political. This gives support to the concept of an "ecology of health" where all human relationships between a community and its environment are health related. Moreover, there is a personal responsibility of the individual for his own health and the health of the community. As far back as the seventeenth century John Donne expressed this viewpoint beautifully when he stated in part: "No man is an Island, entire of itself; every man is a piece of the Continent, a part of the main . . . any man's death diminishes me, because I am involved in mankind."

HEALTH FROM PAST TO PRESENT

Through the years there has been overwhelming support for government and school-community programs designed to raise the health of the citizenry. Strong recommendations have come from such groups as the American Medical Association, the American Public Health Association, the Educational Policies Commission of the National Education Association, and the White House Conference on Health. It was at this conference that both private and public health physicians reported that "educated patients" are much better patients; they understand something about their own health and follow the recommendations of their physicians, and recover sooner from illness.

Man's apparent concern for his health, welfare, and survival has not always been so noticeable and scientific as it appears to be today.

The gradual decrease over the centuries of magic, guesswork, incantation, and superstition, together with the corresponding rise in applied scientific knowledge represents a magnificent process of

slow evolution. Sound ideas were practiced side by side with unsound treatments and rituals. As in all ages of man, only a minority knew the truth, and they had to work uphill in the face of customs, habits, and ignorance. In prehistoric times, and even today in some parts of the world, evil spirits were "scared away" because of the general belief that they caused sickness. Yet these same prehistoric people discovered that certain herbs and other plants were quite good for numerous disorders. As far back as 4500 B.C. along the Nile in Egypt, Imhotep was practicing medicine in Luxor and Karnak. By 2500 B.C., surgical operations were being performed with the "help" of Thoth, the god of medicine. Today, thousands of Egyptians in the same region wear the scarab beetle charm about the neck to ward off disease and encourage fertility.

The constant struggle for light over darkness has been, and always will be, a continuing one. This is well demonstrated by early Hebrew law relating to communicable disease, isolation, quarantine and cleanliness. The books of the Bible—Leviticus and Deuteronomy—are rich in illustrations of early health recommendations and practices. This is further illustrated by a 500 year period of ancient Greek and Roman history (300 B.C. to 200 A.D.). It was Hippocrates who taught that each disease arises from a natural cause. It was the Athenian youth who took good care of their bodies and worshiped the goddess Hygeia under the guidance of priest-physicians. It was Galen, the Greek physician and writer, who experimented widely in physiology but was looked down upon by the Roman citizens of the period. Yet the Romans were really interested in health and developed many practical surgical instruments to be used on wounded gladiators and soldiers. They made more progress in sanitation, plumbing and sewer construction than almost any other civilization over the years. The Roman aqueduct is still considered a masterpiece of engineering.

During the disease-ridden Middle Ages, advancement in hygiene and medi-

[5]Quoted by Theodosius Dobzhansky in *Biological Basis of Human Freedom*. New York: Columbia University Press, 1956.

cine was somewhat retarded. Hospitals were organized for the care of the sick, but it was not until the tail end of the fifteenth and beginning of the sixteenth centuries that scientific advancements began to be noticeable. By the seventeenth century Leeuwenhoek and his microscope opened a previously invisible world to man. Witchcraft reached a new high but alchemy slowly gave way to chemistry. By the middle 1700's all physical and biological sciences were making great strides. Scientists were no longer hidden for protection but were looked upon with some degree of respect. Uncleanliness was everywhere, in the streets, in the hospitals and in the homes.

In the nineteenth century a variety of medical discoveries and changes in hygienic practices took place. In the face of high death rates from infectious diseases, a number of significant discoveries occurred. Some of these were the clinical thermometer, the stethoscope, the x-ray, radium, the antiseptic method and anesthesia. It was proved once and for all that communicable diseases are caused by microorganisms which enter the body from without, that insects carry malaria and yellow fever, and that the universal practice of healthful living not only improves one's resistance to tuberculosis and other diseases but it also improves total health.

The twentieth century, building upon the past, has produced much of what is known and practiced today. Health promotion activities may go down in history as the greatest single contribution of the twentieth century. Federal, state, school, and community health programs have flourished. The man in the street—the common man—has not only felt the impact of this, but has actually taken part in the promotion program. He has had a hand in hospital organization, maternal education, the mental health movements, and school health education. He knows something about heart disease, allergies, psychological stress, cancer, brain surgery, obesity, disease-carrying insects, blood transfusions, the science of nutrition, longevity, streptococcus and staphylococcus bacilli, antibiotics, tranquilizers, sodium fluoride and fluoridation, and countless other items related to disease. His dollars have supported the fight to bring poliomyelitis under control, to pursue the cause of multiple sclerosis, muscular dystrophy, and coronary occlusions. His personal sacrifices on the local level to raise money for the Community Chest or United Fund, or to give blood, have given him an insight and appreciation for the place of health in modern society.

Thus the average citizen is gradually moving from superstitions and ignorance to a somewhat scientific viewpoint regarding health. A democratic education calling for an enlightened citizenry has done much to promote this awakening and movement away from darkness and indifference toward light and understanding. But all the health battles are not won yet. In fact, the battle has just gotten under way. The health needs of the people are extensive, and the implications for educators are great indeed.

THE NEED FOR EDUCATION FOR HEALTH

The more complex civilization becomes, the less valid is instinctive behavior, and the more man must depend upon the processes of education to guide him. He must use modern knowledge and techniques from the health sciences.

It is not difficult to make a long list of the reasons *why there is a need for health education.* Some of the more significant reasons are as follows:

The Changing Times

Nothing stands still. Change, like night and day, is an absolute. And Western civilization, in addition to reaping the sweet fruits of progress, is suffering from the spoils. In a society where speed, status, comfort, and economic success are high marks of achievement, it is not uncommon to find men and women who cannot adjust to the increasing pressures. They keep plugging along, lacking an apparent sense of values. Some become overfed and underactive. And, while others become complacent and simply vegetate from year to year with few goals in life to stimulate the best in them, there are others who literally "burn" themselves out in a life packed with situations generating insecurity, fear, anxiety, worry, jealousy, anger, and hatred. Resulting tensions refuse to stay bottled. They make their presence known in headaches, indigestion, gastrointestinal upsets, restlessness, sleeplessness, irritability, and fatigue.

Society today is anything but peaceful and serene. Even with a careful education for health, it is most difficult to achieve balance in living and to obtain an attitude of mind conducive to total well-being. Western civilization is characterized by the spectacle of man fighting for perfection while knowing little about where he is headed. His efforts all too often do not produce the peace of mind he seeks. Instead they result in more cholesterol to cause coronary disease, increased secretions to cause gastric ulcers, blood pressure to cause cerebral hemorrhage, and frustrations leading to the doors of the mental institution. Reduced to its simplest terms, survival depends on the physical-mental-spiritual balance. Moreover, it depends on how one *travels* toward the goals of life, perhaps more than whether or not he ever arrives.

Value Illness

The concern for health by official bodies and professionals in health-related fields is at an all-time high. This does not mean that the average citizen is well informed or has permitted his value system to be changed to any substantial degree. Although individual health status has improved, there are still thousands of people suffering from what Maslow refers to as "value illness."[6] This is the negative element behind drug addiction, alcoholism, illegitimacy, corruption, graft, and numerous irregularities in all walks of private and public life. The adult citizen *knows* what to do but is not *moved* to the state of doing it. This is illustrated continually in the field of health behavior where the knowledgeable individual is simply indifferent to the consequences of his own acts. He is not actively immoral, antisocial, or destructive in intent; he is simply amoral. His own moral principles and standards of right and wrong actions somehow do not compel him to act in keeping with what he knows is best.

Norman Cousins, editor of the *Saturday Review*, cites an alarming example of this value illness when he discusses a doctor friend who is a heavy smoker.[7] The doctor reports that he did not need all the government publications to convince him that smoking can cause cancer or bronchitis or various forms of heart disease. The evidence was admittedly plain to him in his daily visits to the hospital wards. Moreover, he was able to reinforce his feelings by noting that he had seen enough lung surgery to recognize the difference between the pink healthy tissue of the non-smoker and the discolored tissues of smokers. Yet, he could not give up smoking himself.

Here, says Cousins, is a problem far more serious than the problem leading up to it. Involved here are the ultimate questions a society has to ask about itself. Cousins asks: "What are the basic values of its people? How much sensitivity do they have to the fragility and preciousness of life? What connections do they see between a respect for life and healthy development of the society itself?"

World-Wide Conditions

Ultimately the thoughts of all men must be geared to conditions the world over. More people live in mud huts than in any other type of dwelling; more travel by foot (or by burro) than any other way; most have a life expectancy less than half that of the people in the United States; most mothers see half

[6]Maslow, Abraham H. *Toward a Psychology of Being.* Princeton, New Jersey: D. Van Nostrand Co., Inc., 1962.

[7]Cousins, Norman. "The Danger Beyond Smoking," *Saturday Review,* January 25, 1964.

their children die before reaching maturity; more people get sick without a physician's help available than those who have even rudimentary medical care. In short, most of the world's peoples are in the "have not" stage. It is encouraging, however, to know that evidence is available to indicate that in the long run improved health practices in one area of the globe have a favorable effect on other areas. This is also true in terms of health education ideas, for these ideas spread sometimes as quickly as new vaccines, sanitary practices, and wonder drugs.

The effectiveness of the World Health Organization is demonstrated by the large number of countries embarking upon health protection and education programs. Some of the world goals and accomplishments in a single year's time are impressive.

Improved communication and transportation have brought the people of the world closer together. Consequently, the health and welfare of the other fellow is more the worry of the ordinary citizen than ever before. Man may glory in his individuality, but it does not separate him from the universal self—the oneness of man. In fact the healthiest person alive today owes his enviable status to the practices of his friends and neighbors. In a complex society the welfare of the majority is directly affected by the welfare, knowledge, and understanding of the minority.[8] In short, education for health is the concern of the individual on both a local and a world-wide basis.

American Health Statistics

The health of the American people is well on the rise and has been for some time. Much of this is due to vast achievements in medical research, spectacular progress in the field of antibiotics, and an increase in health maintenance organizations.

In addition to these medical factors, a large share of credit should be given to public health and school health prac-

tices. The reduction in the tuberculosis death rate, for instance, represents one of man's finest accomplishments. At the start of the century the annual death rate in the United States from tuberculosis was 194 for each 100,000 persons. Today it is less than four. Such a favorable picture has been brought about by a number of factors and not solely by medical care and research. It is related to such items as better housing, improvement in nutrition, public health education, and a generally higher standard of living. The significance of education is further illustrated by the death rate from appendicitis; it has been reduced approximately 60 per cent over a 20 year period, due primarily to an enlightened public—a public that does not run for a cathartic every time there is a stomach or abdominal pain.

It is true that health in America is becoming a "social accomplishment." The death and sickness rate for practically all infectious diseases is down. A decline of 80 per cent in maternal death rates was recorded over the last two decades. Life expectancy is the highest ever. Under the mortality rate prevailing around the year 1900, the expectation of life at birth for the total population was not quite 50 years. By 1930 the figure had risen to 60 years; in 1955 it was 69.5 years. According to the National Center for Health Statistics it rose to almost 71 years by 1971. As in earlier years white females have the best record of longevity. In 1955 it was 73.6 years. In 1972 it was almost 75. Thus since the turn of the century almost 25 years have been added to the expected lifetime. Coincident with the reduction in over-all mortality during the present century is the rapid reduction in newborn deaths. In 1900 to 1902, 24 per cent of newborn white males and 21 per cent of white females failed to survive to their twentieth birthday. Now, less than 2.5 per cent are likely to die before that age. However, there is room for improvement in the survival chances of the newborn. Although the United States has the lowest infant mortality rate it has ever experienced—less than 19 deaths per

[8]Willgoose, Carl E. "Health, Welfare and Religious Freedom," *School and Society, 73 (1893)*:198, March 31, 1951.

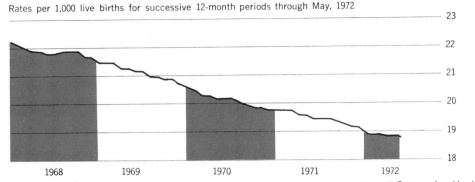

Rates per 1,000 live births for successive 12-month periods through May, 1972

Figure 1–1 U.S. Infant mortality rate continues its steady decline (National Center for Health Statistics).

1000 live births (Figure 1–1) — it still ranks only fifteenth among the countries of the world. The Scandinavian countries rank at the top.[9]

Medical science has made spectacular progress in the last 20 years. The danger of infection through surgery has been greatly reduced. Low cost vaccines are very effective against serious illness. Regular medical examinations and early treatment prevent disease and disability in thousands of individuals. Vast numbers of people leave hospitals well who would have died two decades ago. And the average stay in the hospital for an appendectomy is five and a half days. It was 14 days 20 years ago.

Although much of this presents a pleasant health and welfare picture, there are problems ahead. For one thing, it is expected that the population of the United States will continue to increase, although the birth rate is nearing a point where some demographers are cautiously suggesting that it may be possible to reach a "replacement" level of population growth in this decade. (The replacement rate is the number of children per family required to replace their parents in addition to the children who die in infancy.) And if the trend continues

it might be possible to achieve "zero population growth" within the century. To achieve this, however, a replacement level of births would have to be maintained for about 70 years.

Another consideration is the skyrocketing suburbs, the growth of the cities, and the extensive shifts in population. Currently over 30 per cent of Americans change their address at least once each year. Packard points out that the average citizen moves about fourteen times in his lifetime.[10] Families are repeatedly displaced; one student attended three different school systems in one year. With this comes a decrease in friends as well as in community involvement. But more serious, says Packard, because of this fragmentation of community living, we no longer know our neighbors and so we suffer from crises of individual and social identity. It is not surprising, therefore, that communities find that they have to develop or expand medical and public health facilities and services.

Significant Health Problems

The degenerative diseases of the adult population frequently have their roots in the day-to-day health practices of children and youth. Proper practices, established early in life, tend to reduce mortality and morbidity rates at all age levels. Childhood deaths, however, represent a significant statistic, particularly in the

[9]See especially Metropolitan Life Insurance Company, "Neonatal Mortality — United States, Canada, and Western Europe," *Statistical Bulletin,* 53:3–6, January 1972. See also Helen C. Chase, "The Position of the United States in International Comparisons of Health Status," *American Journal of Public Health,* 62:581–589, April 1972.

[10]Packard, Vance. *A Nation of Strangers*, New York: McKay, 1972.

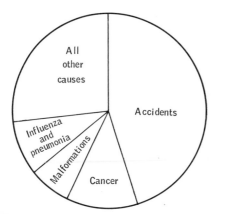

Figure 1–2 Pie graph illustrating causes of child deaths, 5 to 14 years of age.

five to fourteen year age period. (See Fig. 1–2.)

Some of the more prominent health problems are as follows:

Cardiovascular diseases rank first among the leading causes of death in the United States, Canada, and Western Europe. More than half of all deaths each year are attributed to these diseases. The male statistic is higher than that for the female prior to age sixty. (See Fig. 1–3.) Coronary arterial disease is on the rise, but it can be reduced when people know enough to watch their weight and limit their consumption of fats, seek diversion and tension-free recreation to attain a sound attitude of mind, and engage in a moderate amount of physical activity. Mortality and morbidity from heart disease is two to three times as high among people who do not realize the importance of physical activity and fail to get regular exercise. From the Framingham Heart Study, where there has been continuous evaluation of 5127 adults in one community since 1949, it has been shown that there is a clear association of coronary heart disease with age, elevated blood pressure, serum cholesterol, overweight, cigarette

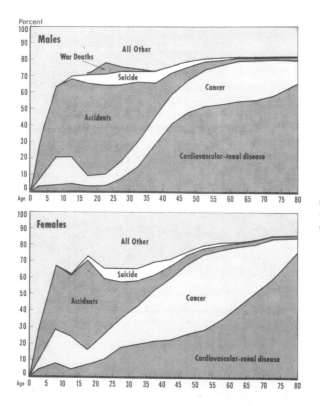

Figure 1–3 Per cent of deaths from specified causes by sex and age—1971 (Metropolitan Life Insurance Company *Statistical Bulletin,* April, 1972).

smoking and lack of physical exercise.[11] This is confirmed by the results of a study of 88 per cent of the entire community of Tecumseh, Michigan, where it was discovered that the maintenance of desirable body weight is an effective method to control blood cholesterol levels.[12] Of major importance, therefore, is the specific role of education. People must learn to recognize the symptoms of heart disease or cancer or any other disease and see their physicians early.

Mental illness is a multidimensional problem which affects people in all walks of life. As a disease entity it extends from those who are seriously deranged to those who are simply unhappy, hard to live with, and poorly adjusted to their world. Mental patients occupy 50 per cent of all the hospital beds in the United States. According to a Harris poll of some 500 physicians, about 90 per cent of their patients suffer from hypochondria and psychosomatic ailments — derived chiefly from such items as loneliness, insecurity, family conflicts, the pressure of raising children, the stress of overwork, burning the candle at both ends, and fear of failure.[13] The same study indicated that boredom and monotony ranked high as an underlying factor contributing to poor mental health.

Another serious outcome of inadequate mental health relates to the all-time high national divorce-marriage ratio — the number of divorces granted per 1000 new marriages. The average figure is now 455; in some states it is well over 500. This rise in broken marriages to almost 1 out of every 2 is considered alarming by many, and dismissed by others as just a trend toward easier divorce due in part to "no fault" laws which recognize "irreconcilable differences" as the only grounds.

Children are especially involved. About 400 out of 100,000 children under age 18 require psychiatric care as out-patients each year. Moreover, mental disorders are considered a significant factor in numerous physical illnesses, are strongly associated with suicide, and are often found to be implicated in accidents. In addition to causing considerable suffering and family disruption, mental illness exacts a financial toll of over two billion dollars a year for health care, and several billions of dollars more in annual loss to industry.

Because of better treatment and rehabilitation, there has been some decline in the number of patients. This advance has been offset by the number of people seeking treatment sooner. Also, the alcoholic, the retarded, and the brain damaged are being served.

Poor health in a society has many manifestations. Suicide, for example, was the cause of over 25,000 deaths in the United States in a recent year, compared with over 10,000 homicides. This fact in itself should prompt more attention to be focused on the type of behavior that leads to an individual's self-destruction. But the suicide figure does not tell the whole story of suicide. For every successful suicide there are ten unsuccessful attempts for various reasons. Because of the moral and religious stigma attached to suicide, many such cases are undoubtedly not recorded. Also, it is difficult to determine what percentage of other violent deaths, including the 60,000 annual automobile deaths, are caused by a conscious or subconscious desire to end life. Medical and safety authorities are almost unanimous in the belief that some percentage of all categories of violent death are in reality suicides. Moreover, almost half the suicides occur within three months of an emotional crisis, and about 40 per cent of the men and 20 per cent of the women kill themselves because of ill health. The

[11]Editorial, "Children Participate in Framingham Study," *Journal of Mississippi State Medical Association,* January 1972. See also Ralph S. Paffenbarger, et al. "Characteristics of Longshoremen Related to Fatal Coronary Heart Disease and Stroke," *American Journal of Public Health,* 61:1363–1370, July 1971.

[12]Montoye, H. J., Epstein, F. H., and Kjelsberg, M. D. "Relationship Between Serum Cholesterol and Body Fitness," *American Journal of Clinical Nutrition, 18:*397–406, 1966.

[13]Smolensky, Jack, and Frank B. Haar. *Principles of Community Health,* 3rd ed., Philadelphia: W. B. Saunders Co., 1972, p. 417.

rising rate has led to the recognition of a major medical and public health problem. Existing suicide prevention centers have been effective in saving lives each year and have demonstrated the importance of public education in detecting the potential suicide. Many suicides can be averted if unusual depression or signs of mental illness are recognized and properly treated.

The suicide rate for younger people has been rising steadily. In California the rate among girls 15 to 19 years old was 8 per 100,000 in 1971—double the rate for the previous ten years. Suicide prevention, therefore, begins by getting at the causes during the formative elementary school years.

The need for a formal educational approach to prevent and reduce poor mental health is evident. Experience has taught that preventive mental health services can reduce mental illness, alcoholism, divorce, suicide, emotional disturbances, juvenile crime, and employment problems. In view of the huge population increases expected in the years ahead, it is obvious that the man of today is faced with a herculean task in building and staffing the hospitals, clinics, or jails which people with these mental health problems would require.

The real solution is to *prevent* the disorders through combined efforts of lay and professional people. This is not easy, for our way of life with its emphasis on personal status, speed, and materialism tends to produce individuals with a disturbed sense of values. Balance in living is frequently difficult to attain. Large numbers of people are basically unhappy. They are looking for relief—"a way out." Only a few years ago the pharmaceutical industry spent more money on developing new tranquilizers, stimulants, sedatives, and analgesics than on any other kind of drug. Even earning a living fails to satisfy large segments of the population, for man is further removed from the goods produced as technology advances. His effort is only a partial contribution, and his identification with the product grows dimmer and dimmer. The frustrations and resentments

that pile up at the workbench move along into the family circle, the neighborhood council, the polling place, and the social gathering. The worker cannot change his personality, his lack of self-esteem, his sense of impotence, his boredom—in short the patterns imprinted on him by his job—as easily as he sheds his overalls.

Alcoholism and drug addiction are primarily symptoms of poor mental health. The nation's No. 1 "drug problem" is alcohol. It is estimated that there are 10 million alcoholics in the United States out of the 95 million who drink. One in every 18 beginning drinkers will become an alcoholic. Untreated alcoholism shortens life 12 years and contributes to many types of fatalities—with at least half of the nation's traffic deaths involving drunken drivers. The heavy drinkers cost the nation some 15 billion dollars a year in lost work time, property damage, health and welfare costs, and do incalculable damage to personal and family life (a leading cause of separation, divorce, desertion and emotional problems).

The alcoholism problem will be helped when there is wide discussion of drinking patterns and the responsibilities of those who drink. As Globetti points out from his workshop at the Murray State University Center for Alcohol Education, cultural attitudes have much to do with practices.[14] Evidence suggests that the behavior which accompanies drinking under abstinence and permissive conditions differs significantly.

Most young drug addicts start with alcohol and graduate to opiates by age 18. Also, it is felt that the management of heroin addiction may be influenced by alcohol use.[15] Faced with the staggering number of 700,000 heroin addicts, many private and public associations are seeking preventive measures as well as controls. In New York City one high school

---

[14]Globetti, Gerald. "Problem Drinking in an Abstinence Setting," *School Health Review*, 2:14–16, April 1971.

[15]Barr, Harriet L. et al. "Alcohol: First Drug Used," *American Medical News*, April 17, 1972.

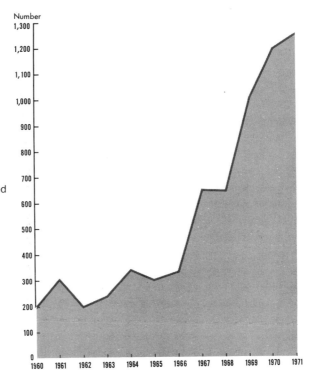

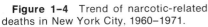

Figure 1-4 Trend of narcotic-related deaths in New York City, 1960–1971.

student in 20 is using heroin—a practice which causes more fatal drug poisoning than barbiturates; this is attributed to acute reactions, overdoses, and diseases directly related to narcotic abuse.[16] (See Fig. 1-4.)

According to the National Institute of Mental Health, marihuana use has increased and amounts to as much as 90 per cent among some groups of high school students. There is an upswing in use among collegians too, with 50 per cent having used it sometime. Actually, some 24 million people have tried the weed, as indicated by a Department of Health, Education and Welfare study. Although the safety margin appears high and the drug seems to be more socially acceptable than other more potent narcotics, research findings show evidence of a number of negative side effects to the individual user. Unfortunately, most users ignore side effects for major effects. Thus in one extensive study by the

National Commission on Marijuana and Drug Abuse about 5 per cent of the youths surveyed had tried cocaine, 8 per cent amphetamines, 7 per cent barbiturates, and 10 per cent hashish. In short, drug-taking has become a recreational pastime—a real challenge to the very meaning of the word recreation.

Cancer, a malignant neoplasm, is killing about 500,000 Americans a year. It is the second most frequent cause of death in the United States, Canada, and virtually all the countries of Western Europe. It is calculated that about six out of every 24 persons will develop cancer; of this number two will be saved, one will die who could have been saved, and three will die who cannot presently be saved. Significantly, the high death rate could be reduced by 33 per cent if proper treatment were started in time. Recent studies show that a high percentage of people treated early for cancer live at least five years.[17] Unfortunately,

[16]See "Drug-Related Mortality," *Statistical Bulletins,* Metropolitan Life Insurance Company, February 1972, pp. 3–8.

[17]Metropolitan Life Insurance Company. "Cancer Survival—First Five Years," *Statistical Bulletin, 52:*4–7, June 1971.

40 per cent of the women with breast cancer do not seek help until it is too late. Thousands could be saved if men, women, and children would have an adequate medical examination each year, and follow up unexplained lumps, sores and discharges. As it is, the reluctant participants in screening programs tend to be the less well-educated, foreign born, and those with lower incomes.[18]

Getting the public to accept the fact of cancer openly and do something about it in time is primarily a health education job. Today, pregnant women discuss it in mothers' classes, and children discuss it in the schoolroom. Posters like the one in Figure 1–5 help to get the message across. In lung cancer, the single biggest problem is a lack of knowledge of how to motivate smokers to stop smoking and to forestall young people from acquiring the smoking habit. Simply telling them that 12 times as many smokers die of emphysema as non-smokers is not the answer.

Educational programs in the schools, coupled with the efforts of the U. S. Public Health Service and the National Clearinghouse for Smoking and Health, may prove helpful during the next several years.

In addition to causing cancer, coronary heart disease, chronic bronchitis, and emphysema, cigarette smoking cuts several years off the life expectancy of millions of Americans. Smokers at every age pay a high risk price—22 per cent of heavy smokers can expect to be hospitalized during any given 24-month period, as compared to only 14 per cent of non-smokers.

Fatalities from ulcers, particularly gastric ulcers, are three times as common among smokers as non-smokers. Less familiar is that mothers who smoke tend to have more premature babies. In one study of 2000 pregnancies, fetal mortality of babies born of mothers who smoked was 79 per 1000, as against 41 per 1000 for non-smoking mothers.[19]

---

[18]Fink, Raymond, et al. "Participation in Repetitive Screening for Early Breast Cancer Detection." *American Journal of Public Health,* 62:328–336, March 1972.

---

[19]Ochsner, Alton. "The Health Menace of Tobacco," *American Scientist,* 59:246–252, March–April 1971.

WHAT ARE YOUR CHANCES OF DEVELOPING LUNG CANCER?

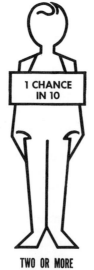

1 CHANCE IN 270

NON-SMOKER

1 CHANCE IN 36

LESS THAN A PACK A DAY SMOKER

1 CHANCE IN 10

TWO OR MORE PACKS A DAY SMOKER

Figure 1–5 Lung cancer and smoking. (Courtesy American Cancer Society.)

Both men and women with long histories of cigarette smoking have more severely wrinkled faces than do nonsmokers. In fact, the association between smoking and the prominence of wrinkles is even stronger than the association between prolonged outdoor exposure and wrinkling.[20]

It was hoped that with the discontinuance of cigarette advertising on television the practice of smoking would drop off. It did for a while, and then it built up again, producing a greater number of heavy smokers. Moreover, the effect on the smoking patterns of youth was not particularly great. This is because the actions of young people are more affected by people around them—their parents, siblings, and especially their peers. If no one in the family smokes, there is a very good chance that the student will not smoke. (See Fig. 1–6.) In the end, smoking for many young children is a positive choice that must be discussed in terms of self-image and social identification.[20a]

The over-all *physical fitness* of youth is another concern of parents and teachers. American youth are physically softer than those in many other countries. Youngsters in general lead a rather sedentary existence. Research indicates that civilization plays strange tricks. Many of the youth of the land are lacking the physical wherewithal to participate in vigorous, growth-stimulating activities. They simply have not been exposed to first rate health and physical education programs. Muscular weakness and lack of physical fitness are linked to a life lacking in muscle-building chores, with rich foods, bus and automobile transportation, more spectator rather than participation activities, more TV viewing, less walking, labor-saving devices, apartment living, and lack of adequate play space. Education to meet the loss of fitness is a constant need.

The need for proper programs of physical activity is of paramount concern to teachers of young children. Adults can hardly be expected to change their sedentary ways of living if in their early years of formal education they did not acquire an appreciation for physical skills and the need for regular exercise throughout a lifetime. Walking and bicycling, according to the eminent heart specialist, Dr. Paul Dudley White, are simple and practical exercises that should be a part of one's plan of normal living.

It has been demonstrated by the President's Council on Physical Fitness and Sports that physically underdeveloped children can be readily identified and given vigorous developmental activity to increase their level of physical fitness. A project involving over 200,000 schoolchildren in five states revealed that where a school had a physical education program prior to its selection in the project, the average physical fitness test failure was 25 per cent. In schools that had no program, however, the average rate of failure was 46 per cent. In all schools, swift improvement was achieved when below-average students were given individual attention.

Millions of people have *poor teeth*. In fact, about 95 per cent of the population suffers from this condition. The average number of unfilled cavities is five per head. Also, 26 million people have lost all of their teeth. Obviously, the American mouth is a disaster area that could be improved if gum stimulators and toothbrushes were properly used. The high rate of periodontal disease, caused by an accumulation of tartar which results in swelling and inflammation (68 million adult Americans have this disorder), is largely due to the fact that early symptoms are ignored and neglected.

Tens of thousands of children have serious difficulties with their teeth. The National Health Survey has indicated that half the children in the country under 15 have never been to a dentist. It is true that poverty, ignorance and indifference have something to do with dental decay statistics, but there are numerous examples of well-educated parents with

---

[20]Daniell, Harry W. "Smoker's Wrinkles," *Annals of Internal Medicine,* December 1971.
[20a]See especially the clear discussion presented by Bernard Mausner and Ellen S. Pratt, *Smoking: A Behavioral Analysis,* Elmsford, N. Y.: Pergamon Press, 1971.

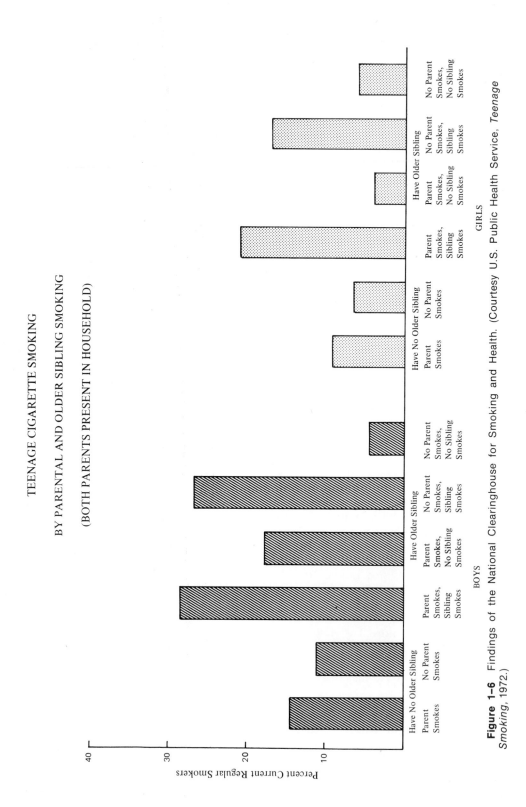

Figure 1-6 Findings of the National Clearinghouse for Smoking and Health. (Courtesy U.S. Public Health Service, *Teenage Smoking*, 1972.)

moderate to high incomes whose children's teeth are no better than the average.

By the time the average child reaches school, he has three carious teeth. At age 12 or 13 he has five permanent teeth attacked by caries. The decay rate rises sharply in the intermediate grades and is associated with poor academic achievement and high absence frequency. (See Fig. 1–7.) It is evident, too, that fluoridation of the water supply is highly significant. Yet, large numbers of people continue to resist a move in this direction because of entrenched beliefs and general misinformation. Although the effectiveness of water fluoridation has been amply demonstrated, this procedure is only now beginning to have the impact that might be expected. When large cities such as New York, Chicago, Philadelphia, Baltimore, Cleveland, Washington, St. Louis, and Detroit fluoridated their water, the impact was significant.

Fluoridation of the drinking water not only reduces tooth decay up to 70 per cent, but it is a tremendous money saver. In ten years Chicago's fluoridated water supply has saved parents more than two million dollars in dental costs for children under 14, and at the same time has reduced tooth decay by 67 per cent. This financial saving is dramatically illustrated by the findings of a two-city study in New York State where the mean cost for dental care per child in Kingston (non-fluoridated water) was more than double that in Newburgh (fluoridated water).[21]

The benefits from public water fluoridation programs greatly reduce the hazard of malocclusion, especially severe malocclusion which may be regarded as physically handicapping. Also, research is beginning to indicate that fluorides slow the course of periodontal disease by retarding bone destruction. Rheumatoid arthritis and osteoporosis—abnormal porousness of bone—are lower in areas where there is a high fluoride content in the water.

The staggering need for dental care, with an estimated backlog of 1,000,000,000 untreated carious lesions in teeth in America would make one feel that the dentists are overworked. Yet surveys have indicated that only 40 per cent of the dentists are reported to have

---

[21] Ast, David B., et al. "Time and Cost Factors to Provide Regular, Periodic Dental Care for Children in a Fluoridated and Nonfluoridated Area," *American Journal of Public Health, 57:*1635–1642, September 1967.

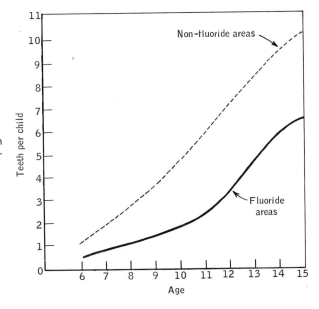

Figure 1–7 Relationship of tooth decay in children to age and fluoridation.

an overload. It has been conservatively estimated that if all the dentists devoted their time exclusively to filling teeth, five years would be required to take care of the backlog alone. Education to get more people to see their dentists regularly must involve both the general public and the school personnel. Only a cooperative effort in the years ahead will improve the situation to any degree.

Accident statistics overwhelm the average reader. *Accidents* are the greatest threat to life and limb in childhood and call for an education of the public through school and community health agencies. This is recognized today as a necessity if man is to survive in a society demanding ever increasing human adaptability. Considerable adaptation takes place at an early age. Adaptation to physical strains, psychological stresses and hazardous situations is to be considered by parents and teachers alike. Here are some impressive findings:

Fifty-two million people a year are injured in some kind of an accident, and another 104,000 are killed.

Accidents are the chief cause of death in children ages five to 14 years.

Over four million non-fatal injuries occur annually in and about the home.

Sports and recreation account for approximately 5200 fatalities and a great many more serious injuries annually.

More than 8000 people die by drowning each year. Over half the people in the U. S. cannot swim well enough to save themselves in an emergency (National Safety Council).

Motor vehicle accidents take over 60,000 lives a year and inflict disabling injuries on an additional 1,800,000 persons in the United States. Another 1,500,000 are injured but not disabled. In this connection, as many as one million drivers have claimed whiplash injuries in a given year from an estimated 3,800,000 rear-end automobile collisions; much of this is due to an indifference to the proper positioning of head restraints by individual drivers.

Socially maladjusted individuals are more likely to be involved in accidents than are those without such difficulties.

The National Safety Council estimates that if seat belts were used consistently by all drivers and passengers, the incidence of serious injury could be reduced by one third and between 8000 and 10,000 lives could be saved annually. However, few parents when driving regularly lock car doors and secure children in seat belts.

Seventy-five million bicycles ridden in the United States today are connected with an annual loss of 800 lives. Four out of five such fatalities are believed to be associated with the disregard of safe practices. Safety authorities estimate that between 120,000 and 150,000 persons sustain disabling injuries in such mishaps in a single year.

Firearm accidents claim a toll of about 2400 lives a year. Snowmobile injuries have increased spectacularly chiefly because of poor judgment by the operators.

Annually some 1500 pedestrians, five to 14 years of age, are killed in traffic. Injuries, which are a better indicator of the seriousness of the problem, show that 50,000 schoolchildren are injured in pedestrian accidents every year.

Medicines cause most accidental poisonings in children, and aspirin heads the list. Children under five who swallowed aspirin were the victims in one-fourth of all cases of accidental poisoning reported in a recent year to the National Clearinghouse for Poison Control Centers.

Tetanus (lockjaw) is almost entirely preventable by vaccination, but only one person in four bothers to get the preventive tetanus toxoid shots. Half of the 450 tetanus patients reported in the United States each year still die unnecessarily.

Animal bites, a significant urban public health problem, represent about half of the total of other reportable diseases in some large cities—with children under 15 years of age being the major victims.

The need for education for safe living is great indeed. It must begin early with children. While adults have a high incidence of motor vehicle and firearms accidents, and often discuss ways of reducing them, it becomes most difficult to talk to the excitement-loving, venturesome youngsters who are repelled by the idea that being safe means avoiding unnecessary risks. So they have needless accidents while pursuing their day-to-day activities.

Childhood curiosity, like childhood enthusiasm, needs guiding. For example, every 24 hour period more than 750 children in the United States are poisoned by their own curiosity, which impels them to gulp aspirin and sleeping pills, sip floor polish and kerosene, and swallow kitchen detergents, rubber cement and cosmetics. Over 400,000 children gnaw peeling paint containing lead; 3200 of them suffer permanent brain damage and 200 die. Children consume pesticides too. Out of 111 deaths reported in one study 51 per cent occurred in children under 10 years of age. Children, it has been said, will eat just about anything—and there are some 15,000 substances which are, to some extent, poisonous.

The *problems of aging* are many. People are living longer; the population is growing older. It is not at all unrealistic to base training of children now in school on the probability that a high percentage will live past 90 and many beyond 100 years. This will place increased value on the continuous application of proper health knowledge all through the years. Interestingly, people who live to a ripe old age have some practices in common. Charlie Smith, a bona fide 130 year old Southerner, uses his body and mind as much as possible and stays clear of stressful situations. Shirali Mislinov of Azerbaidzhan (Republic of USSR) at 167 years of age has never been obese, competitive, over-ambitious, or gluttonous for the delights of food and has always practiced a certain self-control. In America more than two-fifths of all persons 65 years of age and over are limited in activity by chronic conditions, primarily heart disease, arthritis, and rheumatism.

The effects of *environmental pollution* are shocking. As the ecological balance is slighted and technological progress is championed by the many, the pollutants tend to increase, causing huge economic losses and lowered health for mankind. Fortunately, the environmental movement has come of age. The industrialists are beginning to stop further damage to the living space. Large numbers of people are rallying behind the Commoner "laws" of ecology. (1. Everything is connected to everything else, and, 2. everything must go somewhere.)[22] And as difficult as it is to comprehend, the human mind is attempting to understand the complexity of ecological processes.

Partially related to the pollution problems are sheer numbers of people taking up space, requiring certain needs, and creating a number of dysfunctions—a number of which lead to overcrowding, dehumanization, tension, violence, and severely challenge the earth's carrying capacity. The presidentially appointed Commission on Population Growth and the American Future, after two years of detailed assessment, stated in its report that no substantial benefits would result from continued growth of the nation's population. Since then there has been a decline in the population growth rate. Between 1958 and 1972 the fertility rate dropped from 120 births per 1000 women of childbearing age to a figure of 80. Although achieving a "zero population growth" in a decade or two is still questionable, it is estimated that by 1982 there will be 4 to 6 million fewer pupils attending the nation's elementary schools. The ecology movement may be bringing about some of the decrease in population, but much of it is really due to a sharp increase in the number of working wives and more families embracing effective contraceptive practices. Moreover, the decline may be temporary because of the large number of children born during the post-World War II "baby boom."

Although the air is getting cleaner, dozens of large cities suffer from radiation, smoke, smog, fumes and chemicals. Generally, the greater the air pollution the greater the number of deaths. Air sampling stations show that the automo-

---

[22]Commoner, Barry. *The Closing Circle*, New York: Alfred A. Knopf, 1971.

bile is still a top-ranking culprit which produces one-half of the contaminants found in the air. Other methods of transportation rank second, followed by the petroleum industry, combustion of fuels, use of organic solvents, metals, chemicals, incineration of refuse, and minerals.

Severe air pollution triggers illness and may bring about premature death to thousands of people. Even "ordinary" levels of air pollution can cause coughing, sneezing, wheezing, and suffering. Short range discomfort may be followed by long range disease. Bronchitis, emphysema (a deteriorating lung condition sometimes marked by heart enlargement and impairment of heart action), and lung cancer are more prevalent in areas of high air contamination. A careful check of total deaths in New York City by day of occurrence indicates periodic peaks in mortality which are associated with periods of high air pollution. Temperature inversion conditions and low wind speed permit air pollution to build up to high levels.

Although it is known that cigarette smoking and air pollution are separate causes of emphysema, it has now been shown that the combined effect is even more deadly. Smoking, however, has a greater chance of influencing emphysema than air pollution, for it has been found that the percentage of emphysema is higher among moderate smokers not exposed to pollution than among nonsmokers exposed to pollution.

Cleaning up America's polluted waters is a task for government at all levels and for industry in every community. The Council on Environmental Quality reports that rivers and waterways are dirtier than ever. Concentrations of phosphates and nitrogen compounds, which cause lakes to die, have increased. Education of the citizen is required if water pollution control programs are to continue to be implemented. Man has made numerous bodies of water so bacteria-ridden that he cannot drink it, so oily and irritant that he cannot swim in it, so unsupportive of life that he cannot fish in it, and so mal-

odorous and filled with refuse and old junk that he cannot contemplate its once natural beauty.

Today, even noise pollution is a health hazard in industry and in the community. Exposure to severe noise causes hearing loss, changes in cardiovascular blood pressure, pulse rate and breathing, gastrointestinal motility, endocrine gland excretions, and interferes with the process of thinking and learning. Noise does not need to be deafening to be dangerous; exposure to 85 decibels for more than five hours a day may lead to a gradual loss of hearing. A noise of 160 decibels, however, can rupture the ear drum.[23] Only an educated consumer will demand a reduction in noise levels in the home or on the street. Therefore, the problems of air, water, and noise pollution need to be discovered and worked on by children in the classroom if hopeful changes are to occur in the future.

Overweight has been a health problem in civilized countries for a number of years. An individual should know that it is to his advantage to reach his desirable or "ideal" weight and stay there the rest of his life. However, about three out of five men in their fifties are overweight. Half of the women beyond the age of 40 are more than 10 per cent above their desirable weight. Even half the men in their thirties are at least 10 per cent above their optimum weight. Studies at the University of Washington School of Medicine indicate that the teenage population is 20 to 30 per cent overweight and that girls are more frequently overweight than boys. Studies by Harvard University personnel show that young obese girls are significantly less active than non-obese children. Not only are these children underactive and overfed, they do not exert energy to do *anything* often enough. They are passive and altogether too dependent on their parents. Worst still, they are not happy with themselves. This has personality and emotional overtones—particularly as one's self-con-

---

[23]Konopa, Valene and Stanley Zimering. "Noise—The Challenge of the Future." *Journal of School Health*, 42:172–177, March 1972.

tempt and feelings of inferiority lead to poor social relationships and less than adequate school performance. Much can be done through a team-learning approach.[24] Since the production of fat cells occurs more rapidly in early life, it is especially advantageous to control the foods and discuss the topic with younger children.[25]

Absenteeism everywhere has been slowly climbing. The annual rate for industrial absenteeism is approximately 7 per cent, an all-time high. The acute diseases such as colds and upper respiratory illnesses account for half of the current absenteeism; chronic debilitating disease accounts for the other half. Because of this, more than ten billion dollars a year is drained from the economy. Studies among high absentees show that they tend to be unhappy, discontented, egocentric, and generally unhealthy. Conversely, the worker with few absences tends to be happy and contented, outgoing, and reasonably well.

In New York City 65 per cent of school absences are caused by health problems. Preventable school absences in this one city cost upwards of five million dollars annually in state aid.

Sex-Related Problems

There is a massive accumulation of evidence to indicate that one of the foremost health-related problems of the century is the widespread lack of knowledge and understanding of human sex and sexuality.

Since 1958 the venereal disease rate has increased 500 per cent to become pandemic, despite the fact that it should be common knowledge that syphilis and gonorrhea can be cured with penicillin. Reported cases of gonorrhea have more than doubled in the past several years. There were 624,000 cases reported by mid-1971, but the estimate was that there were more than 2,500,000 infections actually occurring. Much of the increase has been among children between the ages of 12 and 19 years. Moreover, in the past decade congenital syphilis in children under 10 years of age rose by 168 per cent. Society has been slow to act. In 1940 the U. S. Surgeon General could not even use the word syphilis in a radio broadcast. Almost 35 years later the word still causes adults to blush, and sixth graders to ask what it is. In New York City, where syphilis doubled among teenage boys in an eight-year period, a study showed that 32 per cent did not know that it could be cured, and 60 per cent did not know that venereal disease is transmitted through sexual intercourse. Keeping sex information "under wraps" has been exactly the wrong thing to do.

Since 1940 teenage marriages have risen 500 per cent, and studies indicate that 50 to 80 per cent of teenage wives are pregnant at the time of marriage. The divorce rate in such marriages is three times as high as that for individuals married after 21. Interestingly, the proportion of brides who are pregnant at marriage decreases as the level of education increases.[26]

Illegitimate births among girls in the 14 to 19 age group are more than double what they were 25 years ago. In 1972, U. S. Office of Education figures indicated that almost one-quarter million girls age 17 and under had a child. One in every 10 school-age girls is a mother. Studies show that very few of these girls understand conception and the sex function. This is also true for most girls with unwanted pregnancies.

The school systems in several of the larger cities have been concerned with the sex education of pregnant and unwed girls. The growing number of such students has caused problems. In a recent year the special school for pregnant secondary school girls in Baltimore had 895 girls and had to turn away 1200 more for lack of room.

[24]See report by Carrie Lee Warren, "Adolescent Obesity," *School Health Review*, 3:19–20, May–June 1972.

[25]Hammar, S. L. "Overfeeding in Infancy: Factor in Adolescent Obesity," *Pediatric Herald*, September–October 1971.

[26]Tillack, Warner S., et al. "A Study of Premarital Pregnancy," *American Journal of Public Health*, 62:676–679, May 1972.

In view of the large number of un-wanted teenage pregnancies, and the in-creasing desire to amend the situation through abortion, one is compelled to support the view of Goldstein from the University of California Medical Center:

The greater good is to be gained in viewing abortion for what it is—a poor, very poor method of remedying a failure of contraception. And generally, failure of contraception is a fail-ure of education, just as surely as delay in seek-ing advice and help to obtain an abortion is a failure of education.[27]

Although unwed mothers and preg-nant girls are being helped and children with venereal disease are being treated, very few school systems are providing a comprehensive sex education curricu-lum for students of both sexes in grades one to 12. This is most unfortunate, for this is a society in which chaperones and supervision of youth are unfashionable, the young people are left on their own with easy access to privacy, children of all ages are totally vulnerable to the on-slaughts of commercial exploitation of sex, news media report all kinds of sor-did sexual occurrences, and sex misin-formation comes from many question-able sources. Until this void is filled with a quantity and quality of factual knowl-edge, the young person will continue to remain very defenseless about sex. Stud-ies show that boys and girls do not want sexual license; they crave information and explanations. They seek standards which will help them understand the role of sex as a part of their total personality. And they want to talk about it—in the way that they talk about any other topic in the school curriculum. Kirkendall, in calling for sex education, makes this need quite clear when he says:

The chief determinant of sexual conduct is not factual information but the general feeling of satisfaction and worth which the individual has been able to develop about himself as a per-son. One's pattern of sexual behavior is a reflec-tion of one's total life pattern. An individual who feels he is accomplishing something with his

life...will not be driven by guilt, anxiety or com-pulsion to engage in sex with little regard for what this means to other persons or to his total situation. In other words, he is in a position to direct and manage his sexuality.[28]

Considerably more attention will be given to program planning in the area of sex and family living education in Chapter 7.

Superstitions

There is a wide variety of superstitions in existence throughout the world. They are based in some cases on old wives' tales, and in other cases on pure magic. Rich and poor alike believe them, and contrary to what might be expected, they are a part of the daily existence of the bright scholar as well as of the dull and ignorant. Superstitions are difficult to combat because they are concealed be-neath the veneer of education. It has been succinctly stated that man surveys the world about him, clutching science with one hand, hoping for its benefits, yet holding firmly with the other hand to the superstitions of the ages. One sees the figure of Samuel Pepys, famous diarist of the 1600's, headed for home with a rab-bit's foot in one pocket and a copy of Hooke's "Book of Microscopy" in the other.

Gullibility

This is a nation of healthy people. It is also a nation of tub thumpers, pill takers, television addicts, neurotics, and help-less individuals. Probably more people are "lost" in terms of what to do for themselves along health lines than most people realize. Newspaper advertising on the one hand and television ads on the other keep heads turning from this prod-uct to that product like a mass of human-ity watching a tennis match. Americans have been accused of buying everything and anything if it is supposed to be "good for you." Nearly 20 billion pills are con-sumed each year. This averages out to about one hundred pills annually for

[27]Goldstein, Phillip and Gary Stewart. "Trends in Therapeutic Abortion in San Francisco," *Ameri-can Journal of Public Health, 62*:695–699, May 1972.

[28]Kirkendall, Lester A. "Sex Education," *Dis-cussion Guide No. 1*, published by Sex Informa-tion and Education Council of the U. S., October 1965, p. 9

every man, woman, and child in the country. Most pills, of course, are taken from necessity and render an important service in conquering or checking disease and improving personal efficiency. Millions of pills and gallons of patent medicines are devoured for imaginary illness brought on by gullibility. Parents are gullible and so are their children; they require a better understanding of health.

Fads, Diets, and Quackery

Mature people are sometimes like the classmates of the little girl in the fourth grade who comes to school with a pretty red ribbon in her hair. Before the week is out, half of her girl friends in the class will be seen sporting attractive ribbons in their hair.

On almost any street in the community friendly neighbors spread the word that something helped them with their aches and pains. Some people subject themselves to such things as vitamin pills, steam baths, spinal manipulations, or blackstrap molasses and yogurt simply because their friends think it good for them. No thought of securing qualified medical attention has entered their minds. Reducing fads cost the public 100 million dollars a year. Too often overweight folks seek only an easy way to lose weight. Instead of exercising they would rather deaden the appetite with an amphetamine pill (which is not an effective treatment for obesity). People want to swallow a pill, suck a skim milk or lemon juice wafer or chew mint-flavored gum, eat what they please and still lose weight. They do not know that it may even be harmful. For example, diabetics and individuals with high blood pressure or heart disease should take tablets only upon the advice of a physician. People are always waiting for the "miracle drug," and, if tranquilizing drugs work for one person's illness, the attitude of the man on the street is often: "Why won't it work for my troubles, too?"

Presently, the extreme example of a public health hazard is the Zen Macrobiotic diet. By avoiding fluids as much as possible and concentrating on the "highest level" diet of 100 per cent cereals, the individual stands in danger of incurring serious nutritional deficiencies such as scurvy, anemia, lack of protein and calcium, emaciation and loss of kidney function. Tragically, the Zen followers believe the cult claim that the diet not only helps one achieve the ultimate state of well-being, but also cures cancer, mental disease and heart trouble.[29]

Cults and quackeries may be more serious than fads, for they tend to confuse the public as to their relationship with science. People practicing certain cults and quackery often believe they have a "cure," and they make what they have to offer sound powerfully scientific, especially to the person who is in need of help. The quack is hard to place behind bars because he often claims that he is not dispensing medicines. As long as he does not prescribe drugs or practice surgery, he seems to be safe in many states today. But his influence in spreading health misinformation is great indeed. Public and school health education can do much to curtail fads, cults, and quackeries.

Misconceptions

"The trouble with people is not that they don't know . . . but that they know so much that ain't so."

—Josh Billings, 1818–1885

People are under all kinds of common misconceptions. Some border on superstitions; others are more acceptable and easy to believe, such as "it is impossible to cure any cancer." One of the biggest misconceptions in our society today relates to the topic of who is qualified to practice medicine. Thousands of unsuspecting people have little idea of the meaning of "Dr." or "M.D." They assume that these letters refer to specialists of comparable ability. Yet, in some places, almost anyone can hang up a sign in his front yard with "Dr." written on it.

---

[29]Council on Foods and Nutrition. "Zen Macrobiotic Diets," *Journal of American Medical Association*, October 18, 1971.

A rather extensive list of harmful misconceptions about health and safety was compiled by Dzenowagis from information given by sixth grade schoolchildren.[30] As in his earlier studies, he points to the needs for health education in a convincing manner. Children in this grade had erroneous beliefs, and they had trouble discriminating between truths, half-truths, and falsehoods. Dzenowagis concluded that certain dangerous misconceptions were prevalent among 28 per cent of the sixth grade children.

Over a 25 year period, Kilander discovered a slight but steady improvement in the level of health information held by children and adults. Here are several examples of the more interesting misconceptions selected from several hundred test items:

Approximately one-third of the students in college believe entirely or in part that "a prospective mother can make her child more musical if she listens to good music." Exactly half of a group of 50 mothers in the PTA were similarly misinformed.

About one-third of the public thinks that water contains calories and is fattening.

About one in five believes that a newborn child's disfiguration may be caused by the mother's fright during pregnancy.

About one out of four students still believes there is some truth to the statement that "fish is brain food." One out of three nonprofessional adults holds this misconception.

The Extremes — Indifference Versus Neurotic Behavior

People seem to vary in their attitude toward health on a scale all the way from a state of indifference with too little concern for health to a state of over-concern to the point of neurotic behavior. Somewhere between the two lies the area of the moderate attitude.

Indifference is closely allied to gullibility and ignorance. It is a negative factor that has always retarded the wheels of progress. It is more common in adults, whose minds are less flexible than in children, who tend to be openminded. It evaporates slowly when human enlightenment takes hold. Indifference to common health practices is illustrated rather well by the story of the nurse-teacher who called on Mary's mother to tell her about the little girl's long standing case of head lice. After the nurse had spoken to her for several minutes, the mother simply gazed out across the fields, shrugged her shoulders as if to dismiss the whole business and said, "Well, everybody has a few."

The other extreme is neurotic behavior. A growing number of adults are becoming almost neurotic about their health. They sometimes join cults, become food faddists, and practice any health fancies which suit them at the moment. These people thrive on all the loose bits of information on psychosomatic illnesses that float about in their community. Moreover, their imaginary difficulties sometimes become real, and then their neurotic behavior relates to something more serious.

Citizenship

In the final analysis, citizenship itself is pertinent to both the health status and the health understanding of the citizen. Health education, therefore, may be considered a vital part of education for citizenship.

Behind disease control and other health practices is the reasonably good community. And the "good community," according to Edward Lee Thorndike, is made better in this country primarily and chiefly by getting able and good people as residents — people who, for example, are intelligent, are reasonably happy, do not contact syphilis, or commit murder, or allow others to do so. In short, an enlightened citizenry goes a long way toward building the utopia of tomorrow.

[30]Dzenowagis, Joseph G. "Prevalence of Certain Dangerous Safety Misconceptions Among a Group of Sixth-Grade Children," *Journal of School Health, 33*:26–32, January 1963.

EDUCATION DEFINED

A proper definition of education includes some reference to aims, purposes, or goals. The word "education" comes from the Latin word *educere,* meaning "to lead forth" or "to lead out." It refers to the drawing out of a person something latent or potential. It suggests a change in some particular direction. Education, therefore, may be defined toward certain preconceived goals. Thus, education is anything but haphazard. There is a well defined purpose expressed through clearly stated aims and objectives.

EDUCATIONAL AIMS AND OBJECTIVES

Principles, not men—when men desert principles, may they be deserted by the people.

—Courier of New Hampshire, 1802

There has always been a high degree of respect in this country for the person with an avowed purpose.[31] One of the most famous remarks used year after year at commencement exercises was made by Leland Stanford who said, "the world stands aside for the man who knows where he is going."

In education, as in other fields of endeavor, one needs to know where he is going. Direction is always important. One must possess a personal philosophy of life that is fundamentally sound. Like Maxwell Garnett, most people believe that human societies should aim toward the fulfillment of some far-reaching purpose.[32] Such a point of view coupled with an interest in education equips the individual with the basic ideas to formulate the aims and objectives of education.

Aims are generally far-reaching pur-

poses, while objectives are usually near-at-hand goals. The proposition to raise the nation's health 10 per cent would be of such magnitude that it would be considered an aim. A lesser proposition to purify the water supply, however, would be a fair example of an objective.

Most purposes of education make a definite reference to healthful living. In 70 b.c., Cicero proclaimed to his subjects in Rome, "In nothing do men more nearly approach the gods than in giving health to men." Centuries later, in 1550, Rabelais said, "The aim of education is not so much to fill thee with learning as to train both thy mind and thy body.... Without health, life is no life." In 1690, John Locke made his much quoted statement: "A sound mind in a sound body is a short but full description of a happy state in this world; he that has these two has little more to wish for; and he that wants either of them, will be but little the better for anything else."

The essential purposes of education have not varied to any great degree in a century of time. What Herbert Spencer wrote in 1860 on the question, "What knowledge is of most worth?" does not depart significantly from modern goals. His ends of education were concerned with life and health, earning a living, family rearing, citizenship, and leisure.

In 1898 Nicholas Murray Butler, president of Columbia University for forty-three years, again asked the old Spencerian question. He acknowledged Spencer's science in education approach and went on to point out that the most enduring knowledge must ultimately relate to things of the spirit.[33] A major contribution of Butler's was that he viewed a proper education as one in which the practical aspects could be linked to the things of the spirit. This means that health education must be both reasonable and emotional if it is to penetrate the mind of the student and be significant in the spiritual life that constitutes humanity's full stature.

---

[31] For a clear-cut illustration of singleness of purpose, see Abraham Lincoln's straightforward letter to Horace Greeley on the Saving of the Nation. (Willgoose, Carl E. "Health: The Fundamental Objective," *Education, 68(8)*:451, April 1948.)

[32] Garnett, J. C. Maxwell. *Education and World Citizenship.* Cambridge, England: The University Press, 1921, p. 315.

---

[33] Butler, Nicholas Murray. *The Meaning of Education, and Other Essays and Addresses,* New York: The Macmillan Co., 1898.

As far as health education is concerned, most sets of purposes stress health as the primary aim. They also point to the need for education for leisure, an item that concerns physical and mental health to a great degree and probably has as much to do with the survival of man as any other aim (Figure 1–8).

THE ULTIMATE SCOPE OF HEALTH EDUCATION

It may be seen in the above objectives of education that agreement has been reached by educational philosophers stressing the need for health education in the schools. The ultimate scope of health education is a broad one. Thus, each person, in order to satisfy his own needs and, at the same time, contribute his share to the welfare of society must possess:

1. Optimum organic health consistent with heredity and the application of present health knowledge;

2. Sufficient coordination, strength, and vitality to meet emergencies, as well as the requirements of daily living;

3. Emotional stability to meet the stresses and strains of modern life;

4. Social consciousness and adaptability with respect to the requirements of group living;

5. Sufficient knowledge and insight to make suitable decisions and arrive at feasible solutions to problems;

6. Attitudes, values, and skills which stimulate satisfactory participation in a full range of daily activities;

7. Spiritual and moral qualities which contribute the fullest measure of living in a democratic society.[34]

If we learn anything at all from the present condition of adult mankind, it should be that the problems, diseases,

[34]Statement prepared and approved by the delegates to the American Association for Health, Physical Education, and Recreation Fitness Conference, September 12–15, 1956, Washington, D.C.

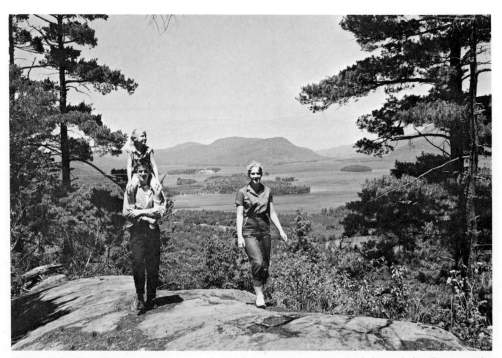

Figure 1–8 The effects of pressure and rapid pace are counteracted through family recreation. (New York State Department of Commerce.)

and inadequacies of the moment did not suddenly appear; rather, they emerged gradually, having had their roots established during the early elementary school years. This is to say that the backaches, ulcers, gastrointestinal pains, hypertension, obesity, chronic fatigue, coronary thrombosis, and the neurotic and psychotic behavior related to anxiety, apprehension, worry, fear, hatred, and jealousy are all tied directly to a *pattern of living* and level of understanding obtained during the formative years. A sense of values early in life, coupled with the proper skills and knowledge, sets the stage in more ways than one. The part played by health education in this period can be most productive.

QUESTIONS FOR DISCUSSION

1. What is the relationship of physical efficiency to total health?

2. How can we get citizens in the community interested in, concerned with, and involved in school health programs?

3. How can we gain greater cooperation in closing the gap between the objectives of the school health program and what is really being accomplished?

4. What is happening in your community relative to the control of air pollutants? Water pollutants?

5. Are there ways in which health professionals in the community can influence health instruction practices in an elementary school?

6. How has the World Health Organization contributed to child health on an international level?

SUGGESTED ACTIVITIES

1. Dobzhansky, writing in *Mankind Evolving: The Evolution of the Human Species* (Yale University Press, 1962, pp. 346–347), points out that "nature and nurture" work together. Hoyman writes about the same thing. So does Dubos. (See references listed at end of the chapter.) Look over an article or two which pertains to human ecology and health. Prepare a written paragraph on what you have read and another one setting forth your comments.

2. Survey a number of persons in health-related professions (public or private) and find out how they feel about education as a means of preventing poor health. Are they concerned about venereal disease or cardiac statistics, or something called "value illness"? Compare your findings with several of your classmates.

3. Compare the several positions with regard to population growth and its bearing on human health and welfare. Do official governmental figures substantiate the views of demographers and ecologists? What is the view of the conservationist?

4. Review the list of nine *Imperatives In Education* set forth by the American Association of School Administrators. Indicate ways and means in which health education can contribute to the fulfillment of these points and help meet the needs of the times.

5. Compare the views of Senator Edward M. Kennedy with those of Marvin Henry Edwards relative to health care in America. (See *Selected References.*) What are your comments relative to the Senator's Federally-financed, cradle-to-grave suggestions as compared with the program of less government involvement of Mr. Edwards?

6. In his utopian book, *The Shape of Things To Come,* H. G. Wells assumed that scientific thinking, modern-day engineering, and public education, by their intrinsic worth, would prepare a kind of future that would be approved of by the educated middle-class citizen. Later, when he wrote *Mind at the End of Its Tether,* Wells became disillusioned as he noted that Nazi Germany scored higher on scientific rationalism, engineering, and public education than did any other European nation. Take a moment to examine this observation. Do educational goals and programs need very careful definition as they relate to a civilization? Write out some specific implications for educators and others who build a society "close to the heart's desire."

SELECTED REFERENCES

Aristotle. "Pleasure and Happiness," in Randall, John H., Buchler, Justus, and Shirk, Evelyn (eds.). *Readings in Philosophy*. New York: Barnes and Noble, 1946, pp. 356–368.

Bucher, Charles A., Olsen, Einar A., and Willgoose, Carl E. *The Foundations of Health*. New York: Appleton-Century-Crofts, 1967, Chapters 2, 14, 17.

Budnik, Dan. "The Restoration of a River." *Saturday Review*, April 8, 1972.

Carrell, Alexis. *Man The Unknown*. New York: Harper & Brothers, 1936.

Commoner, Barry. *The Closing Circle*. New York: Alfred A. Knopf, 1971.

Cutler, Robert. "*No Time for Rest*." Boston: Little, Brown and Co., 1966.

Douglas, William O. "Toward Greater Vitality," *Today's Health*, 51:54–57, May 1973.

Dubos, René. *Man Adapting*. New Haven: Yale University Press, 1965.

Edwards, Marvin H. *Hazardous to Your Health*. New York: Arlington House, 1972.

Hafen, Brent Q. *Self Destructive Behavior: A National Crisis*. Minneapolis: Burgess Publishing Co., 1972.

Hoyman, Howard S. "An Ecologic View of Health and Health Education." *Journal of School Health*, 35:110–123, March 1965.

Kennedy, Edward M. *In Critical Condition: The Crisis in American Health Care*. New York: Simon and Schuster, 1972.

Leff, S. V. *From Witchcraft to World Health*. New York: The Macmillan Co., 1957.

Mark, Norman. "Health Criticism: Curbing Those TV Commercials." *Today's Health*, 50:9–15, August 1972.

McKenna, Ken. "If Creeping Boredom Is Your Work Problem." *Today's Health*, 50:43–46, August 1972.

Millner, Bernard N. "Health Needs of School-Age Children." *Journal of School Health, 36*:276–280, June, 1966.

O'Neil, Brian, et al. "Automobile Head Restraints — Frequency of Neck Injury Claims." *American Journal of Public Health, 62*:399–406, March 1972.

Purdom, Paul W. "The Shape of a National Health Program." *American Journal of Public Health, 62*:12–15, January 1972.

Rosen, George. "Health is a Community Affair," *American Journal of Public Health, 57*:572–583, April 1967.

Schwartz, Harry. *The Case for American Medicine*. New York: David McKay Co., 1973.

Tuck, Miriam, L. *Consumer Health*. Dubuque, Iowa: W. C. Brown Co., 1972.

Vincent, Ronald G. "A Fence or an Ambulance." *Journal of School Health, 37*:369–373, October 1967.

Wattenberg, Ben J. "The Decline of the American Baby." *World, 1*:20–22, August 29, 1972.

Whiteside, Thomas. *Selling Death: Cigarette Advertising and Public Health*. New York: Liveright, 1971.

Willgoose, Carl E. "Recreation: An Attitude of Mind." *Education, 81*:42–44, September 1960.

Willgoose, Carl E. "What Will Health Be Like in 1977?" *Journal of Health, Physical Education, and Recreation. 39*:30–31, March 1968.

Willgoose, Carl E. "Providing for Change: New Directions," in Read, Donald A. (ed.). *New Directions in Health Education*. New York: Macmillan Co., 1971, pp. 1–17.

2 THE ELEMENTARY SCHOOL HEALTH PROGRAM

Grant me the strength, time and opportunity always to correct what I have acquired, always extend its domain, for knowledge is immense and the spirit of man can extend indefinitely to enrich itself daily with new requirements. Today he can discover his errors of yesterday and tomorrow he may obtain light on what he thinks himself sure today.

—Maimonides

School health programs exist in the elementary school because salubrious practices of well-being and the right style of life (orthobiosis) need to be developed early. Even in the primary grades there is a sense of urgency when one speaks of the healthy personality—forming feelings and values which underlie a positive self-image and are foundations for future relationships. Moreover, the expression of Maimonides relative to man enriching himself to meet "new requirements" is especially valid in this century, where it is necessary to learn at an early date how to meet successfully the adaptive requirements created by rapidly changing conditions, and the variety of mental and physical disease states emerging in spite of an increase in health care, comfort, prosperity, and general affluence.

JUSTIFICATION FOR SCHOOL HEALTH PROGRAM

As a society comes of age it strives for excellence instead of quantitative growth. Dubos says as much when he speaks of the "mature society" as one that is not only stable in numbers and in material production, but is also in "ecological equilibrium with the resources of the Earth."[1] Along with this comes the development of a far greater sense of personal and collective responsibility which tends to ensure a proper *quality of life*. As a sensitive historian, Dubos wants mankind to be aware of the past and to consider human welfare in the future in a more humane way. What better justification could there be for improving the health of the citizenry through the creation of well-planned programs of health education in the schools?

There are numerous justifications for a total health maintenance and education effort in the schools. For one thing there is a considerable body of evidence available to support the premise that failure to develop optimum health puts a limit on genius. *Mens sana in corpore sano* is not a new expression. The quality of the mind is made known through the competent actions of the body. A lowered health status reduces one's ability to perform—as a genius or as a moron. Man approaches his potential mental capacity

---

[1]Dubos, Rene. *A God Within*. New York: Charles Scribner's Sons, 1972.

27

only when he is capable of putting his thoughts into action. Likewise in learning, Thorndike's law of readiness simply means that the individual pupil must be ready to learn. He must be organically sound, mentally alert, and emotionally able to receive the most from the total school curriculum. A pain in the stomach, an earache, or some other such bothersome factor is a distracting stimulus. Whereas an adult can, in effect, say to a stomach ache, pain, or emotional problem, "get thee behind me," the primary grade pupil simply cannot ignore it. His ability to learn is directly impaired, and he will not respond as well as his contemporaries, either in the classroom or anywhere else.

The Educational Policies Commission of the National Education Association has stated repeatedly that an educated person understands the basic facts concerning health and disease; the educated person protects his own health and that of his dependents; and an educated person works to improve the health of his community. If these are some of the characteristics of an educated person, the school program must provide experiences that will impart knowledge about and develop proper attitudes concerning health and safety practices.

Social accomplishment is more than slightly related to well-being in the community at large, because charity consists of being able to give of oneself without thought of return. And in the school, social accomplishment as well as academic accomplishment is ever-dependent on good eyesight and hearing, freedom from disease and handicapping defects, emotional stability, and a satisfactory rate of growth. The broadly conceived school health program is concerned with these things just as much as it is with classroom instruction. The focus today is on disease prevention. There is wide acceptance of the concept that the cancers and afflictions of mankind do not represent medical failures but educational failures. Thus, preventive medicine and preventive education have much in common. This idea is well brought out in the following verse:

" 'Twas a dangerous cliff, as they freely
    confessed,
  Though to walk near its crest was so
    pleasant;
But over its terrible edge there had
    slipped
  A duke, and full many a peasant.
The people said something would have to
    be done,
  But their projects did not at all tally.
Some said, "Put a fence 'round the edge
    of the cliff";
  Some, "An ambulance down in the
    valley."
The lament of the crowd was profound
    and was loud,
  As their hearts overflowed with their
    pity;
But the cry for the ambulance carried the
    day
  As it spread through the neighboring
    city,
A collection was made, to accumulate aid,
  And the dwellers in highway and alley
Gave dollars or cents — not to furnish a
    fence —
  But an ambulance down in the valley.
The story looks queer as we've written it
    here,
  But things oft occur that are stranger.
More humane, we assert, than to succor
    the hurt,
  Is the plan of removing the danger.
The best possible course is to safeguard
    the source;
  Attend to things rationally.
Yes, build up the fence and let us
    dispense
  With the ambulance down in the
    valley.[2]

In the School Health Study it was especially well verified that school children display a mass of ignorance about health and well-being in general. This "major weakness in the educational system," as it was called by the writers of the Study, prompted them to say that the best place for health instruction is in the school — chiefly because the school is the only agency that can keep pace with the rapid advance of medical science and can give the child the basis of health

---

[2]Tussing, Lyle. *Psychology for Better Living.* New York: John Wiley & Sons, Inc., 1959, pp. 18–19.

problems so that he can engage in intelligent health practices.[3]

HISTORY OF SCHOOL HEALTH MOVEMENT

The history of public health is as old as the Egyptian and Hebrew civilizations. But the history of school health is much more recent. Certainly, one of the reasons for this is that, in the centuries gone by, man had only a slight regard for the growth and development of youth. It was a man's world; women and children were strictly secondary. Although formal education was fostered in many places, health maintenance and promotion as such were not the concern of the school.

The school health movement has a European heritage. In 1790 Benjamin Thompson, known as Count Rumford, started school lunches for underprivileged children in Bavaria. About this time Johann Peter Frank wrote scientific articles on the topic of school hygiene. Other eminent scientists of the day such as Rudolph Virchow (1821–1902) and Henry P. Bowditch (1840–1911) urged medical examinations of schoolchildren and studies on their growth and development. In England, in 1832, Edwin Chadwick studied child employment conditions and became interested in the schools. Theophile Roussel followed somewhat the same pattern in France. Great writers such as Victor Hugo, Charles Reade, and Charles Dickens were influential in starting a school health movement. It was Hugo, in 1865, who established school lunches for poor children on the Isle of Guernsey. They became so popular that by the early 1900's half the cities in Germany had lunch programs for schoolchildren.

In the United States interest was growing in the areas of school health. In 1842, Horace Mann, Secretary of the Massachusetts Board of Education, wrote in the *Common School Journal*,

"So intimately are all parts of the human constitution connected and so vitally do the mental and moral depend upon the physical power, that we can understand either only by studying them in connection with others. For this reason, the knowledge of laws of structure, growth, development, and health of the body is essential to a comprehension of the corresponding particular in the phenomena of the mind." These words carried a great amount of weight. It is not strange, therefore, that by 1885 the American Association for Physical Education was formed. Prominent medical doctors from this group advocated scientific programs of physical activity and hygiene in the schools. By 1894 the Boston schools were ready to begin the first regular medical inspection program in America. Then followed Chicago, New York, Philadelphia, and others. Interest grew and numerous health agencies were born that in turn had a potent effect on school health efforts. Notable among these was the formation in 1912 of the Children's Bureau of the Federal Security Agency, an organization set up to investigate subjects relating to child life and welfare. Shortly thereafter in 1918 the American Child Hygiene Association was formed.

From about 1900 to 1915 a continued effort was made in the schools to give medical examinations and control communicable diseases. Public health practices improved in many communities and influenced the promotion of child health. Some schools taught hygiene courses consisting chiefly of anatomy and physiology. At first the teaching emphasis was on health knowledge as pure subject matter. It became apparent after a while, however, that the educator must appraise the quantity and quality of the health information in terms of its effect on attitudes and practices of students. As far back as 1910 men like Luther H. Gulick and R. Tait McKenzie stressed the need for appraisal in school health.

Following World War I, school health programs accomplished a great deal. Research was developed illustrating the benefits of properly constituted programs. In 1922, Claire E. Turner, work-

---

[3]School Health Education Study. *School Health Education: A Call for Action.* Washington, D.C., 1965.

ing with Mary Spencer, carried out his now famous Malden, Massachusetts, school health demonstration project. Over a two year period he compared the children of three fourth grades, three fifth grades, and three sixth grades in two school buildings with a control group of similar grade school children in two other schools.[4] Health education was developed with the experimental group and data were collected concerning growth, health status, and health habits. The demonstration was not only successful, but because it was widely publicized it caused other promoters of school health to "take heart" and begin health instruction in the grades.

The most thorough research into the status of health education and the needs of youth was started in 1961 and brought to a head in 1965 by the School Health Education Study.[5] The findings indicated that health content is repetitious throughout the grades without consideration for the problems of youth; universally neglected content areas of interest to elementary teachers are consumer education, sex education, venereal disease, non-communicable disease, smoking, alcohol and drugs, community health programs, environmental hazards, mental health, and nutrition and weight control. Experimental curriculum materials were later tried out in pilot-study communities to test the conceptual approach to learning.

Today, school health is an integrated phase of the total school program. This has come about chiefly from a rising interest in the welfare of children, an increase in associations dedicated to raising the nation's health, White House Conferences, the monetary funds of philanthropic organizations, and the tireless efforts of pioneers such as Claire Turner, Thomas Wood, Haven Emerson, Mabel Rugen, Mabel Bragg, C. E. Winslow, Oliver Byrd, Raymond Fran-

zen, C. C. Wilson, Sally Lucas Jean, Ruth Strang, Sara Louise Smith, and Fred Hein. In addition, considerable credit should go to such organizations as the American School Health Association, American Public Health Association, American Association for Health, Physical Education and Recreation, and the Joint Committee on Health Problems In Education of the National Education Association and the American Medical Association.

LEGAL FOUNDATIONS FOR SCHOOL HEALTH PROGRAMS

One of the first laws created for the protection of schoolchildren was passed in 1833 in France. It made public school authorities responsible for the health of schoolchildren. Other European laws followed in Austria, Sweden, Germany, and Russia.

Horace Mann's agitation for the science of health, then termed "physiology and hygiene," resulted in Massachusetts, in 1850, becoming the first state to require hygiene by law as a compulsory subject in all the public schools of the commonwealth. A number of other legal enactments occurred about the turn of the century. Instruction about alcohol and narcotics was required by 1890 in all states. Many states required physical education before 1900. In 1899 teachers in Connecticut were required to test the vision of their pupils. A school dentist was hired in Reading, Pennsylvania, in 1903. Many laws were made soon after this. By 1933 the Nebraska State Supreme Court had decreed that the control of the pupil's health during school hours was the responsibility of the school personnel. This is indeed a big responsibility, and the schools have accepted it in the spirit of service.

Today most states have legal foundations for their school health programs. Many of these are in the form of rules and regulations of state commissions regarding education. The laws in such states as Minnesota, Pennsylvania, Ohio

[4]Turner, Claire E. "Malden Studies in Health Education and Growth," *American Journal of Public Health, 18*:1217–1230, 1928.

[5]Sliepcevich, Elena M. "Health Education: a Conceptual Approach." Washington, D.C.: *School Health Education Study,* 1965.

and New York are particularly clear in setting forth the need for proper attention to health.

SCHOOL HEALTH ORGANIZATION

Paramount to the success of a health program in any school system is the organization of health activities, personnel, facilities and time. With a school population continually growing, it becomes increasingly difficult to meet all the health objectives with ease. Yet, efforts in most places are regularly intensified to improve health through preventive and remedial measures.

Health education is an applied science concerned with relating research findings in health to the lives of people. It narrows the gap between what is known and what is practiced. It is what Will Durant calls "preventive medicine in the classroom." If we say that *health education is the sum of experiences that favorably influence practices, attitudes, and knowledge relating to health*, it is readily seen that we are dealing with something that occurs at all times and in all places in the school.[6] Hence, the entire school personnel and every area of the curriculum have to some degree a part in health education. The organization of these varied efforts into a sound working program is the job of the school administrator.

School health education is essentially a three-pronged process. It consists of health services, healthful school environment, and health instruction. Definitions of these terms have existed for four decades:[7]

Health services "comprises all those procedures designated to determine the health status of the child, to enlist his cooperation in health protection and maintenance, to inform parents of the defects that may be present, to prevent disease, and to correct remediable defects."

Healthful school living "is a term that designates the provision of a wholesome environment, the organization of a healthful school day, and the establishment of such teacher-pupil relationships as make a safe and sanitary school, favorable to the best development of living of pupils and teachers."

Health instruction "is that organization of learning experiences directed toward the development of favorable health knowledges, attitudes, and practices."

The prevalent point of view is that the term "health education" should be reserved for the teaching or instructional part of the school health program. In this manner the pupil has no difficulty attaching a suitable name to his course; he can call it health education — which indeed it is.

RESPONSIBILITY OF THE CLASSROOM TEACHER

There is no person in the school system better fitted to make a significant contribution to the health of schoolchildren than the classroom teacher in the elementary school. She alone occupies the key position for improving child health. With her interest, enthusiasm, and understanding, the school health program moves ahead. Without her support, however, the program is limited.

The role of the classroom teacher is unique; no other person sees the child as she does. She can readily compare his appearance and actions today with what they were yesterday or a month ago. Or she can compare him with the other 25 children in the classroom who are about the same age. This provides the alert teacher with a vantage point that neither the parent nor family physician can match. Thus, every classroom teacher

---

[6]This definition of health education is the one agreed upon by the Joint Committee on Health Problems in Education of the National Education Association and the American Medical Association. The report, *Health Education*, 6th ed., may be obtained from the National Education Association, Washington, D.C.

[7]Health Education Section, Committee Report, American Physical Education Association. *Journal of Health and Physical Education,* December 1934.

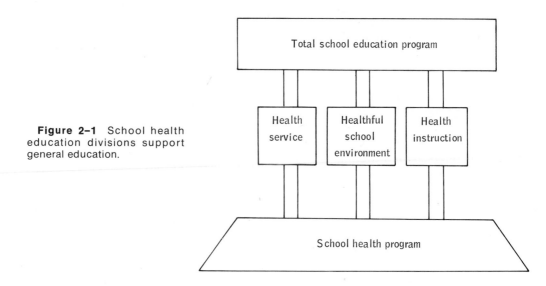

Figure 2-1 School health education divisions support general education.

holds a potentially powerful job for building sound health (Figure 2-1). The extent to which she does this will depend upon many things. She will need administrative support. She will need a warm personality and feeling for children, and she will need to use her powers of observation carefully. To use the words of Frederick Mayer, the teacher should also be an optimist with an attitude of encouragement and hopefulness so that the schoolroom may be "an oasis of hope."[8]

HOW THE CLASSROOM TEACHER PROMOTES HEALTH

Specifically, the classroom teacher promotes health in a number of ways:

By Cooperating with the School Health Services Personnel

Children are properly prepared by the teacher for a visit to the school physician or nurse for periodic physical examinations. Teachers take a positive approach to the examinations by saying to their pupils, "The doctor is coming to see how many healthy boys and girls we have." Learning to visit medical personnel and

come away happy is an education in itself. Any experience that is satisfying or "feels good" to the child is effective in terms of his future behavior. The nurse, the physician, and the dental hygienist should be their friends.

By Detecting Health Abnormalities and Referring Them to Proper Authorities for Appropriate Follow-Up and Correction

The teacher who uses her "eyes to see" can observe a variety of items related to the onset of poor health. The child with frequent colds and sore throats, who is continually sniffling in class, may have any one of a number of difficulties involving the upper respiratory area. Likewise, the child who squints to see or turns his head to hear simple questions may be in need of medical aid right away. Numerous children appear to be well. The child who exhibits signs of emotional upset which may be missed entirely by the parents may be spotted by the teacher as one who behaves differently from the group and needs individual attention. It should be remembered that the younger the person, the more readily he responds to pain or other distracting stimuli. The response may represent a series of incidents leading to poor scholarship. The pupil, for example, who scores well on a test of learning aptitude yet produces work in class that is hardly better than

[8]Mayer, Frederick. "Education and the Good Life," *Education, 78(4):*497, April 1957.

average, is the kind of pupil who bears watching.

By Making the School Environment Pleasant and Desirable for the Pupils

The school, to be at all effective, must be the kind of place a child wants to go to. The classroom is made more inviting by the teacher. She regulates such physical items as temperature, ventilation, lighting, and seating. Her own attitude toward the students has much to do with the health and happiness of the class. There are numerous children who dislike school and show this by coming down with "morning sickness," a real disease of the psychosomatic variety that mysteriously disappears on Saturdays, Sundays, and holidays.

By Providing Health Instruction in the Classroom

Teaching is done both formally and informally. In this respect, the teacher seldom misses an opportunity to refer to the child's health and welfare. Health as a topic is also correlated with other materials. The teacher's task is to teach it with the aim of changing practices and attitudes. Health knowledge as such must lead to the kind of understanding that results in changed behavior.

THE TEACHER'S HEALTH

The effective teacher is one who possesses the vitality to do the job expected of her and has left a little reserve at the close of the day for her own enrichment activities. According to reports and opinions, personality maladjustments are responsible for failure in teaching more often than physical disorders. Even the admirable teacher who loves children, is intellectually alert, and gets along well with others, will be limited in her expression and enthusiasm proportionate to the degree of her physical and mental health.

The health status of the teacher has another significant bearing on education. This relates to the image the teacher presents to her pupils. The sick teacher with a sour personality can hardly practice what she preaches. Whether we care to admit it or not, teaching has long been a process of making little images of the teacher in the minds of the pupils. Very little effective health education can be expected from the image of a teacher suffering from such complaints as chronic fatigue, gross overweight, nagging headache, low back pain, irregular teeth, and a negative, complaining attitude toward life in general. Thus, in teaching young people, the importance of the example of personal health and well-being cannot be underestimated.

RESPONSIBILITY OF THE ELEMENTARY SCHOOL ADMINISTRATOR

Although the alert classroom teacher is worth her weight in gold in any health program, the value of a school administrator who is sympathetic to the goals of school health is highly significant.

The practice of accepting primary responsibility for school health varies in a number of communities. Essentially it boils down to the question of whether the school *controls* all health education or whether it is the responsibility of the local or county health department. In a number of places the city or county health department is responsible for school health services. In fact, county school health planning committees are formed and composed of school people, interested citizens, and county health personnel. These committees, meeting with county school superintendents and county health officers, take steps to initiate desirable health programs in the schools. By and large, however, the trend throughout the country is to place full responsibility for school health and health education with the school administrator and board of education. In the larger cities the administrator may appoint a school health director.

The classroom teacher will find the elementary school principal most helpful, especially if he engages in many of the following activities:

1. Provides for health services and "sets the stage" for the work of physicians, dentists, nurses, psychologists, dental hygienists, and teachers of the handicapped.

2. Is concerned with safe and sanitary building construction, and the activities of the school custodial staff.

3. Is interested in the preparation and personal health of teaching personnel.

4. Promotes in-service education for medical personnel and classroom teachers alike.

5. Obtains adequate funds for the program.

6. Maintains lines of communication between school and community agencies.

7. Arranges for periodic nurse-teacher conferences and meetings of health councils.

8. Meets with parents to secure adequate treatment for all children.

9. Initiates a total school safety program.

10. Assists classroom teachers in securing necessary facilities, materials, and time for health instruction.

11. Provides leadership to school feeding programs.

12. Carries on studies relative to school absences—health problems and school attendance.

It is interesting to note that in one large city school system, the Los Angeles City Schools, the results of an intensive survey indicated several ways in which school administrators could help improve the existing health education effort. For one thing, in planning and coordinating the health program of the individual school, it was suggested that greater use be made of health councils. It was also felt that more use should be made of the school environment in health teaching experiences. Moreover, administrators were urged to develop teacher guides in health education at each grade level, offer more in-service health education, and do a more thorough job of planning the health instruction program.

INNER CITY HEALTH PROBLEMS

In recent years the wide variety of conflicts, frustrations and unhappiness in the urban areas has been uppermost in the thoughts of leaders of government, medicine, social welfare, and education. Hardly an issue or problem is not in some way a health concern.

One thing is for certain: the lowered health status of inner city children, together with other negative variables such as low income and less than adequate family care, frequently results in increased absences and poor school performance. The background for much of this may be blamed on the early years. When, at the infant stage, there is inadequate nutrition, growth is compromised. The brain fails to synthesize protein, and consequently suffers a decrease as great as twenty per cent in the number of cells. Thus, severe malnutrition, which is found frequently in the depths of the inner city as well as in isolated rural areas, results in decreased learning ability, retarded growth, maturation and personal productivity. Moreover, poor child-rearing practices contribute a negative psychological dimension which is closely interwoven with effective learning. It has also been demonstrated that inner city families change their place of residence a great deal; this in itself creates numerous non-utilizers of health care.

Ethnic groups have their problems. The Spanish speaking population needs help. Their ills are often unreported. Illness and premature death is generally higher for blacks than it is for whites. Among the Chinese in San Francisco the incidence of children with vision problems, dental caries, and immunization deficiencies is especially high. Reaching these needy people is difficult to do, for they "hole up" in their crowded, noisy, polluted, insensitive, cold, incomprehensible, inhuman push-button jungle. To reach these groups with the health and education message is, at times, all but impossible because of the breakdown of the neighborhood concept. A return to neighborhoods is needed. There is great merit in preserving an Italian North End, an Irish-Polish South Boston, a Chinatown, a black Roxbury, or any enclave that "feels" comfortable to its residents and has some compatible common denominator, not necessarily ethnic or religious.

One impressive reason that low socioeconomic status and poor health go together, is that there is a lack of concrete information among the disadvantaged relative to the causes and treatment of diseases and the availability of health services. When medical advice is wanted it is generally sought from friends and neighbors rather than a physician or health center personnel. The result is that children are denied medical treatment until a relatively late stage of illness. Blacks by the hundreds know nothing about sickle cell anemia, a genetic disease affecting the red blood cells—for which a medical checkup is a must. Large numbers of families, of all races and persuasions, will listen to some extent to what the schools have to say. Unfortunately, urban bureaucracies are to blame for much of the deterioration of city schools, but the potential for change is ever-present.[9] If some 150-odd compensatory education schemes have been tried and have not worked at all or have worked only marginally or only for a small proportion of the student population, it is probably because the disadvantaged children continue to be *locked into total environments* which are inhibiting models of behavior. It is today obvious that health status and health practices will change very little through the usual hit-or-miss school health efforts. Only a calculated attempt by school personnel to move beyond the school and penetrate the community with innovative health education programs will meet with any measurable degree of success.

CONTRIBUTIONS OF PHYSICAL EDUCATION TO THE SCHOOL HEALTH PROGRAM

Physical education may be defined as a process of changing behavior toward certain preconceived educational goals, primarily through large muscle activity. Health is advanced by increasing the child's vigor, strength, and endurance. Through a broad and varied program of physical activities in the elementary grades, organic growth is stimulated, fundamental physical skills are developed, social efficiency is promoted, and attitudes toward recreation and leisure time are planted like seedlings in the slowly maturing bodies of young people.

Elementary physical education activities such as games of low organization, sport skills, mimetics and story plays, rhythms and dances, and self-testing stunts are full of meaning to the growing child. When properly taught, their contribution to total health, through the avenue of improved physical efficiency and social emotional behavior, is not insignificant.

In recent years President Eisenhower, President Kennedy, President Johnson and President Nixon have made personal efforts to promote a national awareness of the need for physical fitness. The President's Council on Physical Fitness and Sports, through its widely distributed informative publication, "Suggested Elements of a School-Centered Program," has done much to improve existing programs of physical education. Significantly, where programs have been initiated or improved, levels of individual pupil fitness have risen, resulting in an increase in personal vigor and stamina for the many activities of the school day. Moreover, it is not uncommon to find a corresponding rise in levels of achievement and social accomplishment (Figure 2–2).

---

[9] For suggestions for change see Atron Gentry, et al. *Urban Education: The Hope Factor.* Philadelphia: W. B. Saunders Company, 1972.

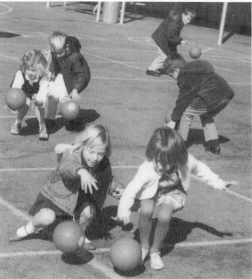

Figure 2-2 Vigorous activity in the elementary school.

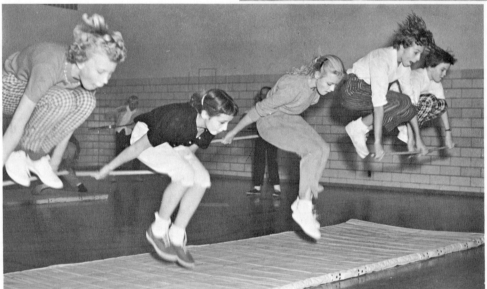

Physical activities, by their very nature, are health teaching activities. They are as much a part of the school health program as food tasting parties or health services. They need to be taught with purpose and understanding. Merely turning children loose on a playground twice a day, day after day, to "blow off steam" is not physical education. In fact, it represents an example of a situation where a unique opportunity is being missed. True, the children will find some relief from the academic activities of the classroom, but they will be denied the chance to learn the skills and develop the attitudes that are so much a part of a good physical education program. This is not to be treated as a haphazard activity, for physical education is not just aimless movement; it is part of the education process. Moreover, physical condition is being increasingly equated with mental efficiency and intellectual productivity rather than with games and sports alone.

Elementary teachers who feel somewhat unprepared in the physical education area, who lack the skill and knowledge to carry on even a partial program of purposeful activity, should do one or two of the following things:

1. Visit a class where a good program of suitable activities is being taught and observe how it is done. In most communities there are at least one or two especially successful teachers in this area.

2. Visit the school or community library and search the existing books for appropriate games, dances, and self-testing stunts.

3. Write the nearest elementary teacher preparation institution for program help.

4. Contact the state educational department supervisor of elementary physical education. Either he will pay a visit, arrange for the teacher to visit a school, or will send written suggestions.

Classroom teachers may feel, therefore, that physical education and health education are cooperative in nature. Both subjects are planned with the purpose of contributing as much as possible to the growth and development of children; total fitness items relating to nutrition, emotional climate, and poor eyesight are the concern of each. In many schools classroom teachers work closely with physical educators not only in the improvement of motor skills, but also on individual pupil posture, muscular strength, and remedial exercises.

PRESENT TRENDS VERSUS PAST PRACTICES IN SCHOOL HEALTH

As education has grown more scientific over the decades, medical and educational workers associated with school health have concerned themselves with the scientific aspects of health status, health knowledge, and health behavior.

For example, at one time the teaching emphasis was on health knowledge as pure subject matter. It became apparent after a while, however, that the educator must appraise both the quantity and the quality of the health information in terms of its effect on attitudes and habits of students. This is reflected in the current trends and practices especially when compared with the practices of several decades ago. Some noteworthy examples follow.

Present Trends

1. Physical examinations of schoolchildren are given in less haste and are more thorough. Better use is made of the physician's time.

2. Screening examinations for hearing and vision losses, together with weighing and measuring of pupils, are popular appraisal activities carried on with objective measures.

3. Classroom teachers cooperate with school nurses, dental hygienists, and other medical personnel in an effort to determine the health status of the child. Many teachers have special training to improve their observation of health abnormalities.

4. Schools have effective health service departments designed to evaluate the *total* school health effort.

5. Health councils operate in a democratic way to determine health status and analyze health behavior. Case studies are frequently run on individual children.

6. The objective is to evaluate the child as accurately as possible and then see that something is done about his needs.

7. Health teaching is done from the viewpoint of a child's needs and interests, and factual information is used to bring about maximum understanding.

8. There is increased use of evaluation techniques designed to measure health attitudes and health practices.

9. Health concepts are becoming far more prevalent than unfounded opinions.

10. Health education is concerned with community resources, and is carried on by concerted action of home, school, and public and private agencies.

11. There is increasing recognition that the emotional health of the teacher influences the emotional tone of the classroom.

Past Practices

1. Physical examinations of schoolchildren were incomplete. As many as 60 to 80 children were examined per hour. Improper organization for health appraisal was common.

2. Screening examinations for hearing and vision were carried on haphazardly with a good deal of subjective measurement.

3. Schools did not use medical personnel to any great extent. Teachers were not prepared to appraise health status and detect abnormalities but did their best by themselves.

4. Schools used physicians only in a limited way. They were concerned only with giving physical examinations.

5. Health committees or health councils were unheard of.

6. Examinations that were conducted often revealed defects and abnormalities which were not followed up and corrected.

7. Health facts were given in a formal way and were essentially pure anatomy and physiology.

8. Tests of health knowledge were made to measure health information only.

9. Health opinions and superstitions were more prevalent than health concepts.

10. Health education was engaged in by uncoordinated groups and agencies. Often one did not know what the other was doing.

11. The health of the teacher was incidental to learning.

As one looks to the future, it becomes quite clear that the impact of professional, public, and voluntary health organizations is such that it will only be a few years before all states implement legislation requiring direct health instruction for all children. There will be a properly *balanced* curriculum with adequate scope and sequence which does justice to all major health problems rather than singling out any one popular problem for overemphasis. The need will be met for greater numbers of school health coordinators or curriculum specialists to work with classroom teachers and for a continuing in-service program to keep teachers up-to-date with rapidly changing health concepts, and to encourage creative teaching. Already, health teaching is moving at an accelerated speed from a "do-gooder" activity to a carefully organized and programmed part of the total school curriculum.

QUESTIONS FOR DISCUSSION

1. In your opinion, how much preparation in the health teaching area should the elementary classroom teacher have? Back up your comments with at least one reference.

2. What is the relationship between physical activity and health instruction in the promotion of health?

3. Observe an elementary school and its health education program. After comparing your findings with others, what are common observations?

4. If health observation of school children is an art as George Wheatley and others believe, do you think it possible to train the elementary teacher so that a high level of proficiency may be obtained?

5. Discuss the role of the teacher's health in relation to teacher employment and retention practices. Should a teacher object to a physical or mental examination?

SUGGESTED ACTIVITIES

1. Alfred North Whitehead wrote that "... you may not separate the seamless coat of learning." In short, every classroom teacher as well as health professional is a health teacher to some extent. What are the implications here for school-community cooperation? Look into this relationship in a specific locality.

2. Look over the nine *Imperatives in Education* set up after a two-year study by the American Association of School Administrators (AASA, Washington: NEA, 1201 16th Street, N. W., 1966). Which of these appear to be implemented the most by improved programs of health instruction in the schools?

3. Find out the health education requirements for your state. Is health instruction required in the elementary or middle schools? If so, how much time has been legislated? If not, is any move being made to bring about a change in state requirements?

4. In the short book by Irene Schram, *Ashes, Ashes, We All Fall Down*, the story is told of some fifth grade children being exposed to terrifying situations (See Selected References). Read the book and compare the story to real-life situations in a city like New York or elsewhere where one must survive under similar or worse threats. Are there health implications here?

SELECTED REFERENCES

American Association of School Administrators. *Imperatives in Education.* Washington, D.C., 1966.

Anderson, C. L. *School Health Practice*, 5th ed. St. Louis: C. V. Mosby Co., 1972.

Aubrey, Roger F. "Health Education: Neglected Child of the Schools." *Journal of School Health*, 42:285–289, May 1972.

Bender, Stephen J. "Health Education in the Elementary School." *School Health Review*, 3:23–26, January–February 1972.

Boyd, William. *An Introduction to the Study of Disease*. Philadelphia: Lea and Febiger, 1971.

Butler, Evelyn. "Thoughts on Health Education in Inner-City Schools." *School Health Review*, 3:12–14, January–February 1972.

Dubos, René. *Man, Medicine and Environment.* New York: Praeger Publishing Co., 1968.

Etzioni, Amitai. "Human Beings Are Not Very Easy to Change." *Saturday Review*, June 3, 1972.

Grout, Ruth E. *Health Teaching in Schools*, 5th ed. Philadelphia: W. B. Saunders Company, 1968, Chapters 1 and 2.

Haag, Jesse H. *School Health Program*, 3rd ed. Philadelphia: Lea and Febiger, 1972.

Hilton, Ernest. "Early Childhood Education: A Sense of Urgency." *Instructor*, 62:15, September 1972.

Hoyman, Howard S. "Bottlenecks in Health Education." *American Journal of Public Health*, 56:957–962, June 1966.

Means, Richard K. *A History of Health Education in the United States*. Philadelphia: Lea and Febiger, 1962.

NEA-AMA. *Health Education*. Washington: National Education Association, 1973.

Nemir, Alma. *The School Health Program*, 3rd ed. Philadelphia: W. B. Saunders Company, 1970.

Oberteuffer, Delbert, Harrelson, Orvis A. and Pollock, Marion B. *School Health Education*, 5th ed. New York: Harper & Brothers, 1972, Chapter 2.

Schram, Irene. *Ashes, Ashes, We All Fall Down.* New York: Simon and Schuster, 1972.

Sinacure, John S. "The Basis of Health Education," *Journal of School Health*, 41:303–308, June 1971.

Sorochan, Walter D. "Health Instruction — Why Do We Need It in the 70's?" *Journal of School Health*, 41:209–212, April 1971.

Willgoose, Carl E. "Don't Just Turn Them Loose." *NEA Journal*, 49:13–14, April 1960.

Willgoose, Carl E. *Health Teaching in Secondary Schools*. Philadelphia: W. B. Saunders Company, 1972, Chapter 2.

Willgoose, Carl E. "Saving the Curriculum of Health Education." *Journal of School Health*, 43:19–23, March 1973.

FUNCTION AND SCOPE OF SCHOOL HEALTH SERVICES

3

Thousands are hacking at the branches of evil to every one who is striking at the roots.

— Thoreau

Where are the roots to the health problems of children? What are the chief impediments to their happiness? To a great extent the over-all task of school health services is to answer these questions so successfully that the student will realize his fullest expectations in school.

No attempt will be made in this chapter to go into all the details of school health services. But it would be remiss of the author if he failed to give the elementary school teacher an opportunity to understand the function and some of the activities of this operation.

School health services are well defined procedures which are established:

1. To appraise the health status of pupils and school personnel.

2. To counsel pupils, parents and others concerning appraisal findings.

3. To encourage the correction of remediable defects.

4. To assist in the identification and education of handicapped children.

5. To help prevent and control disease.

6. To provide emergency service for injury or sudden sickness.

It may be seen from these precise definitions that school health services embrace a considerable amount of school activity. This is to be expected, for the services are educationally sound and defensible. Not only do they contribute to the realization of educational aims, but they help minimize the hazards of attending school and make it possible to adapt school programs to individual capacities and needs. Also—and this is sometimes unrecognized by many teachers and parents—there are potential educational values inherent in health service activities. Through these activities children become informed of their health assets and liabilities, and develop lasting attitudes toward physicians, dentists, nurses, and other health personnel. They also stand to gain two especially important understandings which may have a bearing on future behavior:

1. The need to establish a lifelong practice of having one's health status evaluated at regular intervals.

2. An appreciation of the value of professional services, methods, and techniques.

A COMPREHENSIVE WATCHDOG FUNCTION

The most recent White House Conference on Children placed a high priority on the development of a nationwide network of comprehensive health services for children. Health care delivery systems were to be improved, with an emphasis on the development of preventive and curative health services. Schools and other community agencies were to strive together to improve deficiencies that would otherwise impede scholastic performance.

What is practiced today varies considerably. Big cities with greater resources do more. Even in small school systems much goes on under the leadership of school health services personnel. A good part of this cuts across other school lines and involves considerable cooperative effort between school and community. The kinds of services performed can be extensive. In a statewide public school study in California, for example, the per cent of time given to a wide variety of school health services activities is shown below.[1]

The degree to which a particular health services organization becomes involved in many of these kinds of activities depends upon local understandings and leadership. It requires much cooperative effort in and out of the school. It also depends on the background of the families of the schoolchildren. In one elementary school study of visits to the health office it was discovered that there were significantly greater numbers of visits among older children, black students, children from families in which the mothers had been hospitalized for illness during a previous year, and among those with lowest academic

[1]Hazell, Joseph W. et al. "Intermediate Benefit Analysis—Spencer's Dilemma and School Health Services," *American Journal of Public Health,* 62:500–565, April 1972.

Direct Health-Service Programs	Per cent
Minor first aid	7.6
Vision screening	6.5
Hearing screening	4.7
Major emergency care	3.7
Health communication (information exchange with health professionals, pupils, parents, teachers and community)	3.7
Emotional development (developmental diagnosis, behavioral problems and mental health)	3.7
Absence-due-to-illness (investigation of absence by health-service personnel)	3.4
Dental (screening and care)	2.3
Health services planning and evaluation	2.3
Drug Abuse (resource support of education and management of drug reactions)	2.3
Communicable disease (exclusions, readmissions and immunizations)	2.1
Referral physical examination (as needed rather than as scheduled or required)	1.8
Chronic disease (allergies, diabetes, etc.)	1.5
Periodic physical examination (scheduled or required)	1.0
Immunization identification	

Direct Health-Service Programs	Per cent
(determination of pupil status regarding required immunizations)	1.0
TB screening	0.8
Other health service programs	1.8
Health Service components of other programs for:	
Nutrition (food or food service)	17.7
Educationally handicapped and mentally exceptional (contributions to programs)	11.2
Physically exceptional (components of programs for pupils with hearing, speech, vision, or orthopedic problems as well as for home and hospital instruction)	6.3
Physical education (services for other than athletics, sports, or physically handicapped)	3.4
Health education (personnel as resources)	3.1
Athletics and Sports	2.6
Environment (safety and sanitation)	1.8
Remedial physical education (health service components of programs for the physically handicapped)	0.8
Pregnancy (health service components only)	0.3
Other purposes	2.6
Grand Total	100.0

achievement.[2] Also, those elementary grade pupils less well accepted by their peers tended to make more visits to the school nurse.

The so called "watchdog function" of the school health services crew is helped measurably by cooperative teachers who enthusiastically report what they are able to observe in the classroom and about the school. However, it is made more difficult by examples of ignorance and indifference found in the homes. For instance, in her study of school nursing practices Dorothy Basco found that there is considerable need for parent-education—particularly relative to childhood diseases and important symptoms of illness.[3] Parents will send children to school when they are really ill enough to stay home. In the Basco study it was shown that almost all parents would keep their child at home if there was fever or diarrhea, but less than one-third would do so in cases of respiratory infections causing coughing and sneezing. (See Fig. 3–1.)

Another example that shows the need for a vigilant health services operation is to be found in the resurgence of measles among schoolchildren. Here is a disease which was a serious threat to health for many years, but was greatly reduced over a decade ago because of an acceptable vaccine that is more than 90 per cent effective in protecting against measles. It would have been easy to eliminate measles as a public health problem in the United States if immunization practices had been carefully monitored and encouraged. This was not the case, especially with central city poverty children, and in spite of state regulations requiring vaccinations. The disease, therefore, is on the upswing.[4] (See Fig. 3–2.)

[2]Van Arsdell, William et al. "Visits To An Elementary School Nurse," *Journal of School Health,* 42:142–146, March 1972.

[3]Basco, Dorothy. "Epidemiologic Analysis In School Populations As A Basis For Change In School Nursing Practice," *American Journal of Public Health,* 62:491–497, April 1972.

[4]Hinman, Alan. "Resurgence of Measles In New York State," *American Journal of Public Health,* 62:498–504, April 1972.

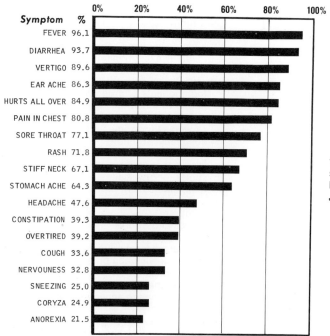

Figure 3–1 Per cent of parents who would keep child home for selected symptoms. (Courtesy Dorothy Basco and *American Journal of Public Health.*)

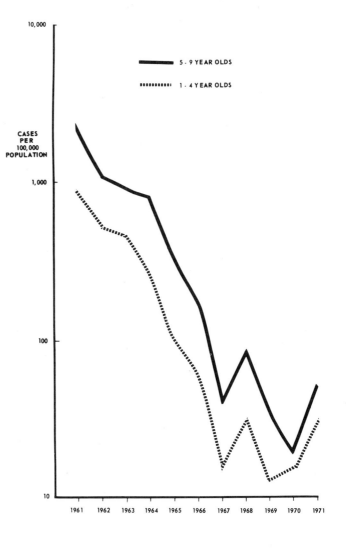

Figure 3–2 Age-specific incidence rates of measles: New York State exclusive of New York City, 1961–1971. (Courtesy Alan Hinman, M.D., and *American Journal of Public Health*.)

HEALTH APPRAISAL

As in all evaluation processes, the more scientific the appraisal, the sooner the purposes of the program may be reached. Total health status of a child may be appraised in a number of ways. Health histories, teacher and nurse observations, screening tests, medical and dental examinations, and psychological examinations represent the more common appraisal activities. These appraisals serve the medical personnel, the classroom teachers, and the pupils. They help the teachers understand their pupils, and they help the pupils appreciate the findings in relation to themselves.

The results of appraisals are also valuable to groups and individuals concerned with health counseling.

Some of the more important appraisal activities will be reviewed:

Health Histories

These are of particular concern to both medical personnel and classroom teachers. Just as history usually helps one to understand the present better, so the past diseases and defects of a pupil help everyone to understand his present status. Good teachers generally ask, "What makes Johnny tick?" It helps to know, therefore, what Johnny has had in the way of communicable diseases, immunizations, major operations, or injuries. In some schools today, classroom teachers help maintain health history records by anecdotally noting pupil health behavior items.

This kind of record is especially valuable when kept up-to-date and referred to when children behave strangely or appear to be in need of special counseling. It is a functional instrument for the exchange of information concerning the pupil's health between the classroom teacher, the school nurse, and the school physician. In California, for example, a particularly useful Health Insert is used with the California Cumulative Record system. It is an integral part of the individual's cumulative record and provides specific information concerning needed adjustments in the school program. It is transferred from school to school and was designed so that a minimum amount of time need be spent in keeping it up-to-date.

Routine Medical Examinations

The chief purposes of these examinations are to determine health status and solve any problems that arise. Their value is recognized in most states by a law requiring periodic examinations of every child in school. When this is not conducted by the family physician, it must be done by the school physician. The compulsory annual medical examination of all schoolchildren, however, has not always been effective. For one thing, the schools have ended up performing the "lion's share" of the examinations, thus missing the obvious advantage of having the family physician examine the child. Another factor is that school health service facilities and personnel are over-taxed when annual examinations are compulsory. This, coupled with the shortage of school physicians, suggests a more realistic approach to giving medical examinations.

The routine medical examination should be a thorough one. To be worth the energy put forth, it must allow the physician time enough to see the whole child: his behavior characteristics, nervous reflexes, speech defects, nutritional status, and temperament, as well as the more typical items. For almost two decades the American Public Health Association has had standards calling for a maximum of 12 examinations per hour—at least five minutes per child. This was brought about by findings that showed as many as 70 children being examined per hour. The idea of "processing" a set number of examinations in a certain amount of time cannot be defended. Examinations, to be worth the time and effort involved, need to be complete from head to toe. Thus, a limited number of students should be handled in one year. Thorough examinations every two or three years are becoming more common, with reexaminations of students possessing definite health problems being given wherever necessary.

The American Medical Association, in conjunction with the National Education Association, has suggested a minimum of four medical examinations: one upon entrance to first grade, one in the elementary intermediate school grades, one at the start of adolescence, and one before leaving school. In some places this has been quite successful. There is general agreement, however, that all pupils entering school for the first time should have a complete medical examination. This has the support of the American Academy of Pediatrics. Moreover, the examination should be done early enough to permit an adequate follow-up on recommendations. June has been found to be the most satisfactory month for children who plan to enter school in September.

As previously indicated, there is a definite advantage in having the family physician perform the examination. He knows the family and background of the child. His examination facilities are usually excellent, and he has quick access to laboratory facilities. Moreover a favorable physician-parent-child relationship generally exists. There are a number of communities in the United States that have no school physician for examinations. Everything is effectively handled by local physicians who cooperate fully with the school nurse. In such cases the family physician is completely informed of what the school desires so that there is uniformity in examinations and reporting. Standard examination forms are used. Also, the family physician is advised to use every opportunity to give effective health instruction just as a school physician would do. This kind of program has been working well in Connecticut where in a recent year over 25 per cent of schoolchildren were examined by personal physicians. There still remains one big disadvantage in using family physicians; there are always some parents who will not take their child to him, or they employ delaying tactics while the child's health is in question. (See Fig. 3–3.)

Another very significant item related to physical examinations of schoolchildren is the growth of specialization in medical practice. In many towns the general practitioner has been disappearing. The family doctor—the man who treated all members of a family, provided continuity of care, and showed concern with the general health of the entire family has been hard to locate. However, there has been a recent upswing in the number of

medical school graduates engaging in family practice; the effect of which is to strengthen physician-family bonds. It seems likely that in the years ahead the health care of the citizen will be a mass cooperative effort in which community physicians and their several assistants will work together in group practice and regional medical centers. In the future such centers will service the schools much more than they are doing at present.

It is a good idea to have the parent or parents on hand during the medical examination to consult with the physician. This is particularly true in the case of primary schoolchildren. Often during these formative years, when growth processes are fairly rapid, it is imperative that the physician and parent see eye-to-eye in their efforts to remedy the situation. The speed with which discovered defects are remedied has an important bearing on health and happiness in the years ahead. Teeth, for example, do much better when repaired at an early date.

Thoroughly screening preschool children is worth mentioning here. Beyond

---

S-15

DEPARTMENT OF HEALTH, PHYSICAL EDUCATION & RECREATION
Roslyn Public Schools

Roslyn, N.Y.

Date

NOTICE TO PARENTS - HEALTH CERTIFICATES

Dear Parents:

Since _____ has not had an annual health examination by your own personal physician, he/she will be inspected by Dr._____ our school doctor, on_____ .

Please sign and return this slip to the Health Office.

School Nurse

Parent's Signature

School Principal

Figure 3–3 Form used when family physician has not conducted health examination.

the discovery of obvious physical handicaps which can limit school success, there is the opportunity to detect other deficiencies pertaining to the special senses, mental retardation, emotional and behavioral disorders and physical, social and cultural deprivation. In Denver and Kansas programs, preschool children are carefully screened relative to immunizations, hemoglobin, urinalysis, and speech and vocabulary.

The emphasis in school health practice today is to give the physician time to interpret his findings to teachers and parents and to make workable suggestions in the health matters on hand. This kind of effort sets the stage for teamwork between teachers, parents, nurses, and physicians.

Special Medical Examinations

Where the school employs the regular medical examination every three or four years, there will be numerous occasions between examinations when it will be necessary to examine individual youngsters. Children returning to school after an absence due to illness may need a special examination, as will those new to the school system. Those pupils in need of special education may need to be examined from time to time. Since physical education and recreation activities must be adapted to the health condition of pupils, it will be necessary to examine boys and girls who wish to compete on an elementary school team. Also, there will be times in the follow-up and remedial aspects of the program when the physician wants to reexamine a certain pupil. Special examinations have value in that they permit a more careful analysis and diagnosis of the particular child.

Screening Tests

These are measures employed by teachers and health services personnel alike to "screen out" or select those schoolchildren who appear to be in need of further attention. The most effective screening tests over the years have been tests for vision, hearing, tuberculosis, and the appraisal of physical growth by the weighing and measuring of boys and girls. In recent years a number of school systems have attempted to screen children for dental defects, physical fitness, and mental health status. Most of these screening tests can be cooperatively engaged in by teachers and nurses. A broader treatment of how the elementary school classroom teacher can screen children for specific weaknesses appears in Chapter 5.

Screening for Vision. As a rule, screening tests are not diagnostic tests. They might well be called processes by which school personnel separate those pupils who are most likely to need further examination from those who are less likely to need further examination. Therefore, in vision testing the teacher is not an expert. She is simply a careful observer who helps during the screening period. (Figure 3–4.) Usually the teacher is aware that sensory impressions gradually develop from a level of discrimination through a perceptual level to a final conceptual level, and that refractive errors, color blindness, eye muscle imbalances, and more serious conditions such as amblyopia need quick attention. She knows that first and second graders tend to be farsighted and that nearsightedness in boys and girls develops at about the fourth grade level.

When a pupil is old enough to cooperate in a testing situation, he is ready to be measured. Thus, even a three-year-old child can respond to the symbols on a Snellen E Chart. Proper advance preparation helps improve the response.

The *Snellen Test*, used for a long time in the public schools to test visual acuity, is quite satisfactory as a crude screening instrument when more valid measures are not available.[5] (See Fig. 3–5.)

It is useful for noting near-to-far-vision. It will tell the classroom teacher whether or not a certain pupil can see the blackboard or wall chart from either the front or back row of seats. The large Snellen Test chart requires reading test

---

[5]The necessary testing equipment and detailed instructions can be obtained from the National Society for the Prevention of Blindness, 79 Madison Ave., New York, N.Y., 10016.

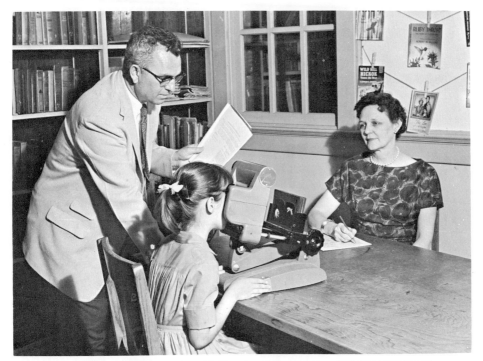

Figure 3-4 Teachers assist with the visual examination (Telebinocular test).

objects (letters, numbers, or symbols) on a chart from a 20-foot distance. The E chart is available for children and illiterates, and the mixed-letter chart is for adults and children above the third-grade level. The largest letters should be read by the normal eye at 200 feet. Because testing is done at 20 feet, this line of large print is designated the 20/200 line. The normal eye should read the 20/20 line at 20 feet; deviation less than normal is recorded 20/200, 20/100, 20/70, 20/60, 20/40, 20/30, and any deviation better than normal is recorded as 20/15 or 20/10. In all probability children below the third grade who cannot read the 20/40 line with each eye should be referred for examination by a specialist.

Although the Snellen Test can be given by a person without medical or nursing training, proper attention must be given to the testing procedure and equipment. Some of the more important items to keep in mind to ensure valid results are the following:

Hang the chart so that the 20-foot line of letters is at the level of the child's eyes.

The heels of the child should touch the line marked on the floor 20 feet away.

Children should be at ease and encouraged to do their best.

Both eyes should be open during the test, the eye not being tested covered with a small card or folded paper resting obliquely across the nose.

Test the child who wears glasses first with them and then without them.

Test the right eye first, then the left, and then both eyes together.

Begin with the 30-foot line and follow with the 20-foot line. If the child fails the 30-foot line, start with the 20-foot line.

Move promptly and rhythmically from one symbol to another at a speed with which the child can keep pace.

Consider a line read satisfactorily if three out of four symbols are read correctly.

Record results immediately in fraction form.

Look for eyestrain, such signs as excessive blinking, frowning, scowling, tilting of the head, and watering of the eyes.

Correlate Snellen Test results with classroom observations.

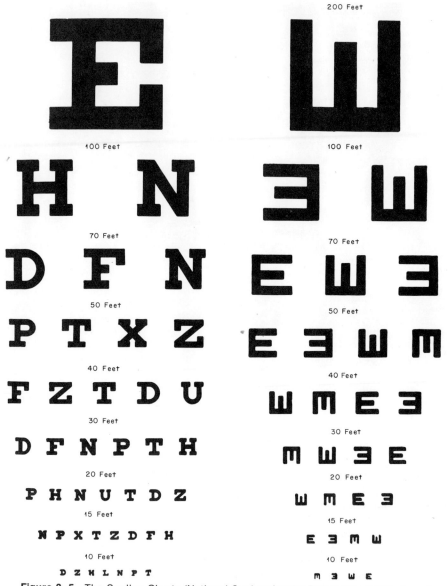

Figure 3–5 The Snellen Charts (National Society for the Prevention of Blindness).

Needless to say there are several more complicated tests of vision that are recommended when a more complete screening examination is desired. These include the Keystone View Company Telebinocular, the Massachusetts Vision Test, the Atlantic City Vision Test, the Titmus School Vision Tester, and the Ortho-Rater.

In recent years considerable attention has been focused on *pre-school vision*

screening and the importance of visual readiness for learning. Studies show that large numbers of children require professional eye care. In New York City, for example, preschool screening examinations discovered that seven per cent of the children had visual defects at 20/50 or worse in one eye. In a study carried on in Minneapolis, Minnesota with a sample of 633 first grade pupils from eight public elementary schools, it was found that over 16 per cent of the pupils required professional eye care. In most communities, therefore, it is advisable to begin the vision screening in nursery schools where the young children are already congregated.[6]

Screening for Hearing. Early and repeated hearing tests are important. Accurate screening is necessary, especially when one considers that an average of two children in every classroom have a hearing problem, that many cases of incorrect speech supposedly due to poor mentality are actually caused by poor hearing, and that there are needless grade repetitions among hard-of-hearing children.[7]

Although whisper tests have been used for years, group audiometers are far more reliable. Six or ten children can be handled very nicely in a pure-tone-audiometer test. Here, each subject has a

set of earphones. Sound intensity is regulated by a knob up to maximum intensity. Different pitches in tone are given (frequency range) by turning another knob. One hundred pupils a day can be tested easily, and it can be used with children of all ages. In Figure 3–6 the raised hands of the children indicate that all of them have been able to hear the first tone produced by the audiometer. Some of the children may not be fortunate enough to hear succeeding tones as the tester lowers the volume on the audiometer. Hearing tests for small children are especially important, because of the fact that early discovery of hearing loss and follow-up can frequently prevent permanent loss of hearing.

Screening for Physical Growth. There is a close relationship between pupil health status, personal growth characteristics, and academic achievement. Learning, in its many forms, depends upon sound health. Children who are small or underweight for their age have a higher proportion of communication problems according to the National Institute of Neurological Diseases and Stroke. Very often a simple sign of retardation in growth, discovered by nurses

---

[6]The booklet *Preschool Vision Screening* and the training film for teachers, *Before We Are Six*, can be most helpful in situations where teachers do the vision screening. They may be obtained from the National Society for the Prevention of Blindness.

[7]In a nationwide study by the National Center for Health Statistics it was found that 16 per cent of 6-11 year old children have a hearing abnormality.

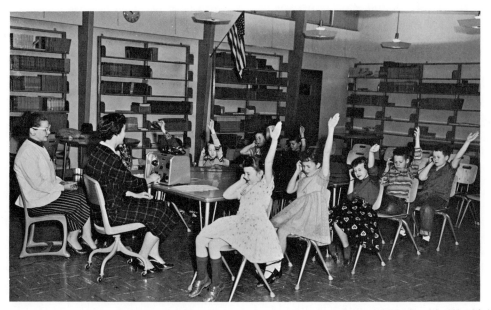

Figure 3–6 A group test using the pure tone audiometer. (Courtesy Oregon State Board of Health.)

or teachers, is significant. Yet the growth period of boys and girls cannot be neatly divided and subdivided into set periods. There is too much individual variation in pupil size, shape, and form due to such factors as heredity, constitutional endowment (body build), and physiological maturation.

A number of screening devices to evaluate over-all physical growth have been developed for school use. These involve age-height-weight measures and are usually handled through the health services department. Frequently teachers weigh and measure their own pupils. The children remove hats, coats, jackets, sweaters, and shoes. Weight is recorded in pounds and half pounds. Height is recorded in inches and quarter inches.

Interestingly enough, the child who fails to gain in height and weight in a four-month period frequently has some degree of ill health. This may be due to a physical defect, an organic strain, a prolonged emotional problem, or perhaps a number of unhygienic health habits.

An easy-to-read and use graph for teachers is the *Meredith Physical Growth Record*. There is a record for each sex, divided into zones (Figures 3–7 and 3–8). For height there are five zones: tall, moderately tall, average, moderately short, and short. For weight the zones are heavy, moderately heavy, average, moderately light, and light. The graphs cover ages four to 18.

The child's measurements are plotted on the graph for any one period. Successive measurements permit the observer to note whenever the points do not fall in *like zones* (that is, tall and heavy, short and light). In such instances the pupil is referred to the physician for examination. It may be that the child is perfectly healthy but of a particular body build. On the other hand, he may have some infection, need an improved diet, or require changes in daily living habits.

Screening for Mental Health. The need for psychiatric services in grade schools has grown faster than private and public psychiatric services can possibly meet. Children coming from a background of environmental depriva-

tion frequently are emotionally immature and harbor a negative self-image. All too often disturbed parents raise disturbed children. This is why Abrams and others make a plea for the employment of full-time psychiatrists to work with students, parents, social workers, school psychologists, nurses and teachers.[8] By observing and talking with individuals and small groups of children this battery of school personnel will be able to effectively screen out those pupils in need of help and facilitate early attention.

Screening for Heart Sounds. When one considers that there are approximately 10 cases of heart problems per 1,000 children it underlines the need for mass heart screening programs. As a relatively new technique, heart sound screening shows promise in school use. A highly sensitive microphone placed on the child's chest picks up heart sounds. These are analyzed by a portable computer which provides information beyond what may be detected with the ordinary stethoscope. Eisner finds the cost low, especially in the large city system, and a chance for the health service personnel to "delabel" certain children.[9]

Whenever a large group of children has been screened, children have been found who actually did not have heart disease, but whose activity had been restricted because someone believed that they did. These children are as much entitled to be considered successful outcomes of the program as are the children who receive effective treatment for their heart disease.

HEALTH MAINTENANCE AND CONTROL

Certainly one of the big tasks of school services has to do with the everyday prevention of illness. This is accomplished through a program of control of personal and environmental factors. Such factors as communicable disease,

---

[8]Abrams, Richard S. et al. "A Suggested School Mental Health Program," *Journal of School Health*, 42:137–141, March 1972.

[9]Eisner, Victor and Allan Oglesby. "Heart Sound Screening," *Journal of School Health*, 42:270–274, May 1972.

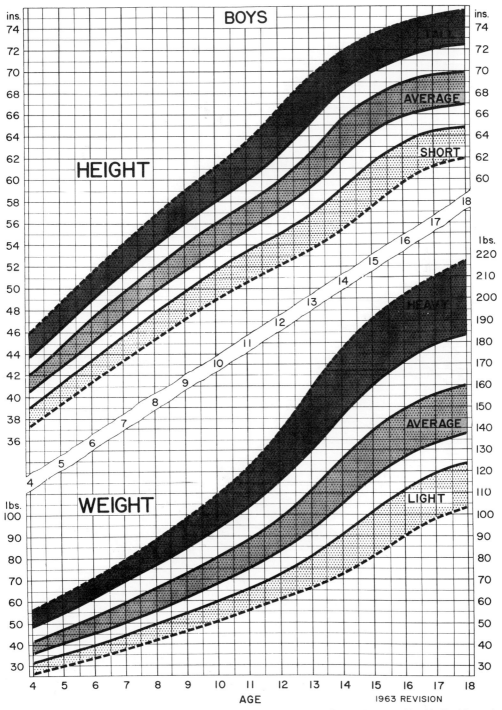

Figure 3-7 Physical growth record for boys. (Courtesy Joint Committee on Health Problems in Education of the NEA and AMA.)

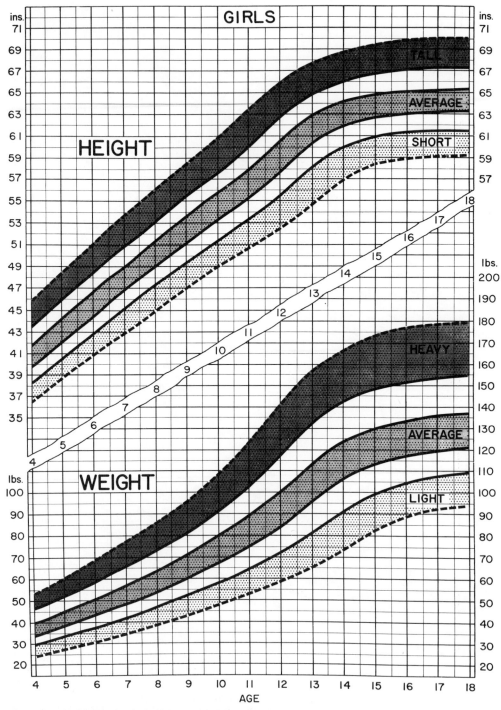

Figure 3–8 Physical growth record for girls. (Courtesy Joint Committee on Health Problems in Education of the NEA and AMA.)

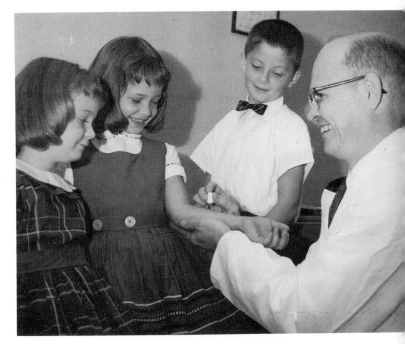

Figure 3–9 Application of TB Tine Test in the screening of school children. (Courtesy Lederle Laboratories.)

emergency care and first aid, accident prevention, and school sanitation are major items.

Communicable disease control involves both the school and the community. The school health services department is generally aware of the sickness rates in the area and is prepared to control disease in the school population through widespread use of vaccination, immunization, prophylactic therapy, and isolation of ill pupils. While children are in school, they must be protected from other children who may be ill. The gathering of pupils in the classroom may set the stage for the transmission of disease. Here, the classroom teacher can be most helpful by observing carefully and reporting quickly those pupils who appear to be ill. (For details see Chapter 5.)

Because of its place in the community, the school is in a position to prevent disease. Measles epidemics, for example, can be wiped out completely in the United States if parents have their kindergarten, first, and second grade children vaccinated. About four million cases of measles a year occurred before measles vaccine became widely avail-

able in 1964. Over 500 children a year died, and hundreds were left with lasting handicaps including hearing disorders and mental retardation. Since young children can spread epidemics rapidly, the school health service personnel must always be alert.

Emergency care procedures for children who become ill or injured while attending school are also the responsibility of school personnel. The school administrator and his staff must always act *in loco parentis,* i.e., in place of the parents; not just any parents, but the wisest and most enlightened type of parents. This can be a sizable job because the figures collected by the National Safety Council indicate that some 60 per cent of the accidents to children of school age occur on the school grounds, in the buildings, or going to and from school. It becomes necessary, therefore, for the health services personnel to cooperate with the teacher and school principal in the event of an emergency.

Children who appear to be ill should be segregated right away. Sometimes an emergency rest room is used. At other times it may be necessary to transport the child to his home. In either case the school physician or nurse should make the decision as to how the sick child will be handled. In the absence of either of these people, the principal and teacher will have to use their best judgment. When the child is sent home, the parents should be contacted so that appropriate action may be taken with the family physician. And when he returns to school after an illness, he should report directly to the health service office for clearance to the classroom. Most local school boards have established a definite policy of readmissions.

The question of *first aid* in an emergency is something that requires careful planning by all school personnel. Ideally, only medical personnel should render emergency care. There will be times, however, when only the classroom teacher is available.[10] What should she do? How far should she go in giving temporary treatment at the site of the emergency? Each teacher should have some knowledge of first aid procedures. She may be able to relieve suffering and prevent shock, or prevent a disability, or even save a life. It is effective school health practice, therefore, to have the school physician discuss this topic at the start of each school year in order that all school personnel will be prepared for the emergency when it occurs.

No attempt will be made here to go into the many details relative to the various conditions of illness, injury, and suffering which may require first aid attention. Familiarization with the standard first aid course material of the American Red Cross would be most beneficial. However, there are several points that classroom teachers should keep in mind relative to helping during an emergency:

1. It is important to note whether the

child is having trouble breathing, or is bleeding profusely.

2. Note also whether the child is in a state of shock. Here the skin is damp and cold, and may be ashen or pale in color. Breathing may be shallow; the pulse rapid and weak, and there may be a vacant, glassy stare in the eyes. The child should be made comfortable, wrapped in a blanket with his head lower than his feet. No liquids or stimulants should be given by the teacher.

3. If the face is flushed, lay the child down on his back with the head raised; if he vomits turn his head to the side.

4. Do not move the child who has had an accident until medical assistance arrives.

5. Always comfort and reassure a child. It is encouraging to know that he will be all right.

6. Do not give food or liquid to ill children. It may cause nausea, vomiting, or strangulation.

7. First aid is always rendered to reduce suffering and discomfort. Remaining with the child until assistance arrives, or until he is with his parents, may frequently be quite essential to his welfare.

Every elementary school should have a well stocked and strategically located first aid cabinet. This should be in the office of the nurse, or if necessary in the office of the principal. The accompanying list of supplies would be considered essential for first aid practice. No antiseptics or medicines are included.

Accident prevention is another health control item that requires some organization. It is closely related to the content of the elementary school curriculum, and it is one that teachers can discuss at length in the classroom. It is also related to the administrator for he sees that steps are taken to prevent accidents, engages in research projects to determine the causes of accidents, and prepares plans to use in case of fires, hurricanes, and other disasters.

School sanitation is a responsibility in health maintenance and control that rests primarily with the school physician. He cooperates with the local board of

---

[10]Practically every major group of educators has recommended that teachers have training in first aid. This includes the American Association of School Administrators, Elementary School Principals, National Education Association, American Public Health Association, and American Association for Health, Physical Education, and Recreation.

First Aid Cabinet Supplies

Items	Use
Absorbent cotton roll	For large pads or dressings
Adhesive tape, roll (widths ½″ to 2″)	To fasten splints and dressings
Aromatic spirits of ammonia	Stimulant
Blades, wood (500)	For depressors and small splints
Eye droppers (6)	To apply oil
Forceps (3″ tweezer type)	For grasping small objects
Glass jars (2)	To hold wood blades
Hot water bottle and cover	Pain relief
Ice bags (2)	Relief of swelling
Mineral oil or petroleum jelly	Relief of irritation
Paper cups (100)	As containers
Roller bandage, 1″ (12 rolls)	For dressings
Roller bandage, 2″ (12 rolls)	For dressings
Roller bandage, 4″ (12 rolls)	For dressings
Safety pins (24)	For triangular bandage
Scissors (blunt)	To cut dressings
Splints (10)	For support
Sterile gauze, 3″ × 3″ squares (100)	To protect injuries
Sterile gauze, 2″ × 2″ squares (100)	To protect injuries
Tincture of green soap	For washing injuries
Toothpicks (500)	To remove particles
Tourniquet (3 ft. ¼″ rubber tube)	To control excessive bleeding
Triangle bandage (4)	For sling
Wooden applicators (1000)	For swabbing and removing particles

health to see that such school items as water supplies, dishwashing facilities, food service areas, and locker and shower rooms are safe and pleasant to use. Occasionally an unsanitary drinking fountain—something that all primary school children seem to like to put their mouths over—will spread a definite disease. The design and installation of fountains, therefore, is of interest to teachers as well as sanitation experts.

SCHOOL ABSENCES

In a number of school systems 15 per cent of all pupils are absent daily. Illness is the major cause. It is also the greatest factor in non-promotion because of the high correlation between illness and poor scholastic achievement.

Respiratory difficulties are by far the largest single group of acute conditions reported nationally. Independent studies in New York and California indicate that close to 50 per cent of all absences are due to respiratory disease, with the com-

mon cold leading the list. Accidents also contribute to school absenteeism—about 2,200,000 school days are lost annually due to accidents.

Good patterns of attendance are cooperatively developed between school, parents, community physicians, and welfare agencies. Both parents and teachers should realize that stressing "perfect attendance" is frequently detrimental to proper school health practice. According to Dr. Carl S. Shultz of the U.S. Public Health Service, the usually healthy child should stay home from school: if he is feverish; if his symptoms (headaches, drowsiness, runny nose, nausea, or diarrhea) are sufficiently severe to be disabling; if he is likely to be disturbing to the class; or if it is improbable, due to his general condition, that he will profit from school. Moreover, the child who is permitted to go to school with a slight fever will probably have more fever later in the day; and the child returning early to school while recovering from an upper respiratory infection may pick up from his classmates other organisms that could produce serious secondary complications.

REMEDIAL OR FOLLOW-UP PROGRAM

Healing is a matter of time; it is also a matter of opportunity.

—Hippocrates

To have an effective school health organization the medical and teaching personnel must do much more than carry out a program of detection and discovery. They must have the time, facilities, staff, and know-how to implement effective follow-up procedures.

The efficient follow-up program begins with careful planning. Once a defect is discovered, one might ask whose job it is to contact the parents. In the small elementary school this may be done by the physician, nurse, or classroom teacher. Notices sent to the parents, notifying them of the suspected difficulty, are generally respected when signed by the school physician. There is considerable logic, however, in having the classroom teacher sign the notice. This is especially true at the primary grade level. Here, the judgment and concern of the teacher are appreciated by most parents, perhaps more than at any other period in the school years to follow. If the teacher says, "Your John needs glasses now," there is a very good possibility something will be done about it right away. Parents, like most people, tend to procrastinate and put off what they know should be done soon. Sometimes they fail to realize the seriousness of the situation. They say to themselves, "After all, John isn't blind, he doesn't walk into the side of the barn." As true as this may be, he still could fail to read the printed page.

Formal notices of medical examinations sent to parents are often like report cards. They are easy to send home but difficult to get back with an indication that something has been done. The larger and better organized elementary schools send out notices that provide space for an answer. Parents have the opportunity to check off whether they have taken their child to a physician or dentist, plan to do so, or need help in doing so. Other school systems use a form with a detachable section to permit parents to acknowledge receipt of the notification.

The success of a follow-up system depends upon the kind of contact school personnel have with parents, the availability of needed services, and the seriousness with which parents view the health abnormality. Cauffman, working with grade school children in Los Angeles discovered several significant parental factors favorably influencing proper follow-up.[11] Among these were 1) higher social status, 2) small families, 3) parent's national background, 4) education beyond high school, 5) non-working mothers, and 6) parental contact involving personal interaction either by telephone or visits. Also, follow-up was more likely when parents received more than one notification, and by more than one person. As part of the same study Cauffman found that children from families carrying health insurance were more likely to receive care for their defects than were children from non-insured families.

If the school nurse has some method of suspense date record keeping, practically all notifications to parents will be accounted for. It will then be possible to keep in close contact with delinquent parents and see that they proceed with the necessary remedial work for their child. In this way the same children with the same defects will not appear year after year in succeeding classrooms with a handicap that might have been corrected.

DUTIES OF HEALTH SERVICES PERSONNEL

The list of duties and responsibilities of personnel connected with the health services department is an extensive one.

---

[11]Cauffman, Joy. "Factors Affecting Outcomes of School Health Referrals," *Journal of School Health*, 38:333–339, June 1968.

Some of the outstanding functions are as follows:

The School Physician

Ideally he is a general practitioner or pediatrician interested in children and their problems and in public health. He helps the administrator coordinate the health services with other parts of the school program. He diagnoses diseases and defects of children but is not responsible for the medical care of individual children. He is familiar with the methods of integrating school health services with health teaching, physical education, special education, guidance, recreation, and lunchroom service. He is responsible for control of disease, sanitation, emergency cases, and safety within the school. He practices the techniques of group work and directs health service as a cooperative enterprise within the school.

Across the country a large number of school systems are unable to employ a full-time physician. In such instances the part-time physician is concerned primarily with basic health services. In 1967 the Committee on School Physicians of the American School Health Association formulated a manual relative to the duties of school physicians. The minimum duties set forth for the part-time physician are as follows:[12]

1. Consults and assists in the direction and implementation of health screening programs. Examines all candidates for interscholastic athletics prior to each season and periodically thereafter. Implements state labor laws in those states requiring boards of education to provide medical examinations for employment certificates.

2. Assists in the coordination of the school immunization programs conducted by family physicians and health departments.

3. Advises on the control of communicable disease within the school.

4. Obtains from family physicians and interprets medical information pertinent to the appropriate classroom management of the child with a physical or emotional handicap.

5. Assumes responsibility for establishing and supervising school emergency facilities and first aid training programs for school personnel. Arranges for emergency care of pupils injured or ill at school when the parent and family physician cannot be reached.

6. Arranges for meetings with groups of community physicians, at which time procedures and communication are discussed to resolve problems to the mutual satisfaction of the school and the physicians.

7. Assists with the planning of parent-education meetings concerning school health problems.

8. Arranges for medical appraisal of pupils who show signs of health problems and whose parents are unable to pay for such service.

9. Compiles reports of the services rendered by the school medical program and of the health problems identified.

Physicians in the larger school systems also handle school employee physical evaluations and school-wide health problems which are staff related. This is part of the total task in which most physicians take a great amount of interest. In fact, next to an interest in children (which is strong), most physicians are motivated to enter school health work because of a broad interest in preventive medicine which involves people of all ages. Most would give more time to the school system if it could be arranged. Unfortunately, because of economic reasons, and because most school physicians are pediatricians and internal medicine specialists, the demands are great upon them to be somewhere other than the schools. However, survey findings are clear that when they are able to be in the schools they do spend their time wisely in the three major task areas: 1) individual evaluations, 2) in-school contacts with nurse, principal, teacher, and parents, and 3) both medical and

---

[12]Report of the Committee on School Physicians of the American School Health Association. "A Manual for School Physicians," *Journal of School Health,* 37:395–399, October 1967.

non-medical contacts in the community.[13]

Since physicians spend more time in schools than ever before, they need to develop, not a bedside manner, but a "schoolside manner" which is demonstrated by a genuine interest and technique for working with teachers and other school-community personnel.

The School Nurse

She is more than a nurse; she is a respected member of the teaching faculty, and, as such, participates with other teachers in school affairs. In many places today she is a nurse-teacher with special skills in health assessment of schoolchildren, coupled with a background in health education, counseling, and the use of community resources.[14] She interprets the school health program in the home and assists in the planning of learning experiences in the classroom. She cooperates with the health agencies in the community that are interested in child health. She assists in first aid and home nursing courses. She assists the physician, organizes teacher-nurse conferences, and follows up with parent-nurse conferences. In addition, she is a consultant to the administrative staff, a participant in curriculum design, a counselor, a member of the team providing for handicapped children, and an environmentalist who facilitates emergency care for illness and injury occurring in school or school-related activities.[15]

---

[13]Wagner, Marsden G., Carl S. Shultz and Marian H. Heller. "A Study of School Physicians' Behavior," *American Journal Of Public Health*, 58:517–527, March 1968.

[14]In some states, public or county health nurses will be assigned to town and city schools. Some of their duties will be the same as those of the nurse-teacher, yet in many respects experience indicates that they do not become as much a part of the school "team" as nurses employed by and responsible to the school administrator. This is due, in part, to the fact that their loyalties are divided between school needs and the public health needs of the community.

[15]For a more complete and detailed breakdown of nursing activities, see *This Is School Nursing* and *School Nursing For The 70's*, distributed by the School Health Division, American Association for Health, Physical Education and Recreation, 1201 16th St., N.W., Washington, D.C., 20036.

The relationship of the nurse to the classroom teacher is of major importance. The success of a nurse's work in school is directly related to the closeness, continuity, and harmony of her association with the teacher.

The clever nurse will involve the children when planning for various screenings. Dorothy Shoobs of Columbia University recalls how the nurse carried out an orientation session for kindergarten children who were to undergo audiometer screening in one school system:

The nurse showed the earphones to the children and asked, "Who wears them?"

The children answered, "astronaut," "pilot," "the man in the police station."

The nurse then had one child try on the earphones. She asked the children to be quiet so he could hear the message she was sending him. The children giggled.

She had the child repeat what he heard. He mimicked the sound. The nurse turned up the volume so that all of the children could hear the sound.

Next, she asked the teacher to select a child, and she instructed the child selected to don the earphones and tap with a ruler when he heard the sound. She selected three children to come to the health office with her, and told the class that when each child finished, he would return to class and choose the next child to be screened. The next child would then come to the nurse's office.

As each child came up to be screened, the nurse asked him what he would like to be (astronaut, pilot, policeman, etc.). She repeated her instructions to tap with the ruler when the child received her message (heard a sound). The children generally wore expressions of pleased anticipation as they participated in the screening.

This is a good example of how to make the screening procedure less threatening. By having the children take part in the task they gained some control over what was happening, reduced their anxiety, and set the stage for a more reliable measurement of their hearing.

The School Nurse Practitioner

A large number of school children in America fail to visit private physicians or utilize the services of neighborhood health centers or hospital out-patient departments. They simply do not get comprehensive care; as a result, numerous conditions affecting the ability to learn go undetected for long periods of time. To get around this problem the *school nurse practitioner* program in pediatric health was started in Colorado with Denver Public Schools personnel.[16]

The school nurse is prepared to assume an expanded role in providing health care to school-age children. She receives extra schooling in order to be able to assess the factors that may operate to produce learning disorders, psychoeducational problems, perceptive-cognitive difficulties, and behavior problems as well as those causing physical disease. Significantly, it is the school facility that serves as the principal setting for comprehensive primary and continuing health care and services since it is the one place where children are regularly and readily accessible.

The School Dentist

Dental health services are under the control of the school dentist. Surveys show, unfortunately, that only about one school in 20 has a dentist that visits the school and participates in the education program.

The effective school dentist likes children well enough to perform dental examinations on each child periodically. He supervises preventive dental work and oral prophylaxis done by dental hygienists. He may take part in a school-sponsored dental clinic. He also aids classroom teachers and nurse-teachers in the preparation of curriculum materials in dental hygiene.

The dental health "inspection" indicates a cursory observation of the mouth and teeth of each child. It includes clinical observation using a mouth mirror and explorer in good light. This is not a diagnostic examination such as would be carried out in the office of the family dentist. It does, however, have certain benefits: it is a fact-finding instrument which serves as a basis for the school dental

health education effort; it helps build a positive attitude toward the dentist and dental care; and the child and his parents are motivated to seek and to accept dental treatment as a part of their total health protection. Moreover, such efforts are effective. In Gary, Indiana, for example, the dental health program yielded a dramatic improvement in dental health in the first four grades of schoolchildren.

Few school administrators realize that the local dental society, with the blessings of the American Dental Association, will gladly conduct a dental survey to determine dental health. The information obtained may be used as a basis for stimulating dental health education. Societies will also provide teaching materials, sponsor in-service education programs for teachers, and assist with the development of teaching guides.

The Dental Hygienist

Despite the efforts in some of the larger states such as New York and California, the dental hygienist as a member of the school teaching staff is still rare.

The dental hygienist may periodically clean teeth, and assist the dentist or school physician in the examination of the teeth. She may make topical application of sodium or stannous fluoride where state law permits her to do this. She interprets dental defects to parents, and helps parents make plans for dental corrections. An increasing number of dental hygienists have a degree in education and are prepared to assist elementary schoolteachers in the area of health instruction. (Figure 3–10.)

COORDINATING PERSONNEL

There are a number of people in the school who have a rather special function to perform which touches upon the area of health services. These specialists are a part of the total school health effort. Their day to day activities may rightly be called health coordinating activities. Moreover, their work comes so close to involving the classroom teacher

---

[16]For details of an early program see Henry K. Silver. "The School Nurse Practitioner Program," *Journal of American Medical Association*, 216:1332–1336, May 24, 1971.

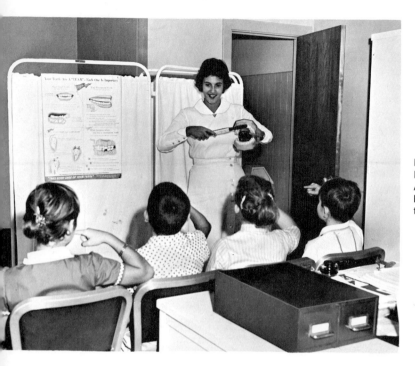

Figure 3–10 School dental hygienist demonstrates how to brush the teeth. (Courtesy American Association for Health, Physical Education and Recreation.)

that brief mention will be made of their duties:

The Health Supervisor or Coordinator

The elementary school health supervisor or health coordinator is a trained school health educator who works with teachers to develop an organized health education curriculum. He coordinates health service activities with classroom activities. He is familiar with the techniques of instructional supervision. He meets with the school health council to harmonize all school activities.

The Physical Educator

The physical education teacher is one of the most popular teachers with elementary schoolchildren. He is concerned with building health, primarily through large muscle activity. He helps the grade teacher develop physical activity programs to meet the needs and interests of her children. He is interested in health safeguards on the playgrounds and in the gymnasium. He cooperates with health services in providing a reme-

dial exercise program for children with postural defects, orthopedic difficulties, and a low level of physical fitness. He provides leadership in recreation for both pupils and teachers. He promotes total health—physical, mental and emotional—through a broad program of individual and group experiences.

The School Nutritionist

She is a trained person in nutrition and home economics. She supervises the school lunch program, cooperates with the kitchen staff, and helps in promoting health primarily through nutrition education.

The School Custodian

The unknown hero in many elementary schools is the man behind the physical environment—the custodian. He is one of the most important health promoters in the school. He is concerned with sanitation, ventilation, heating, cleanliness, and safety conditions in corridors, on floors, walks and exits. He is one of the best friends a classroom teacher can have. Without his help the teacher may have a difficult time with young children.

In a study put out by the United States Department of Health, Education and Welfare, it is pointed out that the schools need trained custodians who, by the satisfactory performance of many duties and tasks, can contribute to the educational objectives of the school.

Mental Health Consultants

Schools are employing psychologists, social workers, school adjustment counselors, and psychiatrists to give more specialized help. The psychologist is able to diagnose individual abilities and personalities. The social worker is the contact between the school and the home and is familiar with available community resources. The psychiatrist, in the few school systems fortunate enough to have one, generally does consultative work with school personnel, and may do diagnostic and therapeutic work with individual boys and girls. A fairly unique characteristic of the Los Angeles program is the wide use of psychiatrists throughout the school health service departments.

THE HEALTH COUNCIL

Health counseling follows health appraisals. The child's health needs can often be served best by combining the thoughts of several interested people. Sometimes a person designated as health counselor plans a meeting where a number of people sit down together to discuss a particular child. In many places the health coordinator is the logical person to head such a committee or council. This type of group in the elementary school may consist of the school nurse, health supervisor or coordinator, the classroom teacher of the child being discussed, the parent, and possibly another person. Working groups such as these are able to make a real contribution to the over-all health program of the school. They solve many difficulties and permit the school to give more than "lip ser-

vice" to the problem of meeting individual needs.

SCHOOL-COMMUNITY HEALTH COUNCIL

There is also another type of council which is timely, broad in scope and affords opportunities for widespread discussion of health problems. Serving in addition to teachers, administrators and parents, are medical and dental personnel from the community, and representatives of public and private health agencies. This provides a voice for all kinds of voluntary health groups concerned with heart, cancer, drugs, mental health, family counseling, and others.

Especially for elementary school-age children and their parents, the school is a natural community center. In a number of cities it has been possible to do things through the school health service as a focal point that couldn't have been done as well elsewhere. The school, therefore, makes a fine location from which the school-community health council may operate. In this manner the local problems dealing with economic issues, crowded housing, hazards to safety, malnutrition, and other deficits of health can be cooperatively aired and pursued. Such items as publicizing and disseminating the importance of blood testing to detect sickle cell anemia, securing community action for drug abuse prevention, fostering preschool examinations and immunizations, organizing to alleviate certain social conditions conducive to poor mental health, and many more multiple interest activities can be carried on. Where there are language problems, for example, the council is able to initiate changes and provide help through appropriate written aids. (See Fig. 3–11.)

Where there is a neighborhood health center located apart from the school facility, the School-Community Health Council can provide the necessary bridge between school and center so that the school health program component

Una Guia Para Comer Bien

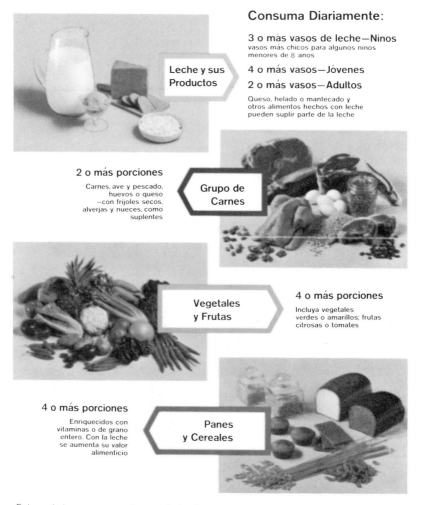

Consuma Diariamente:

3 o más vasos de leche—Ninos
vasos más chicos para algunos ninos
menores de 8 anos

Leche y sus
Productos

4 o más vasos—Jóvenes

2 o más vasos—Adultos

Queso, helado o mantecado y
otros alimentos hechos con leche
pueden suplir parte de la leche

2 o más porciones

Carnes, ave y pescado,
huevos o queso
—con frijoles secos,
alverjas y nueces, como
suplentes

Grupo de
Carnes

Vegetales
y Frutas

4 o más porciones

Incluya vegetales
verdes o amarillos; frutas
citrosas o tomates

4 o más porciones

Enriquecidos con
vitaminas o de grano
entero. Con la leche
se aumenta su valor
alimenticio

Panes
y Cereales

Esta es la base para una buena dieta. Consuma más de éstos y otros alimentos según
sea necesario para el crecimiento, activi-
dad y para guardar un peso adecuado.

12 1972, 3ra. Edición—Propiedad Lit-
eraria de 1958, 1964, National Dairy
Council, Chicago 60606

Figure 3–11 Nutrition information provided for Spanish speaking families. Comes in leaflet or colored poster. (Courtesy National Dairy Council.)

cannot be separated from its neighborhood context.

ADDITIONAL FUNCTIONS OF HEALTH SERVICES

In recent years the services to pupils have been extended in a number of ways.

Working cooperatively with other school personnel, the physicians and nurses are helpful in two important areas:

Detection of Learning Disabilities

The child with learning disabilities requires some interaction with various concerned groups. By definition, he is considered to be of adequate mental abil-

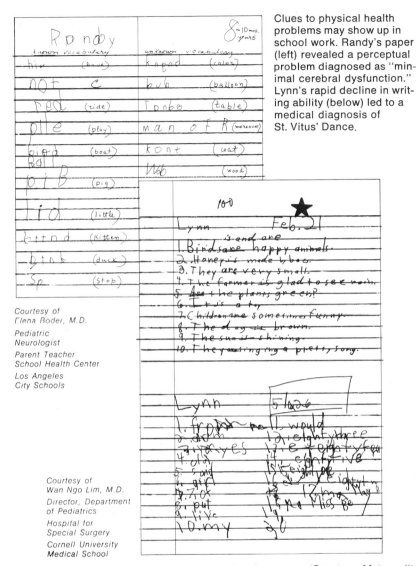

Clues to physical health problems may show up in school work. Randy's paper (left) revealed a perceptual problem diagnosed as "minimal cerebral dysfunction." Lynn's rapid decline in writing ability (below) led to a medical diagnosis of St. Vitus' Dance.

Courtesy of
Elena Boder, M.D.

Pediatric
Neurologist

Parent Teacher
School Health Center

Los Angeles
City Schools

Courtesy of
Wan Ngo Lim, M.D.

Director, Department
of Pediatrics

Hospital for
Special Surgery

Cornell University
Medical School

Figure 3–12 Perceptual problems show up in the classroom. (Courtesy Metropolitan Life Insurance Company.)

ity, sensory processes, and emotional stability. His limitations are perceptive, integrative, or expressive processes which severely impair learning efficiency. Some children need careful observation in order to identify central nervous system dysfunction, which is also expressed chiefly in impaired ability to learn. Needless to say, it is the classroom teacher with the help of a specialist (team approach) that has much to offer. Somewhere between 7 and 10 per cent of school children have need of help in this area. Often this help starts with the neurological examination in order to secure objective findings. This includes an appraisal of gait and posture, motor system-muscle tone, coordination, handiness, right-left discrimination and other motor tasks that may be given fairly quickly. (See Fig. 3–12.) Next comes a thorough look at family history, followed by an appraisal of mental status, vision and hearing, and speech and language.

Administration of Drugs in the Schools

Numerous children have to have their medicine while attending school. A policy, therefore, needs to be in effect in each school relative to the procedure to be followed. The principal should delegate the person to administer the pupils' medication. It may be the teacher in some cases, or the school nurse. Ideally, the school nurse should handle this and be familiar with the particulars. However, the behavior of the child as observed by the teacher needs to get through to the physician prescribing the medication—particularly if drugs are involved. The nurse is probably the best person to facilitate this action.

Certain drugs have a promising effect in the treatment of children with learning impediments. Tranquilizing agents as well as anticonvulsant agents are employed in many places. So are central nervous system stimulants such as amphetamines. Hyperactive (hyperkinetic) elementary school children have been helped with amphetamine drugs, and the Office of Child Development (HEW) has sanctioned this kind of treatment after "very careful clinical analysis." There is great concern over the amphetamines because of their abuse throughout society. Out of twelve million standard doses produced in a recent year, an estimated 50 per cent were diverted to the black market. Surveys among student populations show that fifth and sixth grade pupils are involved in amphetamine abuse. However, with proper school control the hyperkinetic children with significant behavior problems are helped to sit still and give attention to what goes on in the classroom. In this connection, it is especially desirable that there be a regular follow-up program including consultation with school nurses, physicians, parents, and teachers of children who are on behavior-modification drugs.[17]

THE CLASSROOM TEACHER COOPERATES WITH HEALTH SERVICES

Without the help of the sympathetic teacher, the health services personnel would indeed be handicapped. Some of her significant contributions involve the following:

Detection and Referral

The limitations of the routine medical examination of schoolchildren make it desirable to use the classroom more fully in the detection of pupil health problems. To the teacher who is trained to observe children carefully will come many significant signs and symptoms of poor health. Although the teacher is in no position to diagnose, she can certainly detect changes in behavior and refer those to the health services department.[18] It is of interest to note, in connection with these detection and referral activities of teachers, that a great deal of this kind of observation is done across the country in isolated areas where physicians are not plentiful. New York state, for example, is rich in physicians. It has one-sixth of all the country's physicians and one-fifth of all pediatricians. The figures are quite different in New Mexico or Montana. Yet, even in New York state, the vast majority of the physicians are concentrated in big cities, and upstate counties sometimes have difficulty obtaining one. The health observation role of the classroom teacher is further emphasized by the report that many small cities have no school nursing service. And in many places a health examination is merely a brief inspection by the classroom teacher.

Following-up Deviations from Normal Health

The value of an appropriate follow-up program in a school has already been pointed out. The teacher's unique con-

---

[17]Recommendation of *NEA Task Force on Drug Education*, Washington, D.C., National Education Association, 1972, p. 16.

[18]Chapter 5 will show more clearly what the teacher may observe and screen out in the way of disease, growth abnormalities, and behavior changes.

tribution here cannot be overstressed. In this country there are great numbers of children who come from homes where they do not have adequate preparation for school. They lack the sleep, food, or emotional climate that make for satisfactory schoolwork. Poverty, ignorance, and parental indifference are behind this. In the classroom the child falls short of what is expected of him; he may appear listless or lazy, easily discouraged, and show poor scholarship. The alert teacher may be able to notice his dry scalp, sallow skin, poor posture, lack of energy in physical activities, restlessness, and general irritability. It is important that something be done quickly. This situation is not different from one where a child is in need of glasses because he cannot see the blackboard. Expert medical judgment is needed. Follow-up to see that something is done is vital. Here, parents and teachers need to cooperate, but it is the teacher who is in a position of *control*. She actually controls the situation from the classroom, where she has a day by day check on the pupils concerned. Nevertheless, boys and girls still appear year after year with the same defects or difficulties despite the efforts of school personnel.

The following case report from a teacher in upstate New York represents a practical approach to a problem of malnutrition. It is more difficult than most cases, but is the type of case that is present in almost every community. It clearly demonstrates the role of the classroom teacher as a *prime mover* in following up basic health abnormalities. The classroom teacher speaks:

John was an 11 year old boy who lived in a trailer camp. His family consisted of father, stepmother and two stepbrothers, ages one and two years old.

He came to school with dirty clothes, unkempt hair and had been classified for two years as a problem child.

The fourth grade teacher noticed that he was listless, complained of headaches and was retarded in his schoolwork. Then some of the children who brought lunches to school complained that a sandwich, apple, orange, or cooky was missing from their lunches. On inquiry, it was discovered that John was guilty of the misdemeanor. What was the cause? The teacher took John to the school nurse. A confer-

ence of nurse, teacher, and John brought out the fact that he was coming to school without breakfast and going without a noonday lunch.

Since the stepmother couldn't leave her small sons, the nurse arranged for a visit to the trailer. The nurse and stepmother discussed John's physical condition and his meals, but the stepmother displayed disinterest. She said that the milkman didn't come until after John's school bus had gone and that the milk on hand in the trailer had to be used for the babies' cereal. She didn't have time to give John toast or egg or to make him a lunch to take to school.

The nurse contacted the father at the factory where he worked and tried to make an appointment to talk to him. His wife had already mentioned the nurse's visit to the trailer, so his reply to the nurse was, "The wife takes care of the food and the feeding of our family." No satisfaction was gained from him.

The nurse reported the results of the investigations to the principal. The principal, nurse, and school cafeteria manager discussed the case and came to the following decision:

Each morning when John's bus arrived, he went to the cafeteria to perform some little task for the cafeteria manager. In return she offered him juice, a slice of bread and butter, and a glass of milk. He didn't realize that this had previously been decided by the conference.

At noon, tickets were given to the children who purchased school lunches. John had been going without lunch or taking hand-outs from the other children, and was now given a ticket each day with the explanation it was given for doing errands for the principal. This was all arranged without humiliating John.

In June, John had shown a year's growth in achievement over the previous year. This was the greatest achievement he had shown in three years. He was a much happier boy in June than the previous September. Cooperative effort of principal, nurse, teacher, and cafeteria manager improved John's nutritional condition and gave him a new outlook on life.

Assisting in Screening Measures

The grade teacher in most school systems works with the nurse to screen pupils for a number of health difficulties. There are numerous places where screening is done entirely by the teacher; if she does not do it, it will not be done.

In addition to helping with vision and hearing measures, teachers also screen children to determine rate of growth. Growth is usually steady over a long enough period, so teachers weigh and measure their pupils periodically. Sometimes this is done with the aid of the school nurse so that some kind of further appraisal may be made on the spot.

Children are screened for characteristics of poor mental health in some of the more progressive schools. A program, carried out by the teacher, is set up for administering and scoring selected tests and recording the data obtained. Tests measuring the attitude of the child toward school and toward other children, and tests measuring his general behavior are especially useful in combating items of maladjustment.

It should be pointed out that "screening" tests used by teachers are not intended to diagnose. They serve only to select those pupils who appear in need of a diagnosis by a physician.

Carrying Out a Daily Inspection

The principle of observing hands, fingernails, faces, skin, eyes, hair, teeth, and glands, is a good one. The question often asked deals with whether such a daily inspection should be a formal one or an informal one. Certainly the formal inspection is an orderly approach—one which the pupils soon learn to accept.

When teachers are careful not to place *too much* emphasis on health items, the interest of the pupils is just enough to permit valuable learning to take place. Highly competitive morning inspections, however, sometimes force the pupils to be a part of the group "at any cost," even to the extent of being dishonest and reporting that they brushed their teeth when they did not.

Probably the daily inspection can best be carried out on an informal basis. Sometimes during the morning activities the teacher moves about the classroom observing the boys and girls. She obviously will be more interested in noting the appearance of those pupils who had poor health practices the day before. She can still post a record of her observations as a motivation technique for health education. In fact, several companies print daily inspection charts that may be obtained by request. Some teachers, instead of keeping the charts at school, send them home with the children. They are taped to the back of the bathroom

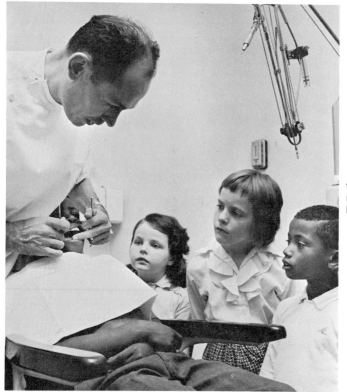

Figure 3-13 Health education is not limited to the classroom. (Courtesy Cincinnati Public Schools.)

door so that the child may keep his own record. This can be very effective for it also serves to keep the parents aware of what is going on.

Health Counseling

Either individually or as a member of a school health council the classroom teacher follows up appraisals by discussing the findings with her pupils. This is most generally planned for, but carried out informally. With younger children the parents are involved right away in the counseling procedure. Some of the finest counseling is done just like good teaching—"as if you taught them not."

Opportunities for Health Teaching

As already suggested in Chapter 2, the classroom teacher has a wonderful chance to educate for health every time the class is scheduled to visit the school physician. If this job is well done, the boys and girls will look forward to going to the physician's office with true delight. Furthermore, having a medical examination can be a most rewarding experience for the youngster in the early grades. These children are curious and, as a rule, they need little external motivation to prepare them for the day when they are looked over by the doctor. The teacher with a pleasant and positive outlook can discuss the why, the what, and the how of such a visit.

Why are we going to have the examination? Will it hurt?

What will the doctor find?

How will all this affect me?

These are good questions. If the pupils are allowed to work on this topic awhile they will come up with a number of other things that have been bothering them—questions relating to the instruments carried in the black bag, or why doctors do not seem to catch the measles or mumps when they visit sick children.

In some classrooms or nurses' offices children have a chance to handle a real stethoscope before the examination, and listen to the beat of their own hearts. Questions are asked and answered so that by the time of the examination the class is practically bouncing with enthusiasm to get started. This kind of ap- proach almost guarantees a *satisfying experience*.[19] Such positive health teaching may be briefly summarized by referring to a story told by a pioneer in health teaching, Mabel Bragg. In a Newton, Massachusetts, school one day, Dr. Emmett Holt stopped a group of children who were skipping merrily down a corridor. "Where are you going?" he asked. "We're going to see the doctor," said a little girl. "Why?" asked Dr. Holt. "Are you sick?" "Oh, no," she replied, "We're going to see how well we are."

THE IN-SERVICE PROGRAM

Orienting teachers and keeping them up to date is the responsibility of the local administration. School health is promoted this way through the in-service program.

A number of school programs have been completely reorganized from time to time because teachers have sat down together to talk about the health of their children. In Indiana, for example, the in-service training of teachers in health education has been successfully carried on for many years. Weekly conferences, under state education department guidance and promotion, have prompted many principals and classroom teachers to modify their existing health efforts. Moreover, in a number of the larger cities, the nurse-teachers speak to all school personnel each year about the health services available in the school and the community. Surveys have indicated that in a number of elementary schools there are numerous teachers who are quite unfamiliar with health centers and the health services available for their immediate use within a few miles or minutes of the school. It cannot be pointed out too often that school health education involves more than the school—it concerns the whole community in practically all of its aspects.

---

[19]An expression used by William James to convey the idea of something that gives deep gratification to the individual, and will be apt to be repeated again because of this.

QUESTIONS FOR DISCUSSION

1. What part should the social worker in the community have in the school health program?

2. What is the current thinking relative to the administration of medication to schoolchildren during school hours? If a pupil must take his pills regularly should he do it in class under teacher supervision or go to the office of the school nurse?

3. To what extent do teachers of your acquaintance engage in "detection and referral" activities?

4. How would you as a teacher feel about keeping anecdotal records on the health behavior of your children? Would it be a chore or something you believe would be useful to other teachers?

5. Are school psychiatrists necessary? Is it not possible that a guidance counselor or school psychologist might be a reasonable substitute?

6. It has been hypothesized by Gabrielson and others (see *Selected References*) that there is a positive relationship between "increased parental perception of seriousness and parent action in school follow-up recommendations." How would you comment on this statement?

SUGGESTED ACTIVITIES

1. Find out what kind of duties school nurses actually perform. Do they do everything this chapter says they do? How do they relate to crippled children? To drop outs? To children who may take advantage of illness? To children who miss classes? To the social workers or health center?

2. Read about preschool health screening efforts. (See Belleville article in *Selected References*.) Aside from the positive elements, what are some of the difficulties found in working with these younger children and their parents?

3. Interview a school nurse, preferably one in a large city and another in a small town, in order to discuss factors affecting school health follow-up practices. This may be organized as a committee project to discover some of the difficulties involved in

following up and in improving the health conditions of schoolchildren. Write out your comments following the interview.

SELECTED REFERENCES

Abrams, Herbert K. "Neighborhood Health Centers." *American Journal of Public Health,* 61:2236–2239, November 1971.

American School Health Association. "The Nurse in the School Health Program." *Journal of School Health,* 37:1–40, No. 2a, February 1967.

Anderson, C. L. *School Health Practice,* 5th ed. St. Louis: C. V. Mosby Co., 1972.

Belleville, Marion and Green, Pauline B. "Preschool Multiphasic Screening Programs in Rural Kansas." *American Journal of Public Health,* 62:795–799, June 1972.

Curry, Marcia F. "Public School Health in Colorado," *Rocky Mountain Medical Journal,* 68:49–60, April 1971.

Dennison, Darwin and Fenimore, Joy A. "A Heart-Sound Screening Program for Elementary Children." *Journal of School Health,* 41:349–351, September 1971.

Eisner, Victor and Oglesby, Allan. "Health Assessment of Children." *Journal of School Health,* 42:348–350, June 1972.

Gabrielson, Ira W., et al. "Factors Affecting School Health Follow-Up." *American Journal of Public Health,* 57:48–59, January 1967.

Gair, Catherine. "What Is School Nursing?" *Journal of School Health,* 36:401–402, November 1966.

Haag, J. H. *School Health Program,* 3rd ed., Philadelphia: Lea and Febiger, 1972.

Lippman, Otto. "Vision Screening of Young Children." *American Journal of Public Health,* 61:1586–1601, August 1971.

Marriner, Ann. "Opinions of School Nurses About the Preparation and Practice of School Nurses." *Journal of School Health,* 41:417–419, October 1971.

National Education Association-American Medical Association. *Health Appraisal of School Children,* 5th ed. Washington, D. C.: National Education Association, 1970.

National Education Association-American Medical Association. *Suggested School Health Policies,* 4th ed. Washington, D.C.: National Education Association, 1966.

National Education Association-American Medical Association Joint Committee. *School Health Services,* 3rd ed. Chicago: American Medical Association, 1973.

Nemir, Alma. *The School Health Program,* 3rd ed. Philadelphia: W. B. Saunders Company, 1970.

Randall, Harriet B. "Use of the School Physician's Time." *Journal of School Health,* 38:116–119, February 1968.

Turner, C. E., Sellery, C. M., and Smith, S. L. *School Health and Health Education,* 6th ed. St. Louis: C. V. Mosby Co., 1970.

4 ASPECTS OF HEALTHFUL AND SAFE SCHOOL ENVIRONMENT

Children attending school near Los Angeles International Airport, and dozens of other large airports across the country, run the risk of suffering permanent hearing damage and are threatened emotionally because of jet aircraft noise. This kind of stressful and disease-producing situation is exactly what Hippocrates referred to twenty-five centuries ago when he talked about the state of the organism which results from reactions to noxious stimuli or disturbing situations. Unfortunately, such negative influences are as much a part of the educational process as the favorable ones. Very often something can be done about it. It is for this reason that physical surroundings and classroom atmosphere are weighed as seriously as curriculum content and teaching method.

IMPORTANCE OF HEALTHFUL LIVING TO THE SCHOOL PROGRAM

The healthful school environment is one which provides for healthful living throughout the school day. It is not a haphazard setup; there is organization to bring this about. The administrator, the physician, and the custodian work together to provide safe and sanitary facilities and such pupil-teacher relationships as are favorable to the best growth and development, optimum learning, and welfare of all.

Concern for the living conditions of students is not new. Most civilizations have given it some attention. Spartan educators realized the importance of favorable surroundings dominated by teachers with strong personalities. Through the years in American schools there have been numerous distractions such as lack of heat in the winter months, poor lighting, inadequate ventilation, unadjustable desks and chairs, unattractive walls, and poor acoustics. Parents sometimes made themselves heard. So did medical doctors who were interested in the schools. At the founding meeting of the American Association for the Advancement of Physical Education, held in Brooklyn, New York, in 1885, Dr. W. L. Savage spoke about "ill ventilated school houses and weary children and of the relief which open windows and physical exercise would bring."[1] Overcrowded classrooms and poor school construction in the late 1800's resulted in several tragic fires which stimulated the popu-

---

[1]Proceedings of the Association for the Advancement of Physical Education. Brooklyn: Rome Brothers, 1885.

lace to look more closely at the school environment. In 1892 William H. Burnham, one of the better known school health pioneers, wrote extensively on "school hygiene" and presented evidence to show the necessity for greater attention to school furniture, cleanliness, growth, schoolhouse architecture, reading, writing, fatigue, and aspects of school health neglected at that time.[2] Gradually, more attention was given to child health, and today educational buildings and programs are continually being modified to provide healthful school living.

No one, however, should be misled into believing that most of the schools are "up to date" just because new buildings are being erected. Teachers still register complaints relative to inadequate drinking fountains, overcrowded classrooms and playrooms, noisy environment, and insufficient janitorial services. In a great number of schools it is possible to discover inadequacies in basic safety measures. School bus transportation is a good example. Despite an increase in new equipment and improved bus regulations, most of the states do not forbid pupils to stand in moving buses.

THE INTERNAL ENVIRONMENT – THE SCHOOL BUILDING

Whether or not the elementary school contributes to the over-all purposes of health education depends in the first instance upon the thinking and planning of members of the Board of Education. Where is the building to be located? Is it to be near main highways, busy streets, noisy factories, or active train yards? Of what is it to be constructed? How will it face? Is there play space within the structure? Are the corridors soundproofed? Are the stairs moderately inclined? What kind of windows does it have? If windows have to be closed, is there air conditioning? Are the classrooms attractive? Is the health examination room adequate in size? Are there locker room and shower facilities? How satisfactory are the lunchroom facilities? These and a dozen more pertinent questions must be discussed by the board members, architects, sanitary engineers and others before the building is constructed. Moreover, it is not uncommon today for teachers' committees to sit down and plan the facilities that to them seem desirable for the maintenance of good health and the promotion of a reasonable degree of individual pupil achievement.

The importance of the internal school environment to the elementary school teacher should not be underestimated. The finest health teaching is done by example. Where there are no facilities for handwashing, for instance, it is pretty difficult to discuss visiting the washroom and washing the hands before eating. There are numerous schools that fit this category. Until recent years the city schools were usually better equipped than the rural schools, but with the closing of many old-time rural schoolhouses and the opening of thousands of consolidated and regional schools serving large areas of the population, the trend for superior facilities is moving away from the large cities.

No matter how poor the facilities are, the classroom teacher owes it to her pupils to strive personally for improvements. She should know that:

1. The water supply must meet the minimum standards for chemical bacterial purity established by the state and local health departments.

2. The common drinking cup is prohibited.

3. The sanitary drinking fountain should be installed in the classroom, or at least one on each floor to serve a minimum of 50 pupils; the height of the nozzle should range from 23 inches for kindergarten to 29 inches for intermediate grade school pupils.[3] The fountain

---

[2]Means, Richard K. *A History of Health Education in the United States.* Philadelphia: Lea and Febiger, 1962, p. 62.

[3]National Education Association, American Medical Association. *School Health Services,* revised 1964. Washington: National Education Association, p. 71.

should be of the modern, slanting type with self-closing valve and mouth guard. Adequate water pressure must be maintained at all drinking fountains.

4. The drinking fountain water should be cool, less than 75° F.

5. The rural schools without running water should use sanitary privies, either the pit privy or septic privy type, or chemical toilets.

6. In the absence of a garbage grinder, food and refuse from the school cafeteria should be disposed of by local collection, burning, burying, or other methods approved by sanitation authorities.

7. Toilet facilities — clean, well ventilated, bright, well-kept, and properly lighted — encourage pupils to maintain these conditions. The dark toilet room, without paper towels and liquid soap, poorly kept, encourages a lack of respect for standards of sanitation. There should be a minimum of one urinal for 30 boys and a split-seat toilet for 25–30 girls.

8. The handwashing basins should range in height from 20 inches for kindergarten to 25 inches for intermediate grade school pupils. There should be one for every 30 children.

9. School cafeteria sanitation must meet the standards of any public or community eating establishment. The cafeteria should also be an attractive place to eat.

10. The school swimming pools and shower room facilities must meet sanitary standards. The use of pupil footbaths is not recommended; instead, individuals are encouraged to practice proper foot hygiene. This involves drying the foot and using foot powder if necessary. It also includes periodic inspection of the pupils' feet for athlete's foot and other skin infections. Floors should be hosed and washed daily.

11. The teachers' rest rooms should be attractive and functional.

12. The school custodian is the teacher's friend and needs the concrete help of the teacher and her pupils.

13. The gymnasium must be well lighted and ventilated and have protective wiring over exposed lights.

14. The halls, stairways, classrooms, and auditorium must be checked for accident hazards.

15. The playground should be clean and level and preferably have an asphalt (blacktop) surface.

16. The school area should be relatively free of disturbing noises, obnoxious odors, and other distractions.

17. School personnel must be constantly alert to observe buildings, grounds, and equipment for possible hazardous conditions:

Broken or splintered furniture or playground equipment
Defective stair rails
Broken sidewalks
Protruding objects anywhere, such as nails
Holes in blacktop surfaces
Sandboxes not properly maintained
Blocked or obstructed exits
Slippery floors
Gas leaks

18. Fire prevention equipment must be conveniently located and inspected at regular intervals.

ASPECTS OF CLASSROOM ENVIRONMENT

The classroom is the teacher's domain. Here are influences too subtle to measure, and here also are influences of major proportion that may contribute to or detract from learning and pupil achievement. These influences, or environmental elements, may be divided into physical factors and human factors. They touch upon all phases of healthful school living, from physical and emotional climate to classroom safety.

Physical Factors in the Classroom

Other things being equal, if the classroom is a pleasant place to live in, the student will find many opportunities for a satisfying experience. One wonders how "satisfying" the Los Angeles experience referred to earlier can be when decibel readings from airport noise are 80 to 96 in the classroom — far in excess of a reasonably quiet neighborhood of 45 to 50 decibels. Worse still, in this situation the classrooms were neither soundproofed nor air-conditioned for pupil comfort when windows were closed. At best it is a struggle to learn in such an environment. No wonder Charles Silberman, commissioned by the Carnegie Foundation to study the schools, termed the quality of life in the classroom "intolerable."

The teacher should know that the physical aspects within the classroom may have as much to do with her success as the motivation techniques and educational methods employed. She should know that:

1. An air temperature not in excess of 68° F. represents an optimal condition for comfort, with a slightly higher temperature of about 70° F. desirable in the primary grades.

2. Such items as humidity, air movement, and children's clothing must also be considered when comfortable room temperatures are being discussed.

3. It is good education for health to have pupils read and record room thermometers at set intervals.

4. Ventilation is as important to comfort as room temperatures; windows should be opened from the bottom to permit incoming cold fresh air to mix with the warm air rising from the radiator, and combined air moves toward the exhaust.

5. Standards of classroom lighting are steadily being revised, both for artificial and natural light. The lighting must be soft, even, properly distributed, and bright enough for eye comfort.

6. The responsibility for checking the operation of window shades and lights is the classroom teacher's.

7. To obtain the best working light from natural sources within the pupil's field of vision and with a minimum of shadows, individual pupil consideration should be given to seating arrangements. The 50° rotation of classroom furniture (in schools with movable desks and chairs) allows for maximum utilization of natural lighting by permitting the light to fall upon the work surface of each child's desk, unobstructed by body shadows.

8. The eyesight of schoolchildren is influenced by differences in brightness. This involves natural lighting, artificial illumination, and the color used to finish the interior surfaces of the classroom. Excessive brightness, which is glare, can be avoided by the type and color of paint used. Upper walls should reflect more light than lower walls and floors. But floors should reflect about 30 per cent of the light; they should not be dark and oiled. Desks should be light enough to reflect 40 per cent of the light, while the chalkboard should not reflect more than 15 per cent. Furniture, chalkboards, and other fixtures should have non-glossy finishes.

9. Uncontrolled sunlight is a fatiguing element that detracts from the total learning process.

10. The classroom should be free from acoustic difficulties.

11. The location and size of desks and chairs should be suited to the pupils using them. Fatigue and tension are often caused by ill fitting classroom furniture.

12. The writing surface of the desk should be at a height which permits the student to write while squarely seated so that there will be no need to elevate one shoulder out of line with the other when writing.

13. The ability of any one pupil to see or hear should be the major point in determining where he sits in the room.

14. Eyestrain may be relieved by alternating instruction involving close eye work with learning activities that are visually less fatiguing.

15. Clean teaching materials, such as maps and books, are desirable. Too often soiled materials are employed on which there is poor contrast between the paper and the print.

Healthful school living is in itself a health teaching item. All pupils must share the load of keeping the school clean and pleasant. By so doing they gain an understanding of the proper use of school property, the rights and feelings of others, and an appreciation for healthful surroundings. It is of interest to note that on many occasions this kind of pupil appreciation carries over into the home environment rather quickly, and is manifested by such actions as cleaning kitchen floors, hanging bright curtains, and helping parents wash windows and paint interior walls.

There are, in addition to the physical factors already referred to, a number of other classroom items that have a bearing upon healthful living. The scheduling of activities and the allotment of time, for example, may be done in such a way that the interest of the class members is kept to a high level throughout the day. This may be ascertained by experimenting with the difficult activities at various hours of the school day. Keeping a rigid time schedule, particularly in the lower grades, does not allow for individual and group variations in capacities and interest. Other classroom environment elements that are of concern here include such things as the length of the school day, the spacing and duration of rest and recess periods, class load, and programs and surroundings adapted to individual needs. (See Fig. 4–1.)

Human Factors in the Classroom

It seems to be a rather common practice to relate all the elements of human behavior, on the part of both pupils and the teacher, to one general category — classroom climate or atmosphere. To be sure, classroom climate does embrace physical surroundings, but it probably is influenced more by individual human factors such as human peculiarities, idiosyncrasies, attitudes, prejudices, likes and dislikes, and health status of the moment.

Few laymen have any idea of the complicated juggling of forces and personalities that is the everyday job of the classroom teacher; it is like trying to stage an important show while trying to keep a dozen billiard balls, knives and forks in the air all at once without dropping or forgetting one.

The role of the teacher is to attempt to maintain an environment for good health, which in turn creates the optimum atmosphere for learning. She must be realistic and deal objectively with pupil relationships. She must think in terms of individuals while operating in the medium of masses of children. She must exercise leadership and be firm with pupils, and at the same time demonstrate cooperation and sympathy for children with personal problems of adjustment.

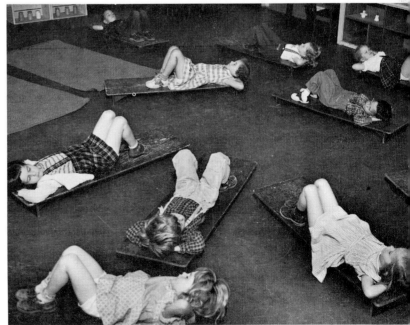

Figure 4–1 A relaxation period fosters healthful school living. (Courtesy Los Angeles Schools.)

Human factors are more difficult to control than physical factors. The elementary schoolteacher is faced at the beginning of each school year with the task of building a mentally healthy environment. She must understand child behavior and recognize that the mentally healthy classroom is one where the children have a high level of self-esteem, are relaxed and at ease, are challenged by the situation to want to learn, are confident they can succeed and receive a personal satisfaction from such success. Furthermore, the teacher must recognize that in adjusting to school the child is making three of the fundamental adjustments to life. First of all, he is making a social adjustment, i.e., to his classmates. In the second place, he is making an adjustment to authority. This is an adjustment made to teachers and principals, which is just and friendly, essential for happy group living. In the third place, the child learns in school to adjust to his own limitations. This, in itself, places the teacher in a unique position, for every child wants to be the best, the brightest and the most productive; the teacher must help him discover his own strong points and live with his limitations.

The teacher does more than recognize these factors. She works to create a school environment that promotes mental health. Such activity on her part is a first-rate example of proper health education. Some of the more specific tasks she can engage in to foster feelings of acceptance, affection and achievement include:

1. Making the classroom a friendly place. "Big Brothers" and "Big Sisters" can be assigned to help newcomers feel at home. Look for the child without a friend and see that he has a chance to sit with an especially friendly person.

2. Showing concern for each pupil. Celebrate birthdays. Telephone the home of the sick child to inquire about him. Welcome him back on his return to class and allow him to talk about his illness to the group.

3. Permitting boys and girls to have a part in planning the class activities.

4. Treating all pupils kindly. Avoid constant nagging, scolding, or correcting. Let children know, without saying in so many words, that you like them, and if they have trouble with something, you will try to see their side of the problem.

5. Accepting children's feelings of the moment. Angry children have their difficulties, but these may be overcome to some extent by directing their attention to some constructive form of expression such as helping the teacher, painting a picture, or talking over the trouble with an older person.

6. Providing for success experiences. Each pupil needs to feel success in at least one area of effort, whether it be sport skills, music, reading, or in picking up paper from the floor! At the same time it should be noted that children learn by their failures. Thus they shouldn't be protected from their failures but should understand them clearly in terms of their successes.

7. Praising individuals and groups for their fine efforts. Praise, properly administered, acts as an effective tonic which spurs pupils on to greater accomplishments.

8. Making provisions for specific student weakness and deficiencies through avenues of adapted instruction and program modification.

9. Helping parents develop a wholesome attitude toward ability and success in the classroom.

10. Recognizing that academic and social pressures may be somewhat offset by "low pressure" teaching and flexible pupil scheduling.

Liking or disliking school has much to do with classroom atmosphere. Needed are more patient teachers endowed with the kind of sensitivity that makes it possible to see how things look from the other person's point of view. Combs clearly indicates that teachers frequently fail to see children's views, and this accounts for most of the failures in human communication.[4] When it comes to children with severe emotional problems, it

---

[4]Combs, Arthur W. "The Human Aspect of Administration," *Educational Leadership*, November 1970, p. 197.

is even more important to see the child's view and resist reacting to a child's hostility on a personal level. Teacher calmness, objectivity and warmth tends to rub off on the pupil.

Teacher's Personal Health Status

The most favorable physical and human factors brought to bear in the classroom may mean very little if the teacher's own health status is below par. Yet various surveys of the mental and physical condition of teachers have produced evidence that a good many of them are ill in one way or another.

Many communities require periodic health examinations. Hypertensive individuals showing some irritability and fatigue and teachers with a history of severe mental illness probably should not teach school. Unfortunately a very small number of teachers are kept from teaching because of poor health. Studies are needed to show more clearly the relationship between classroom-pupil efficiency and teacher health defects and

illness. Certainly no one likes a grouchy teacher. How can she create happiness? Said Ben Franklin in his *Almanac*:

If you would have others merry with cheer, be so yourself or so appear.

It is estimated that *ten per cent* of all teachers in the United States have emotional problems deep enough to merit the designation "seriously maladjusted"; and in the Detroit school system an average of 35 teachers a month seek counsel for emotional difficulties.[5] Withdrawn and depressed teachers are using up their illness days in many localities. In New York there has been a one-third increase in teacher absence since 1960. Research is meager in this area, and when teachers are discovered exhibiting behavior that should keep them out of the classroom, little is done about it. One difficulty is related to defining mental

---

[5] Brenton, Myron. "Troubled Teachers Whose Behavior Disturbs Our Kids." *Today's Health*, 49:16–19, November 1971.

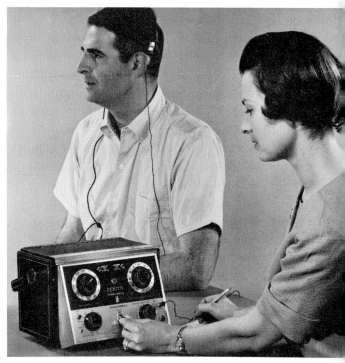

Figure 4–2 Teachers have their hearing checked too. (Courtesy Bausch and Lomb, Inc., Rochester, N.Y.)

illness clearly enough to permit school authorities to label an ill person without risking a legal suit. Another difficulty is teachers themselves; because emotional inadequacy is so threatening the individual frequently refuses to face up and recognize pathology.

It should go without saying that the physical health status of the classroom teacher is related largely to her personal health practices. Teaching is considered one of the vigorous occupations, on a level with medicine, military life, and police duty, and, as such, demands much of the vigor and enthusiasm of the individual. Practices involving good nutrition, dental care, recreation, moderate exercise, and rest are therefore important if one is to sustain an active constitution for effective teaching.

Every day there are untold circumstances that challenge the strength, ingenuity and adaptability of the teacher. Some of these exert pressure on a conscientious teacher and tend to warp her attitude so that she is a little less friendly and appears not to enjoy her job quite as well as before. Teachers need time for enrichment. Just as other people show signs of psychological stress and fatigue from their efforts to make a living, teachers too need relaxation, diversion, and play. Art, music, golf, fishing, photography, and other hobbies provide "just what the doctor ordered" for harassed teachers. The teacher who understands this basic point of view is far ahead of the one with great zest who "pushes" herself until she becomes unbearable to her class.

ASPECTS OF SCHOOL SAFETY

The topic of safety and safety education is an area of study in itself. Actually, safety falls within the school health education domain. It cuts across all fields and involves all personnel that have anything at all to do with the schools. Children learn about safe living through programs of instruction and by well defined

school safety practices that are engaged in by all pupils and teachers.

Needless to say, the school building has its share of hazards to guard against. There are stairways, corridors, lavatories, classrooms, shower rooms, swimming pools, gymnasiums, cafeterias, auditorium stages, and industrial arts shops to worry about. And there are programs associated with these facilities that require constant attention on the part of teachers lest accidents occur that might have been prevented. The same reasoning applies to the external environment. Safety on the playgrounds and playing fields, on the school buses, at the crossings adjacent to the school, and on field trips into the community all relate to healthful school living.

Accidents constitute the major hazard to the lives of children. They account for about half of the deaths among boys and for one fourth among girls. For boys especially, the accident hazard increases rapidly as they reach their late teens. A great many of these accidents occur in the school area.

Research reported by the National Safety Council indicates that 800,000 school injuries occur each year to boys and girls. According to the U.S. Public Health Service, this figure may be closer to four million accidental injuries per year, half of which are due to falls and bumping. In a Louisiana study it was found that "running when walking was required" and "horseplay" were practices strongly contributing to school accidents. In the first six grades the frequency of accidents is highest in the unorganized activities. Serious accidents, as determined by the average number of days lost from school, occur at the bicycle rack area, stairways, athletic fields, doorways, and school sidewalks, in that order.

Obviously there is a need for safety precautions in every school. Administrators, working with teachers, must formulate school safety procedures and establish local regulations. In numerous large city systems such as Boston, Los Angeles, New York, Cincinnati, and Boulder, special policies relative to accident prevention and environmental health have been set forth in administrative handbooks.

An appraisal instrument designed to help teachers and administrators improve their school safety efforts is available from the National Commission on Safety.[6] It is a checklist that encourages action on school safety problems relative to facilities and other environmental considerations, and educational programs.

With over 7200 fires a year in schools, the fire departments carry out inspections, and boards of education are required to implement fire department suggestions with respect to remedying hazardous situations. Police departments frequently study school traffic safety and erect special traffic signals and signs, and order appropriate cross-walk markings. Local civil defense groups also have a genuine interest in school health and safety activities.

Accident Prevention

There are at least four major considerations worth reviewing when an effort is being made to promote school safety. The first of these, which has already been discussed at some length, is the *determination of pupil health status*. The sick child is a hazard to his own safety. His reflexes and responses are slower; he is not as alert; and he lacks the physical capacity that his personal safety demands. Even children convalescing from disease and getting over colds probably should have a modified school program, for it is conceivable that their interaction with children could have some bearing on the safety of others. The second consideration is *concern for equipment and facilities*. Activities in the classroom, on the playground, in the gymnasium, and in the shops involve the use of special equipment. It is the teacher's responsibility to see that this equipment is in proper repair and safe to use. Very often

when a jungle gym frame is loose, or a sliver of wood breaks off a teeter board, or a stone under the swings works up out of the ground, the classroom teacher will complain that it is the duty of the school custodian to do something about it. But in most instances constructive action will be taken in the way of repair only when the teacher personally discusses the situation with the custodian.

The third program safeguard has to do with the *development of activity skills*. In every subject matter area there are specific skills to be mastered. Proficiency in these skills—in the classrooms and laboratories and on the playgrounds—makes the difference between a low and high accident rate. It would be improper for schools to remove every dangerous piece of equipment or condemn all hazardous activities. Children need the experience of meeting challenging situations by developing satisfactory skills. Electric jig saws are not removed from the shops because they can cut off a wayward finger; playground equipment is not dismantled for fear that some child may fall off; and automobiles are not outlawed because of automobile accidents. We learn to live with these things. There is no substitute for skill. The child, for example, who possesses the skill for operating the jig saw, is far better off than the one who has little ability but is closely supervised. This leads directly to the fourth and final consideration, namely, *adequate supervision*. The stairways, corridors, halls, playgrounds, and classrooms need constant supervision, not only because teachers are liable, but also because youngsters are often too busy to look after their own safety. Satisfactory accident prevention involves a combination of all four considerations, especially personal skills and adequate supervision. For example, children boarding school buses, crossing streets, and taking part in fire drills need to practice well identified skills in the presence of capable teacher supervision.

The prevention of school accidents has become one of the major interests of board members, teachers, and administrators. A few of the more significant *ac-*

---

[6] *School Safety Education Checklist: Administration, Instruction, Protection.* Washington, D.C.: National Commission on Safety Education, National Education Association, revised.

cident prevention activities are worth listing, for they have more than a slight influence on school health:

In the classroom:

1. Put sharp objects away.
2. Cover exposed projections such as plant boxes and table corners.
3. Cover exposed lights, radiators and electric fixtures.
4. Play games that are safe for the particular classroom.
5. Move about the classroom in an orderly manner, neither pushing nor running.
6. Use tools at workbench or desk.
7. Keep furniture in proper place.
8. Encourage children to keep feet out of aisle and under the desk.

In the halls, corridors and stairways:

1. Do not leave locker doors ajar.
2. Avoid running and pushing, especially on stairs.
3. Exercise care at drinking fountains.
4. Use care in passing closed doors; they may be opened suddenly and cause serious injury.
5. Report slippery surfaces and worn or broken stairs.

6. Appraise the hall traffic in terms of congestion; rerouting may be advisable.

In the shops and laboratories:

1. Keep floors clean of litter.
2. Look for "shop sloppies" who wave boards wildly around in the air and leave nails sticking up for others to step on.
3. Check and repair equipment each day.
4. Post and discuss safety rules for using laboratory or shop tools and equipment.
5. Provide a minimum of first aid supplies, especially for burns and bleeding.
6. See that gas, water, and electricity are turned off when no longer needed.
7. Stress the importance of good footing and safe clothing. Sleeves should be rolled and ties removed.
8. Use color to denote parts of machinery or chemicals that are particularly hazardous.

In the gymnasium, locker, and shower rooms:

1. Encourage safe play through personal example and discussion with pupils.

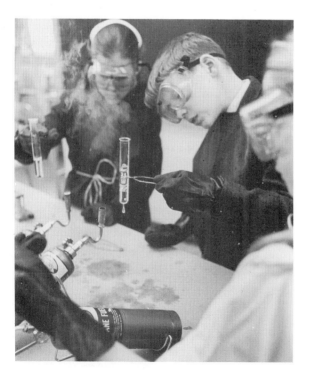

Figure 4–3 Fifth graders study safety in school. (Courtesy National Safety Council and National Education Association.)

2. Stress the rules of the game, point out the boundaries and penalize for infringements.

3. Do not overcrowd the play space. There is danger when groups practice their skills in adjacent areas.

4. Select activities within the physiological and skill limits of the pupils.

5. Seek out the hazards of each game and plan to counteract them.

6. Check exposed projections, gymnasium equipment, lighting, and floor surfaces. Lights should be protected with a heavy wire mesh.

7. Insist that pupils dress in proper uniform with sneakers for all gymnasium activities.

8. Regulate showers from master control panel.

9. Prohibit pushing, wrestling, and fooling around in locker and shower rooms.

On the playgrounds:

1. Enclose the entire playground area with a five or six foot fence.

2. Provide adequate space between pieces of equipment.

3. Mark well and properly space all courts for outside games.

4. Check apparatus for repair items and terrain for foreign objects, such as tree roots or stones.

5. Encourage safe play. Teach the correct use of each piece of apparatus.

6. Carry on team games such as soccer, speedball, and softball in an area away from the apparatus and small children.

7. Reserve one section of the playground that is protected and near the school for kindergarten and first graders.

8. Encourage courtesy, patience, and fair play: they breed a degree of respect for the other fellow and reduce accidents.

Going to and from school:

1. Discuss with children the routes they take home.

2. Encourage parental interest in the safety program, particularly as it concerns going to and from school.

3. Remind children to stay on the walks and in crosswalk lanes, to obey rules, signs, and the traffic directors.

4. Encourage children to report hazardous obstructions along school routes.

5. Cooperate with school bus drivers in the aspects of bus safety.

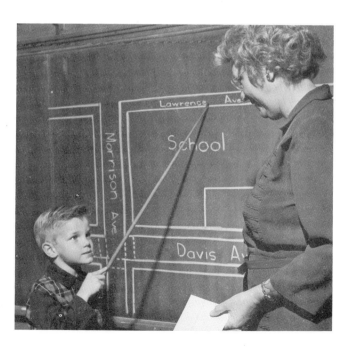

Figure 4-4 City children talk over the best route to school. (Courtesy National Safety Council.)

6. Provide supervision of school traffic patrols.[7]

---

[7]Standard rules governing the operation of school safety patrols have been adopted by states and on a national level by representatives of the National Safety Council, National Congress of Parents and Teachers, National Education Association, American Automobile Association, National Association of Chiefs of Police, and the U.S. Office of Education. Standard rules have been published by the National Safety Council.

What has been said here applies primarily to the classroom teacher. If school living is at all healthful, it will be due in part to the teacher's convictions and alertness relative to hazardous conditions. She will need to stress directly and indirectly what Abraham Lincoln accentuated more than a century ago, i.e., every man has a personal duty to protect himself and those associated with him, from accidents which may result in injury or death.

QUESTIONS FOR DISCUSSION

1. Should apparatus such as swings, slides, and teeter boards be eliminated from the school playground because of the possibility of accidents?

2. Does the expression "healthful living" mean more or less to you than "healthful school environment"? Explain.

3. Would parental education of school-age children be workable? Could child psychology, child safety and other environmental topics be taught in such a way that accidental injuries to children could be reduced? Do you have a better idea?

4. Suppose the teacher's personal health influences learning in a negative way. What should be done in a school system to prevent this situation? To remedy it?

5. Discuss the construction of a check list of items designed to screen the environmental conditions of a school from the viewpoint of health and safety.

SUGGESTED ACTIVITIES

1. Using more than one source, obtain a list of the desirable qualities of the good teacher. Compare your list with those of your classmates. Would it appear that characteristics of sound mental health are significant? Comment on your findings.

2. Read what Charles Silberman has to say about "intolerable" conditions in the classroom (See Selected References). From your experience would you tend to agree or disagree with this Carnegie Foundation writer?

3. Visit several elementary classrooms located in close proximity to a busy airport. Is there evidence that learning is more difficult here than in a quieter environment? Indicate how a study might be arranged in a particular school.

4. Consult the literature of such organizations as the National Safety Council, the National Commission on Safety, and the U.S. Public Health Service, and compare accident statistics for children in the first six grades. Comment on the significance of your findings.

SELECTED REFERENCES ⇐

A School Safety Education Program. Washington, D.C.: National Commission on Safety Education, National Education Association, 1971.

Bidwell, Corrine. "The Teacher as a Listener—an Approach to Mental Health." *Journal of School Health, 37:*373–383, October 1967.

Irwin, Leslie W., Cornacchia, Harold J., and Staton, Wesley M. *Health In Elementary Schools,* 3rd ed. St. Louis: C.V. Mosby Co., 1970, Chapter 3.

Randall, Harriett B. "The Teacher's Responsibility for Mental Health in the Classroom." *Journal of School Health, 37:*448–451, November 1967.

Rosenthal, Etta M. "Dealing With Emotional Problems." *Instructor, 82:*14, January 1972.

Silberman, Charles E. *Crisis In The Classroom,* New York: Random House, 1970.

Stack, Herbert J., and Elkow, J. Duke. *Education for Safe Living.* Englewood Cliffs, New Jersey: Prentice-Hall, Inc., 1970.

Turner, C. E., Randall, H. B., and Smith, S. L. *School Health and Health Education,* 6th ed. St. Louis: C.V. Mosby Co., 1970, Chapter 11.

Willgoose, Carl E. "Educating For Safety." *Instructor, 81:*62–63, February 1971.

Wilson, C. C., and Wilson, E. A. (Joint Committee NEA-AMA). *Healthful School Environment,* Washington: National Education Assn., 1969.

5 NORMAL GROWTH AND DEVIATIONS FROM NORMAL

When Alfred Lord Tennyson wrote that ". . . men at most differ as heaven and earth" he was saying in very few words that there is a certain bit of being normal in being different. There is, therefore, an extensive range of behavior common to man—a circumstance that makes it most difficult at times to determine just what kind of behavior represents poor health or some other inadequacy.

Spotting the atypical or abnormal child in a classroom of essentially normal children is the teacher's business. It is a formidable task, calling for the capacity to discriminate between the pupil who acts differently and is really ill, and the one who acts differently but is simply "marching to a different drummer."

THE CONCEPT OF NORMAL

In discussing normal growth it might be well to refer to a well known quotation from William Shakespeare's *The Merchant of Venice:*

I am a Jew. Hath not a Jew eyes? Hath not a Jew hands, organs, dimensions, senses, affections, passion? . . . fed with the same food, hunt with the same weapons, subject to the same diseases, healed by the same means, warmed and cooled by the same winter and summer, as a Christian is? If you prick us, do we not bleed? If you tickle us, do we not laugh? If you poison us, do we not die? And if you wrong us, shall

we not revenge? If we are like you in the rest, we will resemble you in that.

This quotation is intended to reflect the certain fundamental likenesses which all people have in common. People are never so different that they are not recognizable as human beings, differing only within the limits that human ranges allow. Yet every person differs enough that no two are alike.

What is normal? This question is often disturbing, for in every direction there abounds a multitude of persons and things that are not as they are "supposed to be." A man shuffling along wearing size 13 shoes catches our attention not when he towers well over six feet in height, but when he is only five feet tall. His health may be perfectly normal, but his feet are not; they are too long for a man of his limited height. An appropriate norm table would show this, for a norm is no more than a standard point of reference. It is a kind of average of all extremes of existing characteristics. This may be good or bad, for the norm is in no way an ideal.

A normal characteristic is simply a typical one. It is built around some specific factor or phenomenon and is based solely on generalizations. It considers typical cases and typical behavior and is used for purposes of comparison. If several thousand 12 year old girls have freckles, then freckles are typical and to be expected. If a thousand 12 year old girls, 62 inches tall, generally weigh 90 pounds, then 90 pounds is typical and becomes the norm. We have generalized so that the girls at either extreme, whose weights were part of the several thousand cases, would be below or above normal in weight; they would be labeled "abnormal," "atypical," or "deviants." Yet, there are so many of these deviants in a given sample that they might well represent a large segment of the population.

When an individual is a long way from the norm and is classed atypical, although he is in perfect health, it becomes rather obvious that he is profoundly different and should be treated so if he is to be fully understood. Thus, sociologists, anthropologists, and educators alike think and speak in terms of individual differences for a very good reason. Furthermore, there is almost no such thing as a "normal" human being. Two individuals may compare alike (almost alike) in a certain characteristic, but they may vary immensely in another. It is difficult, then, to say who is normal.

To proceed to the question of what is normal health, it must be admitted that it is quite normal to see people with bad teeth, digestive upsets, nearsightedness, baldness, aching feet, advanced obesity, or mental instability. It even seems normal for more than a million people to succumb to heart disease each year, but these items can hardly be accepted as desirable even if they come close to being within the normal range of what might be found in a cross section of the population. It is imperative, therefore, that we do not generalize all health characteristics and behavior and be blind to the distinctions which make each of us an individual. Healthy people are different. Healthy children are different. Sheldon admirably points this out in his monumental work on the study of body build and constitutional behavior.[1] Sheldon's

findings have been related to educational practice in an article in which it is pointed out that *if children fail to act as we think they should, it is probably because we have not learned to tell them apart.*[2] Williams illustrates it by quoting the Russian novelist, Ivan Turgenev.[3] Turgenev pokes fun at scientists and educators by saying that "a man's capable of understanding anything—how the ether vibrates and what's going on in the sun—but how any other man can blow his nose differently from him, that he's incapable of understanding." (See Fig. 5-1.)

THE NORMALLY HEALTHY CHILD

Educators usually think of the healthy child as one who is well adjusted to his surroundings, is free from physical defects and organic drains, and demonstrates emotional stability. He is not necessarily perfect, but he is well. There are other children who are almost as well, but they are not quite up to average when it comes to some special function such as heart efficiency or hearing. In this respect they are considered atypical and abnormal. Children with obvious individual differences in body build, physical and mental capacities, behavior, and interests may be completely healthy. But *it will take a teacher who is trained to observe children carefully to be able to select from such a group of individually different children those who deviate too far and appear to need medical or psychiatric help.*

Determining whether a pupil is normally healthy can at times be a most difficult job. Some diseases are carried for a long while and are only slightly noticea-

[1]Sheldon, William H. *The Varieties of Human Temperament.* New York: Harper & Brothers, 1942.

[2]Willgoose, Carl E. "Educational Implications of Constitutional Psychology," *Education,* 73(4):225, December 1952.

[3]Williams, Roger J. *Biochemical Individuality.* New York: John Wiley & Sons, 1957.

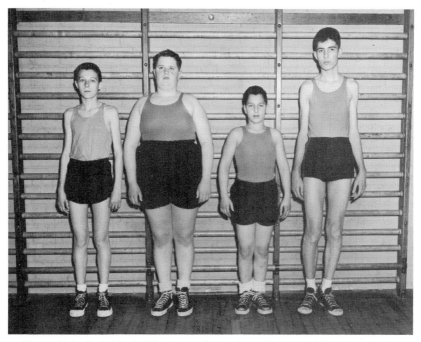

Figure 5–1 Individual differences. Seventh grade boys of the same age.

ble in the early stages. A pupil with a respiratory ailment, for example, may do nothing more serious than cough occasionally for months, thus behaving not too differently from his compatriots in the class. Everyday behavior is a complex process at best and involves an interrelationship of physical, mental, emotional, and social activity. The body operates as a whole; both *psyche* and *soma* are part of the same constitution. A disease or attitude that affects one has a measurable bearing on the other. Thus a malnourished pupil might be irritable and bite his fingernails in class and be mistaken by the teacher for a pupil with an emotional problem. Or a child might actually have a stomach upset because he was concerned over his inability to recite before the class. This might easily be interpreted to indicate that he was making believe he had a pain when in reality it was more likely associated with a defense mechanism wherein he became "psychologically" ill, even psychosomatically ill, because he did not know his lesson and was not prepared to recite before the class.

DEVIATIONS FROM NORMAL HEALTH

To understand thoroughly the concept of normal health and its deviations it is necessary that the beginning teacher have a knowledge of the growth and development of boys and girls. (See Chapter 6.) The extremes of early and late maturation may appear to indicate deviations from normal health when such is not the case. Children do not grow according to a rigid, set schedule; there is no growth pattern to which every child must conform. One must be aware of the fact that mental and social growth may be retarded due to genuine physical difficulties. Inadequate hearing, for instance, may result in poor speech or a reluctance to speak. And because social growth in children is more abstract than physical growth, it will again be difficult to note behavior deviations from normal.

One can learn the characteristics of optimum child health and can also become familiar with the common deviations. Since most people are more familiar with the marks of good health, this chapter will call attention chiefly to the signs and departures.[4]

Teachers may see what is often missed by parents who are too close to their children, and what would be of interest to physicians and nurses if they had access to the child on a daily basis. They may be puzzled if a hitherto cooperative child becomes inattentive, or the otherwise bright child is unusually slow in learning to read, or the ordinarily happy and enthusiastic youngster develops a case of extreme docility. They may wonder about pimples around the mouth, swollen glands in the neck, low shoulders, underweight and malnutrition, or excessive snuffing or coughing. It is when teachers *are* this much concerned with what they have seen that pupils may be helped early and at a time when the greatest good can be accomplished in remedying the situation. In this connection, the excellent thirty-two page booklet, *Looking For Health*, distributed free to teachers by the Metropolitan Life Insurance Company, sets up classroom conditions easily observed by the alert teacher.[5]

What are the signs and characteristics of general poor health, specific physical and mental defects and conditions which can be readily detected in day-to-day contact with boys and girls? Following are some that relate to long-standing defects, chronic illness, neurological disturbances, improper nutrition, and poor health practices.

Important Points for Observation

Height and Weight

Numerous misconceptions exist regarding weight changes and health status.

Maturation and growth are influential variables. Bulk weight is not in itself a sign of health. A pupil of normal height and weight may be suffering from some hidden abnormality or disease. Probably less than 4 per cent of obese or thin children have any glandular disturbances. White and Negro pupils are larger than Mexican and Japanese. Extremes of body build, although somewhat related to nutrition and activity, are quite apt to reflect constitutional patterns passed along from parents or families. The better norm tables allow for individual variations in structure.

Evidence of the wide variation of weight for age was clearly demonstrated by Falkner for white North American children in an extensive study of physical growth. At age ten, for example, boys varied in height (between the fifth and ninety-fifth percentiles) by as much as nine inches and in weight by as much as 40 pounds. Girls at age ten varied six and one-half inches in height and 47 pounds in weight.[6]

Since there is a relationship between the quality of growth and the rate of learning, it is appropriate to weigh and measure boys and girls. Moreover, this is a first-class health instruction activity.

Children should be weighed wearing as little clothing as practicable and without shoes. Although the frequency of measurement varies in different schools, the most effective screening combines weighing with height measurements two or three times a year. This procedure screens out the approximately 10 per cent of elementary school children who fail to gain weight for three successive months between September and May. Failure to realize a weight gain in three to four months is nearly always a sign that something is wrong, either because of poor health habits, disease, or conditions which call for medical examination.

A simple record for each child is suitable for classroom use. Individual growth records are available for each pupil; the

---

[4]The treatment of the topic will be brief, for no attempt is made here to embrace the area of health abnormalities of schoolchildren. Such a topic is broad enough to fill a book. It is referred to here only because observing pupil deviations is a part of the total school health program and is one method of health instruction useful in the grades.

[5]Copies available on request from Metropolitan Life Insurance Company, Health and Welfare Division, 1 Madison Ave., New York, N.Y., 10010.

---

[6]See report, together with growth tables, in *Obesity and Health*. Washington, D.C.: U.S. Public Health Service, 1966, p. 11.

Meredith Tables are useful. (See Chapter 3.) So is the Wetzel Grid for revealing trends in growth.[7]

Deviations in Appearance and Behavior.

Failure to gain in height and weight over a three to six month period
Excessive overweight
Small and underweight for age
Fluctuating weight changes

Skin

The skin shows a great deal to the observing teacher. Pale pupils who appear flushed, and rosy cheeked pupils who appear pale, are usually not up to par. Skin eruptions such as impetigo are very contagious. A number of communicable childhood diseases begin with a flushed or spotted skin. Vesicles appear in chickenpox, red rash in measles, and pallor in malnutrition. Skin deviations are often accompanied by fever, chills, headache, and loss of appetite.

From the pupil's viewpoint skin eruptions are serious in terms of personal appearance; social health seems more important than physical health.

Deviations in Appearance and Behavior.

Pale or sallow
Flushed appearance
Eczematous condition with rashes, scales, and crusts
Persistent sores
Pimples
Acne on face
Boils, warts
Cuts, scratches, bruises, burns
Blueness or pallor of lips
Common skin disease such as ringworm, impetigo, scabies ("itch"), and pink eye
Sensitivity to several substances; allergy
Easily bruised
Itching or burning skin (with frequent scratching)
Fever
Nits (lice eggs) on hair

---

[7]The Wetzel Grid is published by National Education Association Service Inc., 1200 W. Third Street, Cleveland, Ohio.

Teeth and Mouth

The pupil with a foul odor on the breath day after day probably has a mouth, tooth, nose, or alimentary disorder. Decayed teeth and diseased tonsils are often accompanied by enlarged glands. Total body infection, over-all fatigue, and poor appetite may be caused by grossly decayed teeth. Diseased teeth and tonsils set the stage for sore throats, inner ear disturbances, speech disorders, and the more serious viral and bacterial infections. Dental defects occur among children about six times as rapidly as the rate at which they are being corrected.

Deviations in Appearance and Behavior.

Bad breath
Cavities in teeth
Excessive tartar at necks of teeth
Toothache
Malocclusion and bad bite
Irregular spacing of teeth
Protruding and broken teeth
Speech difficulty
Inflamed or bleeding gums
Sores in mouth
Cracked lips, especially in corners of mouth

Neck

Swollen lymph glands are visible as lumps on the side of the neck and below the ears. They are readily seen in mumps and other systemic infections. Glands appearing as small lumps may be large when examined by touch. Swollen and tender glands demand immediate attention.

Enlargement of the thyroid gland is usually accompanied by rapid heart rate, more than normal sweating, and irritability and distractibility in the classroom.

Deviations in Appearance and Behavior.

Enlarged lymph glands
Enlarged thyroid glands on either side of windpipe
Position of neck out of alignment with spine

Hair and Scalp

Dirty children with dirty underclothes often have unclean hair and scalp. The white eggs (nits) of head lice (pediculi) cling to hair while female gray-backs move about. Pubic lice invade the groin area and cause much scratching. Microorganism infections may follow lice and ringworm; both are highly communicable.

Brittle hair and dry scalp often accompany cases of malnutrition. Pride in oneself begins with clean, combed hair.

Deviations in Appearance and Behavior.

Uncombed, uncontrolled hair
Dirty, dry scalp
Signs of vermin and ringworm
Brittle, stringy, and lusterless hair
Small bald spots
Crusty sores on scalp
Excessive dandruff
Frequent head scratching

*Upper Respiratory Tract
(Nose, Throat, Sinuses)*

Nasal and throat abnormalities affect the quality of the voice. Speech improvement comes about when the nasal passage is clear and mouth breathing ceases.

Sinuses and the middle ear may be acutely infected in colds, measles, scarlet fever, diphtheria, influenza, typhoid, and infected teeth. Diseased tonsils and adenoid tissue are deleterious to the whole upper respiratory tract.

Enlarged mucous membranes (hypersecretion) are present with severe head cold and hay fever. Mucous membranes are continuous within eyes, nose, mouth, throat, inner ears, bronchial tubes, and lungs.

Deviations in Appearance and Behavior.

Speech thick or muffled
Mouth breathing
Frequent sore throats
Persistent nasal discharge
Excessive colds
Frequent school absences
Difficulty in swallowing
Sore or scratchy throat
Discharge from ears
Frequent snuffing and coughing
Face or forehead pain (sinusitis)
Fever and bad breath

Sudden sneezing spells associated with allergies

Nutrition

Good nutritional status means much in terms of appearance, vigor, and personal enthusiasm for school activities. The classroom teacher is more effective here than any other person; behavior is so general that one must notice several of the accompanying signs before suspecting malnutrition.

Deviations in Appearance and Behavior.

General fatigue; tires easily
Poor, sloppy postural attitude; postural defects
Frequent and prolonged infections
Restlessness and irritability
Fingernail biting
Difficulty going to sleep
Restlessness during sleep
Lack of ambition
Dark circles or puffiness under eyes
Flabby musculature; possible muscle and joint pain
Poor teeth
Lack of appetite
Dry, scaly scalp, hair, and skin
History of sore mouth, tongue, or gums
Abnormal intolerance of light

Posture and Body Mechanics

Posture is a functional item and involves total body movement, especially standing and sitting, and attitude and gait in walking.

Functional difficulties due to weak musculature, uneven length of the legs, or one's temporary mental attitude may be corrected by exercises and activities assigned by the physician and physical educator, and reinforced by the encouraging words of the classroom teacher. Structural defects (immobile bumps or enlarged joints) need special medical attention.

Even minor postural defects need to be discovered and remedied early in order to obtain the greatest body efficiency in later years.

Many times postural abnormalities are indicative of poor nutrition, organic strains, hidden disease, low physical fitness, sedentary living, chronic fatigue, hearing defects, emotional disturbance, and asthma.

Other things being equal, the way the schoolchild feels at any one moment is often reflected in his posture.

Deviations in Appearance and Behavior.

Flabby musculature
Chronic fatigue
Round shoulders (kyphosis)
Head forward
One shoulder lower than the other
Protruding shoulder blades (winged scapulae)
Pigeon or funnel chest (rickets)
Lateral curvature of spine (scoliosis)
Unequal height of hips
Irregular gait in walking
Arches of feet are flat
Feet toe-out too far in standing and walking
Tendon above heel bone is bowed inward when standing
Heels of shoes wear down on inside borders
Pain in joints of body
Pain in bones of foot

Eyes

The list of deviations is rich in items that the classroom teacher can observe easily, especially in terms of reading difficulties. Some 80 per cent of the work a child does in elementary school is built around visual acuity within arm's reach; it is most important that visual difficulties be corrected just as early in the grades as possible.

Seeing is a process both of optics and brain development. Young children are normally far-sighted and see large objects, large print, and pictures quite well. In most schools students are screened for difficulties involving visual accommodation. Three fourths of all study activities in the elementary school require reading ability. Promotion from first to second grades is often on the basis of reading ability. Yet four out of five retarded readers have normal intel-

ligence. The teacher may notice that the retarded reader often achieves considerable success in those activities where reading skills are not of primary importance.

School surveys show that less than half the children who need glasses actually have them. School follow-up programs need more attention and control.

Early and repeated examinations are important. Good lighting, frequent rest periods, and the avoidance of prolonged sewing, drawing, painting, or reading by primary grade pupils are recommended.

Instruction should be given in how to view television and how to protect eyesight in the home and community. Some 20 to 25 per cent of all schoolchildren have eye defects.

Deviations in Appearance and Behavior.

Complaints of dizziness, headache, nausea
Crusts on lids among lashes
Red rims on lids
Watery eyes; styes
Swollen eyelids
Reading difficulties:
Holds book far away from face when reading
Holds body tense or thrusts head forward at distant objects
Holds face close to page when reading
Inattentive in wall chart, blackboard, or map lesson
Reads but brief periods without stopping
Screws up face when reading or looking at distant objects
Shuts or covers one eye when reading
Tilts head to one side when reading
Tends to look cross-eyed when reading
Tends to make frequent changes in distance at which book is held
Confusion in reading and spelling *o* and *a*; *e* and *c*; *n* and *c*; *h, n* and *r*; *f* and *t*
Apparently guesses from quick recognition of parts of the word in easy reading material

Rubs eyes frequently

Poor alignment in writing

Reversal tendencies in reading

Attempts to brush away a blur

Irritation over work or some emotional display

Strabismus or "squint"

Ear

Children with hearing loss in the classroom account for a sizeable proportion of all people with hearing loss. Two children in every classroom have a hearing problem. Early detection through screening tests permits the parent to obtain treatment reasonably quickly for the child. Pure tone audiometer testing permits quick sweep checks up to the 8000 frequency level. Some pupils fail the 4000 to 8000 high range, others fail the range below 500; but it is important for them to hear in the middle range. With middle range loss the child is experiencing much difficulty. Also, 35 per cent of the failures are in both ears.

Hearing loss varies, indicating a need for constant teacher observation and annual screening tests.

Deviations in Appearance and Behavior.

Discharge or odor from ears

Earache

Failure to answer and misunderstandings

Habit of saying "what?"

Turning head to one side when spoken to

Facial expressions indicating a lack of awareness of all that is going on

Speaking too softly, too loudly, or with an unusual voice quality

Difficulty in locating the source of sound

Unusual dependence on visual cues

Heart

Children with heart defects total about 1 per cent of the school-age population. Most of these children can take part in the normal classroom program. With some degree of restriction, most of these pupils may engage in modified or adapted physical education activities.

Rheumatic fever is declining in incidence and severity, but there are still many children whose heart valves are impaired due to this disease or other chronic infections such as scarlet fever, pneumonia, streptococcus sore throat, measles, mumps, and tonsillitis.

Heart disease in children is prevented by observing and acting on prolonged infections (sore throats or persistent fatigue) and by making sure the child engages in stimulating physical activity, eats nutritious foods, partakes of recreation, and obtains adequate sleep.

Deviations in Appearance and Behavior.

Fainting and dizzy spells

Rapid heart beat

Irregular pulse

Frequent complaints of pain in joints, arms, legs

Repeated nose bleeds

Clubbed fingers

Shortness of breath and sudden flushing of the face on exertion

Early fatigue

Failure to gain weight

Blueness of lips (cyanosis)

Social-Emotional Adjustment

Every young child needs from his teacher a degree of love, warmth, praise, and consistency. He needs gentle and firm guidance and someone interested in his welfare. With these factors he becomes secure, sticks to his tasks, sees himself in relation to his class, is tolerant and creative, possesses an outgoing attitude toward others, profits from his mistakes as well as successes, and, above all else, is a happy pupil equipped to live life with zest, enthusiasm, and hope.

The signs indicating deviations from normal social-emotional behavior are all about. To the observing teacher they are as evident as pimples on the face, and, like many physical ailments, they are best controlled or remedied through early detection and treatment.

Deviations in Appearance and Behavior.

Infantile speech

Foul language; very low, very high, or very loud voice

Unestablished toilet habits

Restlessness, nail-biting, stammering or lip-sucking not due to any discoverable physical cause

Frequent accidents or near-accidents

Over-timidity; seclusiveness, withdrawal, shyness, isolation from the group

Over-aggressiveness; constant quarreling with others

Suspicion and fearfulness; expectation of failure

Excessive day dreaming; inattentiveness not due to any discoverable physical cause

Extreme sensitiveness to criticism; feelings hurt easily; cries easily

Failure to advance in school work at a normal rate in spite of adequate physical health and satisfactory intellectual capacity. Or gradual deterioration or sudden drop in educational achievement; disorderly and careless work

Extreme docility or anxiety to please

Excessive boasting, showing off, attracting undue attention

Resistance to authority, constant complaints of being discriminated against or "picked on"

Poor sportsmanship, some unwillingness to engage in group activities which might result in losing face; playing unfairly or cheating in group games; suffers from being disliked by his classmates

Learning Disabilities

Although health services personnel and the learning disabilities specialist can advise and guide the teacher relative to known cases in this area, much of the early detection, remediation and feedback is accomplished by the teacher. Early classroom detection is significant—in the nursery school, kindergarten, and first grade, before formal learning tasks have been assigned. Perceptual-motor difficulties and motor development problems may occur anywhere in the school. If there is no specialist or clinic available the teacher will likely have to work with the school psychologist and a reading specialist.

Deviations in Appearance and Behavior.

Short attention span

Hyperactivity

Emotional outbursts

Erratic body control

Impulsivity

Distractibility

Poor eye-hand coordination

Hearing and speech disorders

Immaturity

One-sided physical development

Sequencing problems

Language difficulties

Drug Abuse

To the observing teacher of intermediate level and middle-school children there is much to observe in the way of schoolwide behavior that helps in the identification of the drug abuser. Any one of the deviations might be misleading, but when several of these appear in one pupil there is good reason to look more closely.

Deviations in Appearance and Behavior.

Abrupt changes in school attendance, quality of work, and work output

Withdrawal from responsibility

General changes in overall attitude

The Glue Sniffer (or User of Other Vapor-Producing Solvents)

Odor of substance on breath and clothes

Excess nasal secretions, watering of eyes

Poor muscular control

Drowsiness or unconsciousness

Increased preference for being with a group, rather than being alone

Plastic or paper bags or rags, containing dry plastic cement or other solvent, found at home or in locker at school

The Depressant Abuser (barbiturates, tranquilizers, "downs")

Symptoms of alcohol intoxication with one important exception: no odor of alcohol on breath

Staggering or stumbling

Falling asleep unexplainably

Drowsiness; may appear disoriented

A Guide to Childhood Diseases

Disease	Recognition	Prevention	Incubation	Control	General
Common cold	Sniffles, sneezing. Feels poor. Coughing common.	General good health helps.	1–2 days.	Isolate fresh cases for 3 days. Encourage parents to keep child home. Teach proper use of tissues.	Most frequent reason for absenteeism. Potentially dangerous because of ear, lung, throat complications.
Influenza	Cold symptoms, but child is sick, feverish and weak.	Vaccine, particularly effective, protection only 6–12 months.	1–3 days.	Isolate fresh cases for 5 days from onset.	More serious, "grippy" cold with high fever. Occurs sporadically each winter.
Chickenpox (varicella)	Small spots and blisters on body and at hairline. Often fever. Itching.	None.	12–21 days; usually 13–17 days.	Isolate and exclude for 6 days after rash	Common, minor illness, highly contagious among susceptibles.
Diphtheria	Sore throat with white patches; fever.	Effective with 3 doses of toxoid. Boosters every 3 to 5 years.	2–5 days.	Isolate in hospital. May not return until Health Department approves. Classmates and other close contacts receive immunization.	Very dangerous disease —now almost eradicated through mass immunization.
German measles (rubella)	Mildly ill, if at all. Pinkish spots on body, arms, *not* on face.	None, for disease.	14–21 days; usually 18 days.	Exclude case 3 days from appearance of rash.	A common, highly contagious but mild disease.
Measles (rubeola)	Cough, red eyes, fever, followed by blotchy rash on face and body.	Measles vaccine.	10 days to first symptoms. 14 days to rash.	Exclude for 7 days following appearance of rash.	A common, highly contagious acute illness. Most common complications: ear infection, pneumonia.
Mumps (infectious parotitis)	Swelling of cheeks or 1 or more salivary glands; fever.	None effective.	12–26 days; usually 18 days.	Exclude until swelling disappears, or 1 week from onset.	A relatively common and usually mild disease in children, not very contagious.

Table continued.

A Guide to Childhood Diseases (continued)

Disease	Recognition	Prevention	Incubation	Control	General
Streptococcal infections including scarlet fever	Sore throat with fever. Hurts to swallow. Diffuse red rash with tiny spots in scarlet fever.	Antibiotics given promptly.	2–5 days.	Exclude according to pre-arranged school plan. Observe classmates for one week.	A common disease which can be complicated by rheumatic fever, heart disease, or nephritis. "Scarlatina" is the same disease.
Whooping cough	Characteristic cough, with choking, redness of face, and "whoop" on drawing breath.	Vaccine usually given with diphtheria and tetanus to infants. Not desirable for older children.	7–10 days.	Exclude for three weeks after onset of typical cough.	An increasingly rare disease especially among pre-school children.
Athlete's foot	Peeling, cracking redness and occasionally oozing between toes or soles of foot.	Scrupulous foot hygiene. Rigid cleaning of locker and shower rooms.	10–14 days.	Exclude from physical education, locker and shower rooms. Check custodial job.	Mild, very common fungus infection of feet, especially feet which perspire easily, occurring wherever people go barefoot frequently.
Impetigo	Moist patches on skin around mouth, on hands with brown yellow crusts.	Good hygiene.	2–5 days.	Exclude until treatment is started and lesions dry.	Common bacterial infection of skin, mostly in younger children with poor health practices.
Lice	"Nits" seen; itching scalp, "mobile dandruff."	Good hygiene.	1–2 days.	Exclude until treated. Check classmates' heads at discovery and 2 weeks later.	Parasitic infestations of hair, boys and girls, directly related to inadequate brushing and washing.
Ringworm of scalp	Patchy baldness with stubble left.	Good hygiene.	10–14 days.	Exclude until treatment started. Must wear cap, but not take physical education.	Hard to clear up fungus infection of scalp. Rare after puberty.
Pinworms	Itching behind, crankiness, vague stomach pains.	Good hygiene.	4–8 days.	No exclusion necessary, little chance of spread in school. Enforce handwashing.	A common, mild, worm infection, with more unrecognized cases than known.

Table continued.

A Guide to Childhood Diseases (continued)

Disease	Recognition	Prevention	Incubation	Control	General
"Pinkeye" (conjunctivitis)	Reddened, irritated, weepy eyes. Often whitish discharge with sticky eyelids.	None.	1–3 days.	Exclude only in grades K-3. Observe classmates one week.	May accompany cold; more often a mild virus infection.
Poliomyelitis (infantile paralysis)	Headache, stiff neck, fever.	Oral vaccine. Consult physician.	7–21 days; usually 12 days.	Exclude 2 weeks. Observe classmates and give booster vaccinations.	A potentially crippling disease coming in about 7 year waves.
Tuberculosis	By tuberculin test and x-ray	Early detection.	6–8 weeks; occasionally 1 month.	Routine mass testing. Test and x-ray of classmates.	Usually very mild and often unrecognized in school age children. Source is an adult.
Meningitis	Fever, violent headache, stiff neck.	None available. Contacts can be protected by drugs.	Variable, but seldom over 10 days.	Isolate in hospital. If meningococcal exclude from family until treatment starts.	A group of diseases, caused by many agents—some serious, others not.
Tetanus (lockjaw)	Stiffness of face muscles, neck and back.	Mass immunization. Booster doses whenever child is cut or wounded.	4–21 days.	Booster dose for child with dirty cuts or wounds.	Poison from germ in dirty wounds affects nervous system; highly fatal. Not contagious.
Infectious mononucleosis	Persistent fatigue, low grade fever, sore throat.	None known.	4–14 days.	Exclude from school until fever is gone.	A not very contagious virus disease that may take months to get over.
Infectious hepatitis	Jaundice, fever, vomiting.	Clean water and food. Can be prevented in contacts by gammaglobulin.	10–60 days; usually 25 days.	Exclude 2 weeks; or until well.	A virus disease affecting the liver—long recovery period needed.
Cat-scratch fever	Sore at site of scratch, with swollen glands, accompanied by fever.	Avoid cat scratches.	2–8 days.	Exclude until child feels well.	Virus disease from cats. Mild. Not contagious.

Lack of interest in school and family activities

The Stimulant Abuser (amphetamines, cocaine, "speed," "bennies," "ups")

Pupils may be dilated (when large amounts have been taken)

Mouth and nose dry; bad breath; user licks his lips frequently

Goes long periods without eating or sleeping

Excess activity; user is irritable, argumentative, nervous; has difficulty sitting still

The Marijuana Abuser

In the early stages of intoxication, may appear animated with rapid, loud talking and bursts of laughter

In the later stages, may be sleepy or stuporous

Pupils usually are dilated

Odor (similar to burnt rope) on clothing or breath

Remnants of marijuana, either loose or in partially smoked "joints" in clothing or possessions

Usually user in a group, at least in early habit of smoking

Note: Unless under the influence of the drug at the time of observation, marijuana users are difficult to recognize; infrequent users may not show any of the general symptoms of drug abusers.

A HEALTH MANUAL FOR THE CLASSROOM TEACHER

As she lacks medical training, the classroom teacher feels the need of professional guidance to help her face many of the everyday health problems that she meets in the classroom and on the school grounds. A manual gives the teacher in non-medical terms the knowledge she should have about accidents, emergencies, and responsibilities. It also sets forth in detail many of the health deviations in appearance and behavior as well as the symptoms of communicable diseases, which may be seen in and about the school.

A useful health manual for teachers is one which summarizes the symptoms and signs of diseases. The summary on pages 90–92 illustrates the nature of this kind of teacher's guide and should be of value to the reader of this chapter.

SUGGESTED ACTIVITIES

1. Read an article on the mental health of schoolchildren. From this, list the several characteristics of maladjustment that a teacher might observe in a school setting. Comment on the ease with which this observation may be made.

2. Visit a large elementary school and ask the school nurse how many cases there are of serious allergies, heart defects, epilepsy, diabetes, and orthopedic defects. Having determined this, find out how many of these children have restricted programs and to what extent. How do you feel about the adequacies of restricted programs?

3. Arrange for several individuals to solicit from several different school departments copies of health manuals or written instructions to teachers relative to health observations and practices in the school system.

QUESTIONS FOR DISCUSSION

1. From your reading suggest evidence to show that mentally healthy elementary schoolchildren show greater achievement in schoolwork. What are your comments?

2. From your reading and experience, where does the detection and referral program fall down?

3. Samuel Johnson wrote that one should practice ". . . observation with extensive view." He wanted the observer to see many things—even extremes. How might this apply to the teacher in the classroom?

4. Consider the signs of good social-emotional behavior. What are several ways these signs may be developed within the limits of classroom activity? Playground activity?

5. What do you think of the view that prac-

tically every human being is a deviate in some respect? Support your answer with remarks relative to elementary-age children.

6. What can be done to help children of indigent parents receive glasses or hearing aids if they need them?

SELECTED REFERENCES

Anderson, C. L. *School Health Practice*, 5th ed. St. Louis: C. V. Mosby Co., 1972.

Bogle, Marion W. "Relationship Between Deviant Behavior and Reading Disability." *Journal of School Health, 43*:312–315, May 1973.

Bryant, N. Dale. "Learning Disabilities." *Instructor, 81*:49–56, April 1972.

Deahl, Tony. "The Orthopedically Handicapped." *Instructor, 80*:34, February 1971.

Levin, Lowell, et al. "Health Problems of Elementary-School Children As Perceived by School Physicians, Nurses, and Principals." *The Elementary School Journal, 69*:44–49, October 1968.

Long, B. H., and Henderson, E. H. "Self-Social Concepts of Disadvantaged School Beginners." *Journal of Genetic Psychology, 113*:41, January 1968.

Sheldon, William H. *The Varieties of Human Physique*. New York: Harper & Brothers, 1940.

Stuart, Harold C., and Brugh, D. G. *The Healthy Child, His Physical, Psychological, and Social Development*. Cambridge, Mass.: Harvard University Press, 1960.

Turner, C. E., Sellery, C. M., and Smith, S. L. *School Health and Health Education*, 6th ed. St. Louis: C. V. Mosby Co., 1970.

Wheatley, George M., and Hallock, Grace T. *Health Observations of School Children*, 3rd ed., New York: McGraw-Hill Book Co., 1965.

Willgoose, Carl E. "Body Types and Physical Fitness." *Journal of Health, Physical Education and Recreation, 27*:26–28, September 1956.

6 THE HEALTH INSTRUCTION PROGRAM

*Any teacher who responds to love and is capable of giving love,
who is capable of genuine compassion, who finds human
relationships challenging and rewarding, who has limitless
energy and exquisite sensitivity to human needs — plus the
constitution of a professional wrestler — is probably a superman.
If so, then let us go about cultivating supermen. There is
something in the nature of teaching — especially in today's
world — that represents a genuine challenge.*

—Norman Cousins[1]

Most health instruction in the elementary school is carried on by the classroom teacher. It is not done haphazardly; rather, it is a planned program in which the teacher has mastered still another subject matter area. Perhaps he or she is indeed what Cousins would call a superman. Certainly, being familiar with the complexities of health problems and how to teach to this point calls for real ability. Some help is provided in a number of school systems by coordinating or supervisory personnel who have specialized in health education.

It takes skill and enthusiasm to put over the idea that in the long run individual health status has more to do with understanding the advances of medical science than with creating remedies and corrective devices for human inadequacies. This seems logical enough, yet Oliver Wendell Holmes cautioned that "...we need education in the obvious" if we are to discover truth in the less obvious. How else can one close the wide gap between the advent of medical discoveries and the application of medical findings?

THE NATURE OF HEALTH INSTRUCTION

Instructional programs are geared to the principles of learning and carried on in the light of individual pupil differences. These programs are good chiefly because of good teachers. When classroom teachers understand the purposes of health instruction, the program becomes a significant part of the total school health effort.

The broad topic of health instruction in the elementary grades is related to a large number of factors which include program objectives, pupil needs, pupil interests, capacities, and other psychological considerations. Also included are teacher qualifications, educational methods, material sources and aids, and evaluation. Needless to say, instruction becomes a complicated topic, one that must be approached with patience and understanding.

---

[1]From "Norman Cousins Discusses the Human Concept," *Instructor, 80*:58, October 1970.

The general objectives of the health instruction program are about the same for all the elementary grades.[2] But the specific objectives for the primary area will differ from those for the intermediate area. Essentially, this difference is due to the varying capacities and needs associated with chronological age and growth.

Health education may be defined as the organization of learning experiences directed toward the development of favorable health knowledges, attitudes, and practices. It is an applied science and an academic field. Facts, principles, and concepts constitute its body of knowledge. It is derived from physiology, sociology, psychology and the behavioral sciences.[3]

Although the fundamental purpose of instruction is to impart knowledge, there should always be a greater emphasis on the formation of desirable practices and attitudes resulting from instruction. Knowledge of mere facts and mechanical skills is of doubtful value; no knowledge is complete until it is understood enough to be applied.

The desired outcome of health instruction is a change in the behavior of the pupils. This is revealed through daily habits of school and community living, the expression of positive health attitudes, and the grasp of a body of scientific knowledge which provides a basis for intelligent self-direction. To accomplish these outcomes is quite a difficult task. It is relatively easy to impart knowledge in the classroom. Children, for example, will readily learn the names of the vitamins or the rules of bicycle

---

[2]Oberteuffer points out that school health instruction is offered to secure behavior favorable to a high quality of living; to assist in the development of a well-integrated personality; to clarify thinking about personal and public health matters, to remove superstitions, false beliefs, and ignorance; to facilitate the development of security through the acquisition of scientific knowledge; to enrich the life of the community; and to establish the ability in students to see cause and effect.

[3]See the excellent booklet *What Is Health Education?*, distributed by the American Medical Association, 535 North Dearborn St., Chicago, Illinois, 60610.

safety without having it affect their pattern of living in any way. Moreover, it is even conceivable that the same children may have no particular feeling or attitude toward the previously discussed vitamins or bicycle riding. In such a case the knowledge has been "book knowledge" or "test knowledge." It has not been understood and acted upon. The school health instruction program, therefore, must be concerned with certain elements that will *effectively* educate for health.

CRISIS-ORIENTED HEALTH EDUCATION

When pressure builds in a community, as it so often does, to have the schools "do something" about sex, smoking, drugs, and alcohol, the hastily thrown together one-week unit or one-lecture type of activity appears. Frequently it covers a problem—a problem "shot down" this year and forgotten the next. This overemphasis on a health problem resulting in the neglect or omission of a number of other pertinent health problems is inexcusable. To be effective, health instruction cannot be established on the basis of crash programs. This was the position taken by the School Health Division of the American Association for Health, Physical Education and Recreation, in 1970, and given further support later on by the National Congress of Parents and Teachers who called for a comprehensive school health program which avoids "band wagon" approaches and piece-meal efforts relative to health topics.

A unified approach to health teaching, where there is a planned program throughout the school years, is necessary for the formation of positive attitudes and the creation of a healthy life style—the mark of an educated man. Moreover, there is reason to believe that crisis-oriented health programs do not produce immediate results causing a reduction in smoking, drug abuse, or anything else. Behavioral changes in complex socio-psychological areas are seldom accomplished right away; they evolve over a period of time and are influenced by an improved value system.

SCHOOL-COMMUNITY INTERACTION

If you believe as I do, that schools reflect society and that schools can be no better and no worse than the society they reflect, then you may be skeptical as I am, of any educational program that offers to change the schools without first changing society ... Schools are part of society, and society's ulcerations — massive urban hemorrhaging in crime, poverty, population, overarching permissiveness, and the disnesting of the family — overflow by their nature into the educational system. To separate the problems of the schools from the problems of the city is to engage in sloppy romanticism.[4]

There is more truth in the above lines than in a good deal of the educational procrastination that is so often set forth today. There is simply no way to *really* make schools accountable — for the health of the children or anything else — without some soul-searching on the part of the local citizenry designed to find ways of helping the educators. In short, an effective school health education is a two-way street between the school personnel and the townfolk. In numerous towns and cities such cooperation exists and there results a warm feeling about what the schools are trying to accomplish. Local groups and individual citizens volunteer their special skills and knowledges in a semi-organized way so that teachers seeking resource personnel to make their classes more alive know where to go for assistance.

In Rockland, Massachusetts, for example, the question was asked whether parents, clergy, law enforcement officials, educators and health specialists would take the bold steps necessary to meet the varied health needs of children. Would they support community planning as the best alternative available to the problems of illness and wellness? The response was enthusiastically positive. A community health council was formed and proceeded to help the schools through the conduct of open discussion groups; preparation of lists of community sources of health information; establishment of health education materials sections in the town libraries; arrangement of workshops for teachers and others of the "father-son" and "mother-daughter" type; investigation of youth problems in the community; recommendations for possible additions to the school curricula; arrangements for qualified speakers on pertinent health topics, and many more similar activites.

THE ESSENCE OF UNDERSTANDING

The term "understanding" is both a psychological process and an educational outcome. To possess it is to have more than a knowledge of particulars. A pupil does not begin to understand until he is able to react to factual information by moving, feeling, or thinking intelligently with respect to a given situation. Activity is the key word — the kind of activity discussed at length by educational philosophers of the John Dewey era, i.e., "pupils learn by doing." The more activity engaged in, the more senses ... stimulated, the greater the retention and recall of information to be learned.

In recent years it has been emphasized that the way to successful instruction and eventual understanding is to take heed of the following:

1. Factual information must have meaning for the individual if it is to be translated into proper health practices. How a child perceives an item is significant. This is substantiated by the Committee of the Association for Supervision and Curriculum Development in their publication *Perceiving, Behaving, Becoming,* in which it is pointed out that learning is the exploration and discovery of personal meaning in a process that must be a highly personal one.[5] To struc-

---

[4]Dan Pinck in "Education Backdate..." *Saturday Review,* October 14, 1972.

[5]Association for Supervision and Curriculum Development. *Perceiving, Behaving, Becoming—A New Focus on Education.* Washington, D.C.: National Education Association, 1962.

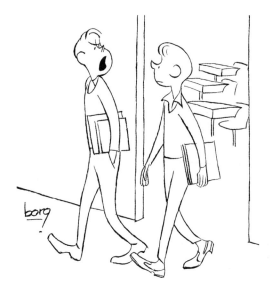

"What gets me is when someone comes up with the answer before I understand the question."

ture personal experiences in a curriculum is difficult, for the schools are part of the society that has made a fetish of the elements of objectivity—facts, figures, and phenomena.

2. Life in school must be stimulating and rewarding. In the early school years it is more important that pupils develop a liking for learning and for the school environment than that specific subject matter be remembered.

3. Relationships and principles are more important than scattered and rote information. In perceiving what they are learning, children may respond more to specific questions involving personal discovery than to the traditional questions so frequently used to initiate a unit of work. In short, it is not uncommon to ask children the wrong questions.

4. Although verbalization has weaknesses, most understandings should be verbalized.

Symbols such as words, numbers, or formulas are examples of verbalized understandings. In all areas of instruction they have to be used sooner or later. "Vitamin A" is symbolic of a body of information, but it is meaningless unless it is associated with the realities for which

it stands. In health education there may be many empty verbalizations that are recited parrotlike by children in dozens of classrooms around the country. Children are taught too often by rote learning. They sing "My country *tears* of thee," and recite that "the circulatory system is composed of arteries, veins, and *artilleries.*" Why does this happen? It seems that there is too much emphasis on isolated items rather than upon wholes and relationships; too much memorization of what has been brought to one's attention, and undue attention given to individual recitations as contrasted with cooperative group activity. Also, there is at times in all classrooms the tendency to make instruction an artificial item by divorcing it from the ordinary activities of life.

5. The student's understanding is inferred from observing what he says and does with respect to his needs.

What the pupil says and does, or fails to say and do, about health situations confronting him, determines the amount and kind of understanding he has developed as a result of a particular program of health instruction. The child who fails to register any particular attitude is sometimes as bad as the child who takes on a negative one. In fact, the child who fails to react to all may be much worse off. Teachers of health, therefore, should continuously appraise their instructional programs. This is especially necessary in the elementary grades where children are not yet mature enough to put distractions aside and fare well under the lecture method.

In addition to what has been said about understanding, there are other guiding concepts which should be considered when health instruction is being examined. Some of these concepts are so sound that they border on being principles. They apply not only to the health area but to all subject matter areas. For example, the laws of learning apply to health instruction, and readiness to learn is a highly prized characteristic when a new topic is brought to the attention of the pupils; motivation influences behavior and sets the stage for optimum learning; interests and needs influence learning, and they may be cultivated; children are taught positively what to do, not what not to do; provisions for individual and group differences improve instruction; rewards are superior to punishment in promotion of learning; interest in the activity provides the drive to engage in it; attitudes manifested in several situations become real—"wide use favors habit"; socializing the activity promotes retention and recall; and success in a subject matter item breeds security in a subject matter area. Needless to say, this is only a partial list of generally recognized concepts relative to learning and understanding. Health instruction can never quite succeed where psychological factors such as these are ignored or treated haphazardly.

FACTORS THAT DETERMINE WHAT TO TEACH

Everything cannot be brought to the attention of schoolchildren. There simply is not enough time. How then does one determine what to teach? Where does a teacher begin?

Determining Pupil Needs in General

What children need to receive from the elementary school is pretty much what society wants children to have. Since the child grows up in an American culture, the culture molds him and influences the nature of his needs.

A Child Needs:	Society Wants Every Child:
1. Interpersonal and intergroup relations.	1. To understand and practice desirable social relationships toward individuals and groups, and within the many varied groups of which he is a member. To be a good neighbor and good citizen of the world.
2. Understanding of the world and people and things.	2. To appreciate and participate in worthwhile activities with others at home and abroad.
3. Self-development.	3. To discover and develop desirable individual aptitudes, interests, and abilities. To develop powers of creative expression. To have sound physical and mental health.
4. Control of the communicative arts and skills.	4. To cultivate the habit of constructive, careful thinking. To gain command of common integrating knowledge and skills.
5. Moral and spiritual values.	5. To develop sound emotional attitudes and habits. To appreciate and accept for himself moral and spiritual values.

The foregoing basic needs of elementary schoolchildren were set forth by the Bureau of Elementary Curriculum Development in New York State.[6]

To determine what to teach, Ragan and Shepherd studied the needs of children and set up seven categories of needs:

1. Biological needs
2. Achieving status in changing social groups
3. Growing gradually from dependence to independence
4. Security and satisfaction
5. Getting and giving affection
6. Developing appropriate communication skills
7. Learning to face reality.[7]

Whatever phase of health is taught must be done in the light of these needs for these are bona fide requirements that children have—even if they are not aware of them. The interrelationship of these needs is impressive.

Determining Pupil Health Needs

Prior to setting up the health curriculum it is necessary to ascertain the child's characteristics for a certain age, his health needs, and his health interests. Children vary in constitution, growth and development, health status, and background of experience. Some have health problems that others know relatively little about. If, however, there are enough children with a particular health problem, then there is a need in the curriculum for instruction in this area. Sometimes a problem is school-wide. Hookworm and intestinal parasites, for instance, are always of concern in certain southern states and have to be discussed regularly.

It is safe to say that there has been considerable difference of opinion as to the amount of emphasis that one should place on different types of needs. All are important to some degree, but in the interest of economy, some needs must be considered more vital than others. Furthermore, there is a strong point of view that it is not the school's responsibility to meet all of the needs. There are numerous agencies, institutions, and individuals which share this responsibility. The home, the church, scout organizations, 4-H clubs, libraries, recreation centers, radio, television, and summer camps all play a part in meeting the needs of children. The school must do its share, but not attempt to carry the whole burden by itself. Dispensing health information is an example of a shared responsibility, for other community organizations do it too. Many schools cooperate in 4-H and scout work and set aside time for religious instruction.

It is quite easy to say that most growing children have about the same health needs. They all need good nutrition and proper eating habits, protection against illness and disease, avoidance of accidents, sleep and rest, regular elimination of body wastes, continuous care of eyes, ears and teeth, good body mechanics and posture, good emotional adjustment, the right attitude toward the opposite sex, and an understanding of themselves. It is not uncommon to find states and larger cities that have excellent courses of study in health which have been carefully prepared over a long period of time to meet the health needs, interests, and capacities of children. Such courses of study are made available to classroom teachers as a basis on which the program can be planned. No one will quarrel with this. But, as good as these courses of study are, they should be used only as guides, for much of the material contained therein will require amplification or adjustment in some way to fit the needs of the local community and the particular pupils.

When one considers the whole child in a society that is continually changing, it is readily seen that needs are something

---

[6]The Bureau of Elementary Curriculum Development. *The Elementary School Curriculum*. Albany: New York State Education Department, 1954. p. 13.

[7]Ragan, William B. and Shepherd, Gene D. *Modern Elementary Curriculum*, 4th ed. New York: Holt, Rinehart, Winston, Inc., 1971, pp. 89–93.

more than psychological, social, intellectual, and emotional; they are also individual, moral, and spiritual. Thus the conscientious teacher has quite a task ahead of her as each school year begins. It will be necessary to seek the answers to some of these questions on needs before arranging the course of instruction in final form:

Question 1. What are the characteristics of my children at specific age levels? In short, what are the signs of growth and development in terms of physical, intellectual, social, and emotional behavior? What are the health needs?

Growth is a continuous process—an unfolding as children move toward adulthood. It is difficult to subdivide the growth period into specific age levels, for the child never abruptly completes a particular stage of development and begins the next. Moreover, there is never a time when all children in a class are at the same growth stage. Chronological age and physiological age (maturation level) may be quite a distance apart.

The following chart, depicting some of the growth and development characteristics of elementary schoolchildren, is a simple device to help answer the question of characteristics of children at specific age levels. The subdivisions used serve only as convenient labels for periods of growth.

Question 2. What am I able to observe in the way of the health practices of my children in specific situations? How do the children behave in respect to food handling, play and rest, handwashing and toilet activities? What do they eat? What kind of lunch do they bring to school? Is the home health teaching in keeping

Characteristics and Needs of the Elementary School Child

General Characteristics	Health Needs
1. Physical Characteristics	
Large muscles are better developed than small ones. Can run, jump, skip, climb; enjoy simple tag games, group singing and singing games. May frequently be clumsy and awkward, and continuous activity brings on early fatigue.	To experience basic body movements involving the arms, legs and trunk, with and without music and rhythms.
	To participate in games with simple rules and boundaries.
Eye and hand coordination not well established.	To have quiet periods of activity; to have rest periods.
Farsightedness prevails.	To have large pictures and large print to read.
2. Health Characteristics	
Usually healthy except for occasional colds, digestive upsets, and "children's diseases."	To be aware of colds and sore throats and how to act with them.
Accidents are the leading cause of death.	To understand how to safely use school equipment indoors and outdoors; to know fire drill procedures; to know about the existence of poisons and neighborhood hazards.
Burns off considerable energy in short periods of time.	To eat mid-morning food, milk or juice.
3. Mental-Emotional Development	
Shows curiosity over a short period of time.	To have experiences beyond the home.
Proud of possessions, proud of clothes.	To gain confidence in himself as a person.
Often brags to others, likes to hear stories.	To have freedom to scrawl and scribble and finger paint.
Capable of self criticism (Gesell).	To engage in rich, stimulating activities.
Active imagination with shifting of ideas as he paints.	To learn what is right and wrong, permitted and forbidden.
High interest in dramatizations. Speaks and acts spontaneously.	To love a warm, friendly, reassuring teacher who understands them.
Amazingly ignorant of many facts of life.	
Very vulnerable and sensitive, quick to feel hurt or humiliated.	
Naturally "mother-centered" and self-centered.	

Table continued.

Primary School Age (Early childhood, Ages 6 to 8 years)

General Characteristics	*Health Needs*

1. *Physical Characteristics*

Growth is relatively slow during this period as compared to the early period. Large muscles of the trunk, legs and arms are more developed than the smaller muscles.

Hand-eye coordinations are incomplete, but developing. Eyes slow to focus and usually far-sighted at start of this period.

Bones are hardening. Heart and lungs are small in proportion to body weight and height.

The loss of temporary teeth begins at five to six years and continues up to eleven or twelve years of age.

To experience many kinds of vigorous activities involving many parts of the body. This will increase heart action and respiration and help build endurance. It will also improve skills of body control.

To have instruction in habits of personal hygiene, such as using the handkerchief, covering coughs and sneezes, the selection of clothing appropriate to weather, etc.

Relaxation periods to follow periods of physical activity. Continued emphasis on posture in all activities.

2. *Health Characteristics*

Quite susceptible to infectious diseases at beginning of this age period. Respiratory difficulties common in winter. Toxins and bacteria may damage heart, especially if protection is not afforded during convalescent stages of contagious diseases of childhood.

Alimentary tract difficulties common in summer and fall.

Endurance may be poor. Fatigue is "enemy of childhood," but recuperation from fatigue is usually good.

Accidents are leading causes of death, especially for boys.

The healthy 5 to 8 year old has bright eyes, color in his face, great vitality, is happy and radiates enthusiasm and an exuberance for most activities.

To be checked regularly for signs of disease and defects.

To have twelve hours' sleep a night.

To have constant teacher supervision to reduce risks of accidents and to have proper instruction in the hazards of home and school.

To have the chance to express himself through many activities that stimulate physical, social, and mental-emotional growth.

3. *Mental-Emotional Development*

Short span of attention.

Individualistic and possessive, egocentric after age six.

Dramatic, imaginative, and highly imitative. Curious about things in general.

Wide variety of emotional reactions.
Enjoys rhythm and rhythmic sounds.

Reasoning ability present, but with little experience upon which to base judgment. Concern for sex differences made known by pertinent questions.

Increase in vocabulary. Language grows with experience.

When approaching age eight he wants his chances to act on his own and is sometimes annoyed at conformity. More sensitive to judgment of peers together with a decrease in concern for adult opinion.

To engage in a number of health activities all of short duration.

To learn to share with others, to play alone and with small groups, and to play as an individual in larger groups. Needs recognition for his personal abilities and to shift gradually to more group activities.

To create and explore, and identify himself with persons and things. Primary grade health stories appeal to the imagination.

To receive guidance in social development.

To respond to rhythmic sounds such as drums, rattles, voice, etc.

To have a chance to discuss and relate personal experiences in classroom health topics.

To receive just enough information on sex as is necessary to answer questions of the moment. Best handled at home.

To visit new places, discuss health implications and stimulate growth in vocabulary of words with a health meaning.

To make own choice in selection of health projects, films, plays, and to help evaluate results of activities.

Table continued.

General Characteristics	Health Needs
A group most eager to learn and most eager to please the teacher.	To see own work displayed.
Interests are now, not later; will accept things on "faith," less interested in explanations and reasons.	To cooperate at home and at school in play and other group activities.
Somewhat self-dependent toward end of this period. Brushes own teeth and hair, dresses self and ties shoes; cleans table, dries dishes, empties wastebaskets, sweeps floors, watches younger children for parents.	To taste some success, carefully sprinkled with enough defeats to provide a stimulus for greater effort and sound adjustments.

with accepted health practices? The observing teacher can tell a great deal about what her children need, and these needs are different. Children, for example, in rural communities sometimes lack health information that may be quite familiar to city children. The teacher, in such a case, who moves from the city to the rural area will often be surprised at the needs that are evident on the local scene. In one first grade class a teacher found one of the boys drinking from the urinal. The boy came from a part of the town where outside privy toilets were used and water was hauled by bucket from a nearby property. School needs, therefore, relate to home needs.

The direct statements of classroom teachers who have observed children over the years are very useful in gaining an understanding of health needs together with implication for what to teach. Some of the pertinent statements, recorded just as they were made, are as follows:

"Many children come to school improperly fed. Results in early fatigue and loss of energy."

"Some of my children have been drinking coffee since they were old enough to hold a cup."

"Inadequate lunch. Child brings money for full lunch and buys only soup, saving rest for candy. Hastily made, poorly balanced lunches. Gulping food to get out to play earlier."

"Many of our children lack emotional security because working mothers have no time for them."

"In our school, we have problems of emotional malnutrition such as a child's hunger for affection, status with his peers, and hunger for success."

"Parents send children to school when they are ill . . . parents are working or too busy to have them 'underfoot'."

"Dripping noses: How to care for the common cold? . . . Certain children will not blow their noses often enough or will not wipe them when necessary. I keep Kleenex available to all, but still some have to be told, 'Blow your nose before we can go on with our work.' "

"Head lice — We have had difficulty in controlling the spread of pediculosis."

"Sleep — television — child acquires spectator attitude — child overstimulated comes to school sleepy."

"Lack of proper sleep and rest at home...waiting for mother to come home from working on second shift at the mill, or sleep being interrupted by a parent going to work on the second shift."

"Some of our children live in run-down, rat-infested, cold water flats. Nothing about this environment in which they live is conducive to good health. This overcrowding often makes it necessary for children to sleep near a kerosene stove, the only source of heat. Such children come to school with a strong odor of oil. . . ."

"Body odor . . . This odor is more evident during the winter months when heavier clothing is not changed when necessary."

". . . older children have to sleep with others who wet the bed. . . . The odor is carried on the clothing of the older children."

Intermediate School Age (Middle childhood, Ages 9 to 11 years)

General Characteristics	Health Needs

1. *Physical Characteristics*

A noticeable growth spurt at end of period which continues into adolescence. This differs with individual levels of maturation.

Sex differences appear, with girls more mature and taller. Sex antagonism gradually appears. Sexual modesty is seen.

Rough and tumble activities highly enjoyed, often by the girls.

A few girls begin menstruation by ages eleven and twelve.

Muscular strength is behind physical growth, postural habits vary.

Some girls may be more developed in motor skills than some boys.

Coordinations are good. Many physical skills are now automatic. Reaction time is improved.

To engage in strenuous activity that taxes the muscles, heart, lungs and other organs to the limits of healthy fatigue.

To engage in wholesome corecreation and coeducational relationships both in the classroom and on the playing fields.

To participate in those physical skills which properly utilize elements of roughness to build motor skills and physical fitness.

To be recognized as different individuals.

To have instruction in body mechanics, fatigue, nutrition and factors influencing growth in height and weight.

To have chance to appraise self through self-testing activities. To relate success in motor skills to personal health habits.

2. *Health Characteristics*

Eyes function well but nearsightedness (myopia) may develop at ages eight or nine.

Resistance to contagious and infectious diseases is much better than in primary grades. Tuberculosis is a threat.

Endurance is improved. More rest is needed for the more mature child.

Permanent dentition continues with incisors and lower bicuspids appearing. Bad teeth begin to appear in large numbers.

Accidents are on the increase for this age group, with burns, automobiles and bicycles heading the list.

Increased interest in foods together with improved appetite. Fewer food refusals and a wider range of preferences.

Girls interested in appearance; boys in developing strong bodies.

To have periodic eye screening tests to determine need for eyeglasses. This should be coupled with health instruction in this area.

To learn about personal and community health practices which have direct bearing on their welfare.

To get as nearly as possible eleven hours' sleep a night and not to play beyond the point of great fatigue. Girls tire more readily than boys, and because they are usually more mature, they require more rest and food.

To have attention directed to dental care. This is a period when many children's teeth are neglected.

To understand the nature of personal accidents at school, en route to school, and in the community.

To discuss nutrition and the role of the four basic foods in maintaining optimum health.

To talk about personal grooming and nature of physical fitness.

3. *Mental-Emotional Development*

They like a wide variety of activities, have a longer span of attention and greater interests.

Strong sense of rivalry and noticeable craving for recognition.

An increasing attitude of independence coupled with a desire to help.

Strong sense of loyalty to groups, teams, or "gangs." Some children are now in a period to be influenced unfavorably. Greater concern over group approval than teacher approval.

Enjoys competition, whether physical or essentially mental, but may become angry when tired, or easily discouraged.

Interest in opposite sex indicated by teasing, hitting, chasing, etc. Girls are more interested in older boys.

To participate in a wide range of health activities involving several methods of teaching and material aids.

To succeed often in a variety of health areas, and to do so through some degree of cooperative effort which affords individual satisfaction.

To have a chance to formally plan, lead, and execute certain projects and to check the progress made. To assist the teacher in the preparation of health exhibits, specimens, posters, etc.

To participate in those activities in which achievement is recognized in the eyes of their group. To gain respect and approval of others.

To compete fairly with others, obtaining an understanding of the place of personal cooperation in the process.

Table continued.

General Characteristics	*Health Needs*
Broadening intellectual horizons. Interest shifting from the immediate environment to the wider world.	To work coeducationally in those health activities which broaden social relationships and obtain answers to questions involving the opposite sex.
Strong interest in collecting things. Love of pets.	To study world health conditions and what they mean in terms of personal, everyday existence.
More critical, need to be shown why. Adventuresome; interested in all kinds of experimentation.	
Girls are clearly superior to boys in language development, especially toward end of this period.	To be given a chance to seek detail in a wide variety of health activities.
	To stimulate improvement of the health vocabulary, a number of meaningful field trips, projects, or dramatizations may be engaged in.

"Our greatest cause of absence is toothache.... Ninety per cent of the primary children have never been to a dentist."

"General fear of dentists that results in harmful neglect of teeth."

"About 20 per cent of the children in my school did not own toothbrushes at the beginning of the year."

"One teacher in the first grade informed a mother that her child was doing failing work because he was unable to hear, and that he should be given a hearing test. The mother said, 'John is not deaf; he is just naughty, and does not want to listen.' "

"A child in kindergarten was very hard of hearing. Not until an examination by the school nurse was it known that he had infected tonsils. The tonsils were removed and the child's hearing was much improved. The loss of hearing had affected the child's speech so that it was hardly understandable."

It is hard to believe in this day and age that home living conditions can be so different. Unless the teacher actually invades the inner city or tours the countryside, seeks the out-of-way places, gets into the apartment buildings and sizes up the community health situations, she is apt to have little real knowledge of pupil health needs. Where a child in one home has his own room and bed, another child in another home sleeps with three others in the same bed; and it may be in a one room dwelling. Numerous places exist where a family of eight, ten, or more live under one roof in one room. Here they eat, sleep, play, and exist in unclean surroundings and without respect for personal privacy. Even today public health workers find it necessary to visit homes on the outskirts of a number of communities from Maine to Georgia, attempting to get the people to provide themselves with better toilets.[8] Attitudes and practices formed in this kind of environment can hardly be modified overnight, and they are most difficult to change right away in the schoolroom.

Question 3. What are the health and safety hazards in the local community? What are the special health problems? Are there hazardous obstacles such as rivers, waterfalls, open sandpits, or automobile traffic, and are there hazardous activities being carried on near by?

These questions are partially related to the previous question dealing with the observed health and safety practices of the children in school. The questions go together because local conditions *do* affect classroom behavior and point to the necessity for certain kinds of health instruction to meet existing needs.

Local statistics relative to the prevalence of certain communicable diseases, the purity of drinking water, the cleanliness of local eating establishments, and

---

[8]Two thousand years ago in the days of the ancient Hebrews, personal health practices were a concern. The Bible says, "Thou shalt have a place within the camp...and it shall be, when thou will ease thyself abroad, thou shalt dig therewith, and shalt turn back and cover that which cometh from thee." (Deut. 23:12–13.)

the safety of milk are fundamental considerations that should be understood by the teacher. If, for example, a community is bothered by black flies or mosquitoes, this should become one of the health topics covered during the year. Moreover, such a topic is probably somewhat familiar to all pupils in the class, and very little preliminary motivation work will be required to provoke discussion and get some action. Several years ago in one Georgia community the sixth grade class became so interested in malaria mosquito breeding that they set out to personally initiate a mosquito control program. They drained small ponds and put oil on stagnant waters. In fact, they became so active with enthusiasm which blossomed as the job progressed that the townsfolk appropriated money and joined in to make the mosquito control project one fine example of community cooperation. Health instruction directed along lines such as these becomes a magnificent force not only for the personal health and welfare of the children and adults, but also for the promulgation of such worthy objectives as social efficiency and civic responsibility.

Question 4. What are the health problems and safety hazards in the state? Is the state in question any different from any other state? What do recent statistics, collected and made available by the county health department, reveal? Is it conceivable that Alabama might have problems different from Montana?

How does the state compare with the National Health Survey which indicates that pupil deaths from accidents lead the list, followed by cancers and leukemias, influenza and pneumonias, and congenital malformations? What about disabling difficulties? Usually respiratory disturbances rank first, followed by infections and parasitic disorders, and injuries.

States, as communities of people, differ in many respects. Some are more agricultural; others are more industrialized. Some are reasonably warm all year round, while others are faced with an annual adjustment to cold and inclement weather. There are watery noses, sore throats, and cloudy skies in Cleveland, Ohio and Oswego, New York, while the sunshine blazes overhead in South Carolina. Farm safety is taught in the cornbelt states and industrial safety in Detroit. Water safety is of paramount interest in Minnesota, Wisconsin, and along the shores of the Great Lakes and seacoast states.

In Florida, hookworm is a major health problem of schoolchildren. Many individuals have contact with it some time or other. Children who go barefooted appear to be everywhere—and so are hookworm and other internal parasites. Vast numbers of elementary age children are treated by their county health unit through the schools. They stay free from the worms for only a short while following the cure, then they become infected again. And the chief reason for this is that they and their families will not put into practice certain beneficial health habits that have been brought to their attention by public health and school personnel. *The need, therefore, continues to exist for more effective health instruction. In fact, most of these children have more than enough knowledge on the subject to pass a written test with a high grade. What they lack is an intelligent understanding deep enough to create positive attitudes and changes in health behavior.*

The educational needs of many of the children of Mexican-American descent are greater than in other American communities. The same thing relative to needs could be said for the Puerto Rican-American area of New York City or the Italian-Chinese-American sections of Boston. In fact, health problems are more frequent among people of low economic standing in almost any part of the country.

Socio-economic backgrounds, climate and weather, prejudices and superstitions—even the terrain of the countryside—affect what is taught. In New Hampshire—a rugged state of forests, mountains, lakes, and streams—hunting and fishing are as much a part of one's education as any single subject in the public school curriculum. Every spring, on the first day of the trout season there is a school holiday throughout the state. Practically every boy and girl who can walk or hobble along goes fishing. During the year, and especially in the fall, great numbers of children and youth carry rifles and go hunting. This is not without educational implications. Firearms safety, initiated at the State Education Department level, has spread as a special sixth grade health instruction topic to almost every city and rural school in the state. This is a concrete example of how a particular health and safety need can be met. It not only serves the immediate needs of the elementary age children, but also carries over to the older age groups.

Question 5. How does the local school environment furnish leads for health instruction? Are there poor physical facilities that may represent a school safety hazard? Do children wonder why they are required to take physical education? What kinds of food do primary grade pupils choose in the school cafeteria? Do food selections differ for intermediate graders?

Opportunities to teach health topics in keeping with health needs and interests abound in the school environment. There are hardly two schools alike in facilities and equipment. Every laboratory, lunchroom, gymnasium and classroom suggests health items of interest and value to pupils. The cleanliness of corridors, walks, and rooms, the lighting, ventilation, temperature, playground equipment, and space all furnish leads to the observing teacher. And one should not forget the number and types of school accidents. Where do they occur and what can be done about them?

Question 6. What are the findings of medical examinations and screening tests? Do health histories and cumulative health record cards indicate any special findings which the instructional program may be able to remedy or improve? Do some children show a slow rate of growth?

Children with slight cases of malnutrition, postural defects, and similar deviations from normal need two kinds of attention. Primarily, they need to have remedial work started quickly, and secondly, they need information about themselves and their difficulty. There is no need to keep children in the dark about personal deviations, especially when their attitudes can be improved so much by a little understanding. Also, other elementary schoolchildren are generally very interested in the health problems of their classmates and how these may affect them. Furthermore, the child with a problem may become a real member of the group and feel quite at home in the class by being singled out as, for example, the teacher's helper for a lesson on posture and body mechanics. In one northern New York State elementary school the teachers have agreed among themselves to have children, returning to school after an absence due to illness, speak to their classmates and tell them about their experiences while ill. Very often the pupil who has been absent a few days with something like strep sore throat will stimulate a real show of interest in the broad area of upper respiratory diseases. Moreover, intermediate grade children want to know what they can do about it.

Question 7. Are there major student interests that relate to health education? Young children are vigorous. Sometimes they are rough and adventuresome. Their play is serious, full of meaning— their way of life. Such children are too often unaware of the things they do that may influence their health and safety. Large muscle activities such as running, jumping, climbing, and wrestling are play activities that are at times hazardous. Climbing out on tree limbs, frolicking in the water in the summer, and testing the ice in the winter are potentially dangerous yet powerfully stimulating forms of recreation. Even interest in becoming Brownies or Cub Scouts presents leads for meaningful health instruction.

Student interests rise and fall according to school and local happenings. A major traffic tragedy, a local epidemic of Asian flu or scarlet fever, or a severe water shortage are current health events that may heighten pupil enthusiasm to the point where the alert teacher can take advantage of it and "make hay while the sun shines."

Current and immediate interests of children can be readily determined in a novel way by providing them with the opportunity of asking questions through a device such as the question box. This makes a bit of a game out of it. The teacher who is observant can determine children's health interests rather well by:

Taking note of what they do before and after school.

Talking with them.

Observing their actions in and about the classroom.

Listening as they talk together.

Watching their activities during leisure moments, unassigned periods, or at play.

Evaluating the stories and materials they bring from home.

Studying their paintings, drawings, crafts, stories, and letters.

Noticing their choices of books, clothing, and other materials.

Studying records of pupils of the same level, such as cumulative records, personal diaries, and class folders of the year's work.

Discussing them with parents and former teachers.

When young children are carefully observed one finds that they are interested in radio, television, movies, play activities, people of other lands, picture magazines, plants and animals, machines, the care of pets, their own body, and many other factual and creative items.

Health interests may also be checked through the use of a teacher-constructed questionnaire or pupil check list. Questions pertaining to medical and dental care, food habits, cleanliness, rest, and posture indicate a great deal in terms of pupil behavior and needs. A survey of individual health practices can be revealing not only in terms of curriculum needs, but also in terms of health guidance. In the primary grades, direct questions which may be asked by the leader will indicate and stimulate interest in health. For example:

1. Do you wash your hands after going to the toilet?

2. What foods do you eat between meals?

3. Do you stay home when you have a cold?

4. When were you to the dentist last?

5. At what time do you usually go to bed at night?

6. How do you sit in your chair? Do you lean over or slide down in the seat?

In her study of kindergarten through third grade children in Pennsylvania, Rashkis discovered an early sustained awareness of many restrictions upon health.[9] Even healthy children were well aware of the potential threat of illness. Eating was the area in which there was the most interest, and as one grew older there was increasing interest and trust in the physician.

Perhaps the most impressive study of children's health interests in recent years was the one entitled *Teach Us What We Want To Know,* completed by the Connecticut State Board of Education.[10] Techniques were used to *get at* the true concerns of students by asking them for advice and suggestions as to what should be taught about health in schools. Through such means as discussions, role-playing, observation, and tape recordings it was possible to gather authentic information. The 180-page paperback book has to be read to be fully appreciated, but a few sample pupil responses relative to interests and picked at random are as shown at the top of the opposite page.

Question 8. Have the pupils had experiences in other areas of learning which provide leads for needed health instruction? It takes many ideas from several study areas to educate for health. Experiences from one subject matter area carry over into another and enrich health instruction. The teacher plans for this in advance by correlating her materials

[9]Reported by Marjorie A. Young in *Health Education Monographs,* No. 28, New York: Society of Public Health Educators, 1968, p. 30.

[10]Byler, Ruth, Lewis, Gertrude and Totman, Ruth. *Teach Us What We Want To Know,* Hartford, Connecticut: Connecticut State Board of Education, 1969. Available from Mental Health Materials Center, 419 Park Avenue, New York, New York 10016.

Grades

K–2	3–4	5–6
How does my body get made?	What shape are my bones?	Why do we have hair?
How does my heart beat?	Why are people so different?	How does a baby grow?
How does God get your heart in there?	How does your mind think?	Why was I born male, not female?
What makes people cry?	What makes you sweat?	How do you get a cold, measles, chicken pox, etc.?
How can I tell if I have a fever?	If a nerve were cut in your arm, could you feel?	What else besides smoking causes cancer?
How can you tell which is a cow or bull?	What goes on inside my body?	Why do people take drugs?
What makes your finger move?	What are the right games to play?	Why don't people stop killing and start loving?
	Where does a baby come from?	What makes it a boy or a girl?

with the content of other areas and the activities of other teachers.

Physical education games, dances, and stunts can be directly related to health instruction topics such as strength, vigor, nutrition, rest, and social health. In fact, for children to have physical education activities and fail to learn why they are important to their health and welfare is indeed a shortsighted kind of education. Yet many opportunities are overlooked to explain why exercise, physical skills, and social contacts are necessary. The same may be said for the special areas of music and art. Do children know that healthy people, free from worry and organic drains, sing and paint better because they are happy?

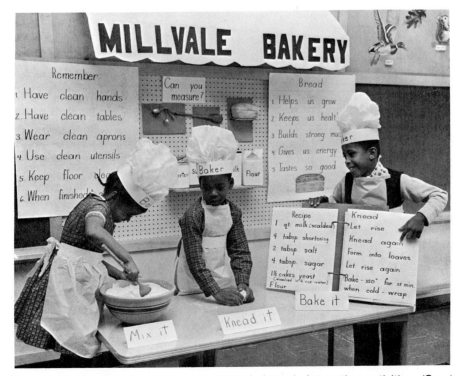

Figure 6–1 Permanent attitudes are formed through interesting activities. (Courtesy Cincinnati Public Schools.)

TEACHING FOR ATTITUDES AND PRACTICES

From an instructional viewpoint, what can be done with the rank and file of elementary school students to develop a proper attitude toward managing oneself and one's environment? And even more important is the question of how this attitude can be extended to decision-making and the action domain. This, of course, is the very meat of this whole book. It has never been an easy topic to resolve, despite much research and an extensive literature. Gordon Allport spent a lifetime struggling in this area. He made it clear, however, that personal feelings are so ingrained, so carefully protected, and even hidden from the holder that a valid appraisal of attitudes following a certain period of instruction is most difficult. To further complicate the matter is the fact that attitudes are frequently more than a feeling—they represent a predisposition to act or a potential behavior—which makes it even more difficult to consider them accurately.

Teach a lesson and ask a pupil how he *feels* about something; it may produce a reliable answer if the setting is right. There may be a response from the heart—especially if there is a feeling of comfort with instructor and class members alike. In a warm, friendly question-discussion situation, for example, accurate inner feelings and beliefs may emerge. However, appraising attitudes on a mass basis, and in overcrowded and occasionally impersonal classroom settings is an impossibility.

What has been said about teaching attitudes applies as well to behavior change. For decades teachers have taught useful health information, yet the world is full of people who failed to apply what they apparently learned. Often the pupil who receives an "A" in the topic of dental health grows to adulthood harboring a mouth full of decaying teeth greatly in need of care. The sixth grader who creates the finest project depicting the relationship of diet to overweight sometimes grows up to be a heavyweight with an attitude of complete indifference to-

ward weight-gaining foods. And every social misfit in our country has been exposed to the influence of a number of reasonably good teachers. Add to this the millions of cases of people involved in vocational failure, chronic unemployment, marital unhappiness, emotional instability, and other expressions of failure, and it becomes quite evident that teaching to create attitudes and behavior change is a most difficult task requiring the best in curriculum, methodology, and teaching.

One way to assess behavior change is to seek the cooperation of the students. An anonymous questionnaire can be employed to find out what action students have taken following the teaching of a number of health topics. For example, one might respond to these three considerations in terms of decision making:

1. Having studied this topic, my *attitude* toward the improvement of health practices is (—better, —worse,—unchanged).
2. Having studied this topic, my *actions and/or activities* in this area are (—better,—worse,—unchanged).
3. Having studied this topic, I (have—, have not—) helped someone else improve a personal health practice.

When this kind of analysis of decision making is made it is possible to discover a number of individuals with improved attitudes and practices. Also, there are many students who will admit having tried to help someone else improve a practice. This happens more often with the older and more mature students who, for example, speak up in favor of automobile seat belts and encourage others not to start to smoke.

Health Teaching

Instructional programs become effective in promoting pupil achievement when they have good teachers behind them. The finest fashioned course of study, carefully modified at the local level to consider immediate needs, is but words on a sheet of paper to the incompetent and unsympathetic teacher. Fortunately, however, most elementary schoolteachers like children and make an effort to understand and work with them.

Teaching has been defined in many ways, but in general it may be considered a procedure involving leadership. If education may be defined as a process of changing behavior toward certain preconceived goals, then teaching is the act of exercising leadership in this process. Good teaching can be so effective that children are taught numerous things without even being aware of it. "We are," wrote Lord Chesterfield, "more than half what we are by imitation. The great point is, to choose good models and to study them with care." This has a profound meaning for educators. Someone has said that "teaching is a process of making little images of the teacher in the minds of pupils." If such is so, and it appears to be, then teachers of impressionable youth and eager-to-learn children might well tremble at the thought of how much power they wield for good or evil. The thought of their responsibilities should shake them to the core and cause them to dedicate themselves more sincerely to the tasks ahead.

The Competent Teacher

A writer once asked Dr. Albert Schweitzer if he did not think that personally setting a good example was one of the best ways of influencing people. Dr. Schweitzer replied, "No! It's the *only way*." The implication is clear that in order to really influence others in developing good health, teachers must be fit themselves.

"Each honest calling, each walk of life," says Conant, "has its own elite, its own aristocracy based on excellence of performance."[11]

There is little question that the teacher must be much more than an ordinary person. Needed are the characteristics, vision, and understanding of the clergy,

the zeal and devotion of the medical worker, and the earthly human qualities of the missionary. The teacher must be an idealist and aim high with enthusiasm for teaching that might well ring out the immortal words of Robert Browning: "Ah, but a man's reach should exceed his grasp, or what's a heaven for?" In short the *real* teacher has everything. This is demonstrated time and time again by the testimony of successful men and women who pay tribute to their teachers of earlier years.

Competency as a teacher is not something which automatically accompanies being hired to teach school. Almost anyone can get a job teaching. The question is, what constitutes a competent teacher?

It has been said that the competent teacher is neither a poem nor a paragon. Assets overcompensate for his liabilities, and his liabilities do not occur in crucial areas.

There are many excellent characteristics that might well describe the competent teacher. Certainly this individual should possess a number of superior traits — personally and professionally. Here are six earmarks or minimum essentials of the competent teacher:

1. A Person with a Personality. Certainly the personality of a classroom teacher, who is aiming toward the successful teaching of health, must be one capable of registering a deep personal concern for the welfare of every pupil in the class. Children, influenced by the attitudes and practices of the teacher's warm, unflagging interest in them, receive an object lesson in what can be done by the teacher who really cares about the mental, physical, emotional, and social well-being of her students. Several years ago a Harvard University graduate study indicated that this *feeling* of warmth and understanding (empathy) was the quality more instrumental in good teaching than anything else. Yet, one cannot legislate or command this quality by decree. Given a little help, it may be developed, especially among teachers who profess to like children.

[11]Conant, James B. *The Education of American Teachers.* New York: McGraw-Hill Book Company, 1961, p. 183.

Dr. James B. Conant, president emeritus of Harvard University, lists two top characteristics of first-class teachers: a contagious enthusiasm for the subject being taught; and a thorough enjoyment of the process of teaching.

Not all teachers have the personality that is desirable for school teaching. It has been stated that the chances are seven to one that in the course of 12 years of school a child will come under the thumb of at least two teachers with personality maladjustments. They may be unstable and neurotic or even seriously psychopathic. This is a most serious problem, not only for the health of teachers but also for the children they teach. The atmosphere of the classroom cannot transcend the mental health of the teacher. Inappropriate emotional response, faulty personality reactions, and devastating character maladjustments are invited and can be spread under bad classroom as well as bad home conditions.

2. A Person with a Significant Store of Useful Knowledge. A limited knowledge of the science of health cannot be offset by a broad understanding of educational philosophy and method. A balance of both is required.

Teachers of health need increasing knowledge. New medical discoveries and public health practices are occurring all the time. The well-informed teacher is one who has sought extended instruction.

3. A Person Who Has Considerable Success in Selecting Important and Strategic Things to be Learned. The key word here is "select." Competent teachers, through study and training, know what they should select to teach, but because there is so much variety to choose from today, the selective function becomes an art. The fourth grade teacher, for example, knows that her students are interested and need some work in nutrition. With few exceptions, there is probably more written material available for classroom teachers in this area than for any other area in the field of health. It is conceivable that many materials are good. Some are better than others chiefly because they have been appraised and found to be more effective in the promotion of desired food practices and attitudes. Thus, the teacher's success in the selection of materials is somewhat related to her ability to evaluate them in terms of their contribution to preconceived pupil goals.

4. A Person with Decided Skill in Arranging What Pupils Do in Order that Learning Will Take Place. The key word here is "arranging." The ability to arrange the teaching situation so that children get the most out of it is high level skill. Today, with the many teaching instruments available — movies, field trips, libraries, and outside speakers — it takes a competent teacher to move from one to another so that all children receive maximum benefits. This holds true whether one teaches health or English.

5. A Person Who Has Success in Establishing Constructive, Stimulating Relationships with Individual Pupils. Although most personal contacts with children are made on a mass basis, the competent teacher knows how to go beyond the mass approach. Individuals are reached. Sam is helped with his problems. Sally has a brighter outlook toward school work. A trip is engineered to the dental clinic for Mike. This characteristic in the competent teacher is the quality *par excellence*, for it gives meaning to teaching as an art.

6. A Person with at Least One Well-Developed, Useful Specialty. It is good for a teacher to be well-rounded, with many abilities useful in education. At the same time, however, excellence in some phase of educational endeavor seems to be a common characteristic of the competent teacher.

Faith in the Worth of Teaching.

No discussion of the competencies of teachers of health would be complete without mention of the teacher's personal attitude toward teaching. This attitude may have more to do with successful health teaching than any other single factor. The teacher who likes the work and approaches the lesson with a pleasant and enthusiastic manner demonstrates a positive approach to the topic that sets the stage for optimum learning. The great New England pioneer in health teaching, Mabel Caroline Bragg, taught her teachers-to-be that the teaching of health—perhaps more than any other subject—calls for a teacher with dynamic vitality, an inspired interest in the welfare of children, and a faith in the worth of teaching. Miss Bragg herself was the magnificent example of this faith, for wherever she went, in college or grade school classrooms, she created an atmosphere of radiant, positive health. One must, therefore, possess a profound conviction of the worth of his work. There must be a sense of greatness in one's profession.

Finally, this faith in the worth of teaching is expressed through service. Through the basic concept of service the individual teacher establishes a place in the group. And through service the group takes on more significance. Unless man can be guided by a motive of service, selfishness and materialism eat at the roots of individuals and nations. Antoine de St. Exupéry attributes the fall of France to this lack of concept of service. In his *Flight to Arras* he says that if man insists upon giving only to himself he will receive nothing, for he is not a part of anything. Later when he is asked to die for something he will refuse to die, for his own interests will command him to live. There will be no deep love for something else strong enough to compensate for his death. Men do not die for tables and walls; they die for a home.

They die for something bigger than themselves. Says St. Exupéry, "Men die only for that for which they live."

HEALTH GUIDANCE

Pupils with health problems have a much better chance to improve when the sympathetic and understanding teacher sits, like Mark Hopkins, on one end of the log with the pupil on the other. In the quiet of the teacher's office much can be accomplished. There is time to talk personally about cleanliness, foods, rest, pimples, or home life. This is health instruction at its finest. The teacher may listen, discuss, and make concrete suggestions. The pupil is relaxed, pleased beyond words that the teacher is interested in him, and is usually most willing to try what is suggested.

The number of schoolchildren who need this kind of assistance is increasing. There have always been a number of children with minor physical deviations needing attention, but in recent years more and more children have problems of adjustment on the mental-emotional plane. Although there are school psychologists, guidance counselors, and in some places school psychiatrists, there are nevertheless far too few dedicated teachers who are both interested and capable of sitting down and talking at length with children in need of special consideration.

SUGGESTED ACTIVITIES

1. In a recent book, Ryan and Cooper describe the "New Teacher" (See Selected References). They feel that elementary teachers have been prepared as universal superteachers with all the skills, whereas in the future teaching should consist of teams of people with differential skills. Survey a number of teachers and see if they subscribe to this view, even to the extent of having a health specialist come to the classroom.

2. The pupil's learning process, the teach-

ing method, and the health education course content are intricately related. Review the philosophy of Jerome Bruner relative to the "discovery method" in teaching. What do you think could be the influence of this method on health instruction?

3. Discover if research carried on in a school health services department is used in some way by teachers. Some cities, for example, survey tooth decay and relate it to a number of school variables. How is this accomplished? Are those who teach children involved in any significant way?

4. Study the list of nine *Imperatives in Education* set forth by the American Association of School Administrators. Discuss ways and means in which health education can contribute to the fulfillment of these points and help meet the needs of the times.

QUESTIONS FOR DISCUSSION

1. What evidence is there that we are bridging the gap between health knowledge and health behavior? How can we better apply what the psychologists have learned about human motivations?

2. High-level conferences frequently recommend better health services, a higher quality of health care, and a more equitable distribution of health manpower. Very often missing is a solid recommendation for more meaningful health teaching. Why does this happen? Is the obvious overlooked, or is there a lack of faith in what education can provide?

3. To what extent do you believe parents receive health education through the health instruction program in schools?

4. From your experience, what seems to be the most effective way to tie up health instruction with physical education at the elementary school level?

5. What health instructional activities are suggested by the prepubescent growth spurt?

6. Youth tend to live in an intense present:

"now" is real, and it relates to exploring and feeling the forces for optimum health. What are the several ways a teacher can respond to this need?

7. As civilization becomes more complex, is there a tendency for education to become somewhat divorced from life? Is this true for health education as contrasted with other subject matter areas?

SELECTED REFERENCES

Brownell, William A., and Sims, Verner M. "The Nature of Understanding." *NSSE Forty-fifth Yearbook,* Part I. Chicago: National Society for Study of Education, 1946, Chapter 3.

Mallan, John T., and Hersh, Richard. *No G.O.D.s In The Classroom: Inquiry Into Inquiry,* Philadelphia: W. B. Saunders Co. 1972.

Oberteuffer, Delbert, Pollack, Marvin, and Harrelson, Orvil. *School Health Education,* 5th ed. New York: Harper and Row, 1972.

Ryan, Kevin, and Cooper, James M. *Those Who Can Teach.* Boston: Houghton-Mifflin Co., 1972.

Wenner, George. "Crisis-Oriented Health Education." *American Journal of Public Health,* 62:1043-1044, August 1972.

Whitehead, Alfred North. "In Deciding What to Teach." *Project on the Instructional Program of the Public Schools.* Washington, D.C.: National Education Association, 1963, pp. 27-28.

Willgoose, Carl E. "Health Education in Elementary Schools." *Education, 82:*131-133, November 1961.

Willgoose, Carl E. "Sequential K-12 Courses Replace Old Style 'Health'." *Nation's Schools,* 85:78, March 1970.

7 PLANNING THE HEALTH CURRICULUM

If you have built castles in the air, your work need not be lost; that is where they should be. Now put the foundations under them.

—Henry David Thoreau

If curriculum is an outgrowth of one's philosophy of health education, how is it possible that more than a few programs of health education appear to be "thrown together"? Can it be blamed on local school indifferences and foot-dragging? In many cases the answer is no; most schools today are really interested in school health and the instructional area. The problem is that far too many school systems fail to perform a conscientious job of *planning* the health curriculum. Quite often there are viewpoints and sound ideas in the minds of school people—and even on paper—but in the words of Thoreau there are no foundations under them. They lack a solid structure for implementation. Missing is a *reasonable* plan that translates remote goals and near-at-hand objectives into a workable program—a program that can be started gradually, subjected to pilot studies, and evaluated with comment from school and community groups.

THE NATURE OF THE CURRICULUM

Curriculum is a word derived from the Latin *currere*, which means "to run."

Where it was earlier associated with race courses and the running of races, it is now commonly defined as a "work schedule" or a "particular body of courses." It is generally linked with an orderly plan and progression.

In recent years the word curriculum has taken on an all-inclusive meaning which refers to the total school program. It has emerged from the time when educational offerings were conceived in terms of the "trained mind" and isolated teacher goals, to a child-centered curriculum.[1]

In any subject matter area it is important to note where curriculum stands in relation to other educational influences. As a body of experiences, it commands a central position between one's philosophy and objectives on the one hand, and teaching methods and evaluation practices on the other. The degree to which it is implemented, therefore, depends not only upon how it is put together but on how well it is taught and appraised.

---

[1]Curriculum and course of study are not the same. Curriculum applies to a larger web of influences, whereas a course of study is more specific—performing the function of a guide to help teachers in planning and carrying out activities.

115

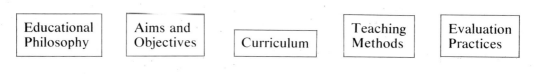

Types of Elementary School Curricula

Curricula are designated in a number of ways. The *separate-subjects curriculum* is regarded as the traditional curriculum. It is often called by such other names as the subject-matter curriculum and the scientific-subjects curriculum. Students study each subject that the school has to offer for a certain amount of time each day. Little attempt is made to relate one school subject to another. For example, physical education is taught without reference to health or social living. Health is taught as a subject by itself. Critics point out that the artificial separation of subjects and the extreme fragmentation of the curriculum are inconsistent with the integration of knowledge and full intellectual development. A multi-disciplinary approach to education is needed.

Since 1925 the trend has been to employ the *broad-fields curriculum* in which closely related subject-matter areas are grouped together. Subject matter is organized, but the emphasis is on large fields or areas rather than on separate subjects. This type of curriculum may group such items as spelling, writing, reading, language-grammar-oral communication, and literature under the broad topic (field) of language arts. Health, safety, and physical education are often grouped together for they possess several things in common. Health may also be taught in the broad areas of science or social studies. This curriculum helps students to see relationships between several things learned in one general area. For example, students learn from the broad field of health and social living that vitamins are more than something to be concerned about for personal health at the moment; they learn that they are related to historical accomplishments. The sailors who manned the ancient ships in the days of Columbus, Magellan, and Sir Francis Drake were somewhat limited in their capacities by vitamin deficiencies in the form of beriberi and pellagra.

Other types of elementary curricula include the *life situations curriculum* based on the problems of everyday living in the home, school, and community—a program established on needs of the moment; the *emerging curriculum* in which no preplanned program is arranged; and the *correlated-subjects curriculum* in which two or more subjects are articulated and relationships between and among them are made without destroying subject boundaries. More recently Goodlad has pleaded for a greater concentration on human values and interests. Because it involves the requirement for a warm, human approach to learning, it is called the *humanistic curriculum.*[2] Goodlad would abandon the system which is organized so that each child would advance a grade a year, and introduce a non-graded system designed so that each child will advance at his own best rate. In building this curriculum unifying principles are stressed rather than specific bits and pieces of information.

There is much agreement that the contemporary elementary school curriculum should stress the relationship of experiences to the learning process. The key word is *experiences.* The curriculum is organized for living and learning. These two words go together. No longer do we educate just for "later life." Education *is* life. It is concerned with the improvement of living—a better life for children and adults at the very moment—because

---

[2]Goodlad, John L. "The Educational Program to 1980 and Beyond," in *Designing Education for the Future*, No. 2, Edited by E. L. Morphet and C. D. Ryan, New York: Citation Press, 1967.

of the *kind* of living that goes on in the school.

More and more curriculum theorists are calling for a curriculum which is organized into a planned series of encounters between the pupil, the teacher, and the wide community of persons and things.

CURRICULUM DEVELOPMENT

Leadership in curriculum development has gone from the subject specialists and university and college professors to the "grass roots" of the community — to the teachers, supervisors, psychologists, specialists, and parents working together. The curriculum, in a sense, is part and parcel of the society, the local community, the classroom, and the pupils and teachers. All of these persons enter into the planning of the program so that the curriculum is viewed in the light of total influences. Materials and topics are carefully selected and developed cooperatively; supervisors and classroom teachers work together to rethink the curriculum periodically in terms of current problems which confront teachers in the school, the classroom, and the community. Where there is a need to make a change, a real effort is made to implement the findings rapidly.

Too often in the past programs have not been properly updated to reflect a changing emphasis on health needs. More recently, it has been popular to be associated with change — even to the extent of believing that change is automatically equated with a seldom defined "progress." Change=Progress=Benefit represents a concept of change that becomes regarded as an unqualified good. Certainly there is merit in the expression, "We must adapt to a changing world," but it frequently gives rise to a doctrine of over-enthusiastic adaptability which advances the assertion of "change for change's sake." When this happens it raises the question as to whether the traditional or existing curric-

ulum has been fully evaluated in terms of its usefulness in modifying health behavior, or if it is being discarded simply because it is "old" and not subject to the seemingly new charm of "innovation" and "creativity." Although local research is frequently given a low priority, there should be some sincere effort to appraise existing programs before entirely new organizations for learning are explored. In short, it is good curriculum development practice to inquire and explore both the new and the old, with comments solicited from many sources. For example, it is possible that a more appropriate health program can be planned in a particular school by upgrading materials in the separate grades. Consider the possible action that might be taken following three findings from the Connecticut study, *Teach Us What We Want To Know*:

1. Children have acquired a large amount of accurate information about health and are more mature in thought and judgment, and at an earlier age, than adults generally think.

2. Young people wish they had been taught about health and often recommend that such information should be given to younger children.

3. Children are capable of making valid suggestions about how and when health topics should be taught.

Most of the larger schools have committees that are responsible for improving the program of studies, articulating it so that all elements of the school's offerings complement each other. This kind of planning guards against unnecessary duplication or gaps in the child's learning experiences. A good amount of preplanning is necessary.

This can be accomplished if the following points are kept in mind:[3]

1. If a program is to succeed, it must have the commitment and support of the community, administration and staff.

---

[3]Adapted from the report of the Curriculum Commission of the School Health Division, AAHPER, *School Health Review*, 2:35–38, September 1971.

2. The personnel involved is important for success.

> *Steering* (In-school) *Committee* — representative from each facet of the school.
> *Advisory Committee* — representatives from the community (could be the School-Community Health Council — see Chapter 3).

3. Basic considerations in developing a curriculum need to be outlined. (See *Elements That Affect the Teacher's Planning for Health* at bottom of page.

4. A philosophy must be developed in order that value judgments may be made and educational objectives selected.

5. Controversial areas must be considered carefully; methods, materials and content must be reviewed in reference to their legality, educational validity, and social acceptability.

6. A work schedule should be developed early with target dates for assignment completion.

The School Health Education Study

The inadequacy of health education has been the concern of many groups and individuals for a number of years. In 1960 the NEA-AMA Joint Committee on Health Problems in Education recommended a survey of the nation's school-children to determine the status of health education in the schools. Under a grant from the Samuel Bronfman Foundation in 1961, the School Health Education Study (SHES) was begun. Its purpose was to discover the status of health instruction and gain public support for reform measures.[4]

Large, medium, and small school systems were studied. Health behavior questionnaires were submitted to the students in the sixth, ninth, and twelfth grades in order to secure information which would reflect the accumulation of health experience in the years prior to graduation.

The findings at all grade levels indicated serious misconceptions about health. Only one in five sixth graders brushed his teeth or rinsed his mouth regularly after eating. Sixth graders also scored poorly in safety education. This was not a strange finding, for it was discovered that health instruction practices were of poor quality throughout the country.

The School Health Education Study undertook a project to bring together health education specialists, supervisors,

---

[4]Sliepcevich, Elena M. *School Health Education Study: A Summary Report*. Washington, D.C.: SHES, 1964.

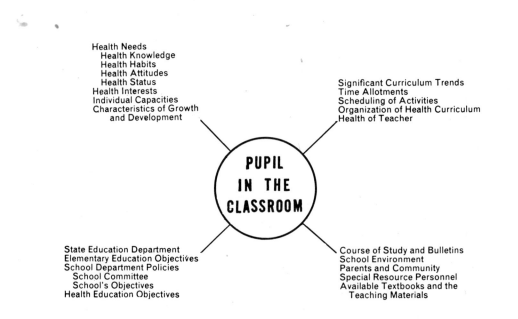

Health Needs
  Health Knowledge
  Health Habits
  Health Attitudes
  Health Status
Health Interests
Individual Capacities
Characteristics of Growth
  and Development

Significant Curriculum Trends
Time Allotments
Scheduling of Activities
Organization of Health Curriculum
Health of Teacher

PUPIL IN THE CLASSROOM

State Education Department
Elementary Education Objectives
School Department Policies
  School Committee
  School's Objectives
Health Education Objectives

Course of Study and Bulletins
School Environment
Parents and Community
Special Resource Personnel
Available Textbooks and the
  Teaching Materials

and classroom teachers to develop sample experimental curriculum materials based on a concept approach. These were carefully prepared and tested during the 1964–1965 school year in try-out centers in Alhambra, California; Evanston, Illinois; Great Neck–Garden City, New York; and Tacoma, Washington.

Beginning in 1966 SHES received support by the Minnesota Mining and Manufacturing Company (3M) to continue the development and publication of curriculum materials. In 1967, packets of materials pertaining to the concepts were available commercially.[5] The ten curriculum concepts developed by the project are:

1. Growth and development influences, and is influenced by, the structure and functioning of the individual.

2. Growing and developing follows a predictable sequence, yet is unique for each individual.

3. Protection and promotion of health is an individual, community, and international responsibility.

4. The potential for hazards and accidents exists, whatever the environment.

5. There are reciprocal relationships involving man, disease, and environment.

6. The family serves to perpetuate man and to fulfill certain health needs.

7. Personal health practices are affected by a complexity of forces, often conflicting.

8. Utilization of health information, products, and services is guided by values and perceptions.

9. Use of substances that modify mood and behavior arises from a variety of motivations.

10. Food selection and eating patterns are determined by physical, social, mental, economic, and cultural factors.

The Health Concept Approach in Curriculum Development

It is appropriate at this stage of curriculum planning to consider outcomes of learning. In recent years, the two terms frequently employed to denote learning outcomes are *concepts* and *competencies*. Although they share a common ground, they are not the same. The concept is a point of view or idea held about something, whereas a competency is a solid ability or proficiency. Both are necessary in health education. Ultimate health behavior starts with one or more health concepts and culminates in a skillful and appropriate action – a health competency.

The concept approach offers the program planner a realistic pattern for the development of curriculum materials in health education. The topic has been well explored. (See especially the references to Bruner, Darrow, Phenix, and Woodruff at the end of this chapter.) Also, there have been several national curriculum studies that have used this approach quite successfully.[6]

A concept is a generalization about something. It is usually built from a number of related sensations, precepts, and images. Concepts range from ideas about very simple things to high-level abstractions. Woodruff has phrased a definition for curriculum planning which states:

A concept is a relatively complete and meaningful idea in the mind of a person. It is an understanding of something. It is his own subjective product of his way of making meaning of things he has seen or otherwise perceived in his experience.[7]

To the individual pupil, a concept is a personal organization of a number of interpretations of things to which he has somehow been exposed. In this respect concepts cannot be taught as such. How-

[5]Teaching-learning guides, together with the basic document (*Health Education: a Conceptual Approach to Curriculum Design, Grades K-12*) and printed originals for preparing overhead projection transparencies, are available from Visual Products, 3M Co., Box 1300, St. Paul, Minn., 55101.

[6]See especially Pennsylvania Department of Education, *Conceptual Guidelines for School Health Programs in Pennsylvania*, Harrisburg, Pennsylvania: Department of Education, 1970.

[7]Woodruff, Asahel D. "The Use of Concepts in Teaching and Learning," *Journal of Teacher Education*, 20:81–99, March 1964.

ever, teaching is directed *toward* concepts. This means that the instructor is working with pupils in terms of whole ideas, even though pieces and bits of knowledges are being employed along the way. More specifically, the concept approach to learning is one in which all the facts, skills, and techniques are interdependent and interrelated. For too many years teachers of health have taught isolated vitamin facts in about the same fashion as history teachers have taught places and dates. The pupil learned his facts by rote memorization or repetition without seeing them as a part of a whole—a part of *his* life. They did not become a part of his value system. The dates, places, and vitamins were soon forgotten.

Therefore, the writers of the School Health Education Study materials realized that all health instruction activities must ultimately be related not only to the individual, but to the family and community at large. Health education attempts to unify man physically, mentally, and socially by developing health education behavior in the form of knowledges, attitudes, and practices with a dynamic focus on the individual, family, and community.

In a conceptual framework there are broad key concepts which represent the highest conceptual level of the health curriculum. In the School Health Education Study the three overriding concepts or processes affecting health behavior are:

Growing and Developing: a dynamic life process in which the individual is in some ways like all other individuals, in some ways like some other individuals, and in some ways like no other individuals.

Interacting: an ongoing process in which the individual is affected by and in turn affects certain biological, social, psychological, economic, cultural, and physical forces in the environment.

Decision Making: a process unique to man of consciously deciding to take an action, or of choosing one alternative rather than another.[8]

Practically all health education experiences can be fitted to the pattern of growing and developing, interacting, and decision making. In the SHES project these key concepts were established as the three unifying threads of the health program from which the ten major curriculum concepts emerge. There are also subconcepts which were developed by elaborating on the basic ten concepts. These sub-concepts were set up in terms of physical, mental, and social dimensions. From this the long range goals were formulated in three domains. (See table below.)

Finally, the progression and sequence for the teaching-learning experience were developed. These were set up as four levels of progression rather than by the more traditional grade level approach.

A number of school systems have used concepts in the development of their local courses of study. *The Health and Safety Resource Guide, Kindergarten and Primary*, of the Waterloo (Iowa) Public Schools is especially well constructed with selected concepts for teaching and learning prepared for immediate teacher use. Of particular merit is the *Health Education Guide to Better Health*, grades K-six, for the state of Washington. All units of study are set up in terms of one to six competencies, each

---

[8]School Health Education Study. *Health Education: a Conceptual Approach to Curriculum Design*. St. Paul, Minnesota: 3M Education Press, 1967, p. 20.

Cognitive Domain	Affective Domain	Action Domain
Understanding	Awareness	Improving
Comprehending	Appreciation	Modifying
Realizing	Consciousness	Developing
(Knowledge, intellectual abilities, skills)	(Interests, attitudes, values)	(Application of knowledge and attitudes)

supported by several well prepared concept statements. (A list of these competencies, together with the respective concepts, may be found in Appendix B.) This admirable design of concepts warrants a thorough study by the reader, for it is especially valuable for anyone about to begin the organization of a health instruction program.

Since teaching can be directed toward concepts, this fosters a striving for goals that are pupil-oriented instead of teacher-oriented. It also gets away from the objectification of factual information and improves the chances of building larger generalizations. There is nothing automatic about this; it requires work to help students conceptualize. Marion Pollock speaks well to the point when she says, "Conceptualization is a natural process, and the difficulty is not in arranging for it to take place, but in arranging for the kinds of perceptions that lead to positive, constructive concepts."[9] In this connection there is some research to indicate that the concept approach to learning is not sufficient to produce a

substantial number of significant changes in student-reported health behavior patterns.[10] It would seem that the approach is only as effective as the teacher's ability to use it.

An example of how concepts may be set up so that they influence curriculum planning and implementation follows. Note the clarity of the concepts.[11]

BEHAVIORAL OBJECTIVES AND DECISION MAKING

Currently a fair amount of discussion is being given to behavioral objectives. These are student objectives at the instructional level, as opposed to the general objectives of an institution or a society. Moreover, the behavioral objectives are stated in such precise fashion that they describe a behavior. If it is realistic

---

[9]Pollock, Marion B. "Speaking of Concepts," *Journal of School Health,* 41:283–285, June 1971.

[10]Allen, Robert E. and Owen J. Holyoak. "Evaluating the Conceptual Approach to Teaching Health Education," *Journal of School Health,* 42:118–119, February 1972.

[11]From the State Education Dept. *Strand IV Environmental and Community Health*, Albany, N.Y.: State Education Dept. 1970 (Grades 4–6).

Environmental and Public Health (Grades 4–6)

Outline of Content	Major Understandings and Fundamental Concepts	Suggested Teaching and Learning Activities	Supplementary Information for Teachers
1. The Environment and Health Status	Man is in constant interaction with his environment which is capable of improving his health or harming it.		
A. History of Environmental Control	Man improves his health status when he understands his environment and uses it wisely.		
	We must constantly adapt to environmental conditions because our environment constantly changes.		
	Many of the devices we have created to improve our way of life have resulted in environmental destruction.		

First Aid and Survival Education (Grades 4–6)

Outline of Content	Major Understandings and Fundamental Concepts	Suggested Teaching and Learning Activities	Supplementary Information for Teachers
1. Introduction to First Aid	First aid involves immediate temporary care and not treatment.		
A. Definition	First aid is the immediate and temporary care given to an injured or sick person until the services of a physician can be obtained.		
B. Values of First Aid Training	Having knowledge of first aid will give a feeling of some competency to care for oneself and others and will serve to make one aware of preventable safety problems.		

it can be achieved and measured. It is noticeably different from the usually stated goals and concepts in that it is not written in terms of understandings and feelings, but in terms of action. It is as if someone took the verb to *do* and applied it generally. Thus words such as the following usually preface the objective:

identifies	distinguishes
analyzes	relates
evaluates	modifies
describes	improves
applies	performs
gives	makes

By stating educational aspirations in terms of behavioral objectives the focus is on action and behavior change from the beginning. Note the difference:

Grade 3

Example 1 *Traditional objective:* To understand that certain foods build strong teeth and bones.
Concept: Certain foods build strong teeth and bones.
Behavioral objective: Identifies foods that build strong teeth and bones.

Example 2 *Traditional objective:* To know that a program of physical activity and rest contributes to well-being.

Concept: Physical activity and rest contribute to well-being.
Behavioral objective: Describes how physical activity and rest contribute to well-being.

In the State of California guide, *Framework for Health Instruction*, both grade level concepts and behavioral objectives are a part of each of the major health units. One small part of the Exercise, Rest and Posture unit follows as an example. (See table on p. 123.)

In the School Health Education Study curriculum program behavioral objectives were developed for each of the 10 concepts. This permits the teacher to focus on certain behaviors during daily classroom activities. Progression in behavioral objectives in the K-3 and 4-6 levels is nicely illustrated on pages 124 and 125.*

A careful look at the wording of these traditional objectives, concepts, and behavioral objectives indicates considerable similarity. The real difference, therefore, must come in *how* the teaching is accomplished. If one does not teach for *decision making* the usual knowledge

---

*Some materials on these pages reproduced by permission of Minnesota Mining and Manufacturing Company, copyright 1970.

Exercise, Rest and Posture

Concept		Primary	Intermediate
I PHYSICAL FITNESS IS ONE IMPORTANT COMPONENT OF TOTAL HEALTH	*Grade Level Concept:*	Play which includes physical activity is healthful as well as fun.	Regular physical activity is beneficial to one's body.
	Objective:	*Lists* the benefits of play and physical activity.	*Identifies* benefits of physical activities to one's body.
	Content:	(1) helps one get along with others; (2) helps one feel better; (3) helps one grow in strength and agility; (4) helps one sleep.	(1) aids in personal appearance; (2) helps to develop strength and coordination; (3) helps maintain weight control; (4) improves circulation and respiration; (5) improves muscle tone; (6) improves appetite.

will be obtained and little action beyond that will occur. This is exactly why the relevance of utilizing behavioral objectives in the classroom has been a source of debate among educators since 1918 (see Ebel research in *Selected References*).

Interestingly enough, pupils seem to enjoy focusing on objectives and learning activities that provide a choice of one alternative rather than another. Inquiring and making a decision rather than simply accepting information on a health topic tends to keep one alert. Inquiring about a topic, seeking answers to a problem, and experimenting boosts specific values which are instrumental in decision-making. The emphasis is on teaching the valuing process and not specific values. Without such involvement any action would be impulsive. (See Fig. 7–1.)[12]

Curriculum Scope and Sequence

Curriculum development deals specifically with the scope and sequence of the total program. When developing a program of health instruction for the pri-

mary and intermediate grades, one must also consider scope and sequence.

The word "scope" is used to define the breadth of the health curriculum. It tells *what* should be taught at all grade levels. The scope is wide or limited, according to the persistent and identifiable wants and desires of boys and girls. Sequence, on the other hand, refers to the *when* of the curriculum and determines the grade placement of the health learning experiences. It defines the curriculum vertically, whereas scope defines it horizontally.

Determination of Scope. The basis for the scope of a health course is found in the necessities of life as revealed by close analysis, not by peremptory judgment. *The scope should present as great and as rich a selection of ideas as possible. Teachers then do their own organizing. This is the modern elementary approach of stressing experience rather than subjects.* The better school systems are steadily moving in a direction beyond and above a static course of study and to a wealth of documentary materials based upon the needs of the group.

One who understands children will select, eliminate, and adapt experiences and materials to meet all their needs. The scope of the health curriculum, there-

---

[12]From "Swing Toward Decision Making" by Theodore Kaltsounis, *Instructor, 80:*45–54, April 1971.

	CONCEPT 1	CONCEPT 2	CONCEPT 3	CONCEPT 4	CONCEPT 5
	GROWTH AND DEVELOPMENT INFLUENCES AND IS INFLUENCED BY THE STRUCTURE AND FUNCTIONING OF THE INDIVIDUAL.	GROWING AND DEVELOPING FOLLOWS A PREDICTABLE SEQUENCE, YET IS UNIQUE FOR EACH INDIVIDUAL.	PROTECTION AND PROMOTION OF HEALTH IS AN INDIVIDUAL, COMMUNITY, AND INTERNATIONAL RESPONSIBILITY.	THE POTENTIAL FOR HAZARDS AND ACCIDENTS EXISTS, WHATEVER THE ENVIRONMENT.	THERE ARE RECIPROCAL RELATIONSHIPS INVOLVING MAN, DISEASE, AND ENVIRONMENT.
LEVEL I — APPROXIMATE GRADE LEVELS K-3	**A** Relates good nutrition, adequate sleep, and physical activity to optimal growth and development. **B** Names major body parts and organs and their related functions. **C** Explains that body types and other factors determine differences in height and weight. **D** Defines the meanings of heredity and environment. **E** Identifies ways in which plants, animals, and children resemble their parents.	**A** Cites examples showing how people of the same age differ and yet are similar while growing and developing. **B** Explains why differences in the rate of growing and developing among children of the same age are to be expected. **C** Identifies ways in which one grows over a given period of time. **D** Describes how each person becomes unique.	**A** Defines the meanings of health and of community. **B** Describes the relationships of health and community. **C** Identifies familiar health problems which are the joint responsibility of individuals and groups. **D** Recognizes local community efforts designed to meet common health needs. **E** Is aware of the variety of health personnel involved in solution of community problems.	**A** Describes what accidents are and the need for their prevention and control. **B** Detects environmental factors which affect health and safety. **C** Indicates hazards existing in the home, school, and community. **D** Identifies procedures which help protect personal health and safety and that of others. **E** Is aware that groups exist to help prevent accidents and eliminate or control hazards.	**A** Distinguishes between being ill and being well. **B** Identifies factors which affect wellness. **C** Discusses ways in which disease-causing organisms can be transmitted from person to person. **D** Identifies ways in which a person can protect himself and others from disease.
LEVEL II — APPROXIMATE GRADE LEVELS 4-6	**A** Describes the basic structure and function of the human organism as it relates to growing and developing. **B** Concludes that although each organ and system has a special task, each is dependent on the other in meeting body needs. **C** Identifies ways in which girls are both physiologically ahead of boys and different in behavior and interests at some stages of growth. **D** Explains the importance of certain personal health practices as they relate to the process of growing and developing. **E** Illustrates the effects of heredity and environment on growth and development.	**A** Describes how growing and developing occurs unevenly for body parts, systems and functions. **B** Identifies different ways children grow physically, mentally, and socially. **C** Differentiates among the variety of influences which continually affect growing and developing. **D** Predicts the kinds of changes that may occur during adolescence.	**A** Explains why some health-related efforts are common to all communities while others are unique to certain communities. **B** Identifies factors that influence the nature of community health activities. **C** Compares health programs, facilities, and services provided by organized segments of society. **D** Describes skills and techniques required to meet existing and emerging community health needs. **E** Explores functions of and the range of career opportunities in health-service professions and allied fields.	**A** Cites authoritative data related to the occurrence of accidents. **B** Illustrates relationships between accidents and human behavior. **C** Reports the effects of environmental factors on the health and safety of individuals and groups. **D** Relates precautions to the reduction of hazards and accidents.	**A** Names various methods by which disease can be prevented, controlled, or cured. **B** Identifies various sources of disease. **C** Concludes that immunization prevents and controls some diseases. **D** Cites examples of the effects of disease upon individuals, families, communities, countries. **E** Recognizes that a concern for wellness motivates individuals and organizations.

CONCEPT 6

THE FAMILY SERVES TO PERPETUATE MAN AND TO FULFILL CERTAIN HEALTH NEEDS.

A Describes the role and responsibilities of individuals within the family.

B Describes how family members contribute to the health of each other.

C Lists similarities and differences between boys and girls in appearance, interests, and activities.

D Discovers that all living things come from other living things.

A Illustrates relationships within a family that influence the degree of health and happiness of all members.

B Is aware that families in present day society display a wide range of characteristics.

C Describes personal qualities which affect peer group relationships.

D Explains body changes which occur during puberty.

E Is aware of the reproductive process and how life begins.

F Defines heredity and is aware of inherited and acquired characteristics.

CONCEPT 7

PERSONAL HEALTH PRACTICES ARE AFFECTED BY A COMPLEXITY OF FORCES, OFTEN CONFLICTING.

A Tells why personal health practices affect participation in life activities.

B Identifies practices which affect oral health.

C Is aware of the influence of growing and developing on personal health practices.

D Discovers that decision making is involved in personal health practices.

A Discusses why guidance is necessary in determining a balance of sleep, rest and activity.

B Distinguishes between practices that promote and those that hinder development of the oral structures.

C Illustrates ways in which personal choices affect health practices.

D Identifies conflicting forces affecting personal health practices.

E Illustrates relationships between personal health practices and well-being.

CONCEPT 8

UTILIZATION OF HEALTH INFORMATION, PRODUCTS, AND SERVICES IS GUIDED BY VALUES AND PERCEPTIONS.

A Names familiar people who promote, protect, and maintain health.

B Is aware that there are differences among health products and among health services.

C Identifies various sources of health information.

D Recognizes that laws and regulations exist to protect the consumer.

A Is aware that emotions, family patterns, and values influence selection and use of health information, products, and services.

B Compares and contrasts health information, products, and services.

C Identifies different kinds of medical, dental, and health related specialists and their role in health services.

D Cites examples of agencies, groups, laws, and standards that protect the health consumer.

E Applies the knowledge that harm can result from self-diagnosis, self-medication, and the unwise use of drugs, medicines, devices, cosmetics, and dietary supplements.

CONCEPT 9

USE OF SUBSTANCES THAT MODIFY MOOD AND BEHAVIOR ARISES FROM A VARIETY OF MOTIVATIONS.

A Identifies substances commonly used by many individuals in society that modify mood and behavior.

B Names ways common mood and behavior modifying substances are used in homes and community.

C Is aware that there are differences between alcoholic beverages and other beverages.

D Realizes there are differences in family practices and feelings about use of tobacco and of alcoholic beverages.

A Describes the range of substances used by man to modify mood and behavior.

B Differentiates among controls on purchase, possession, and use of substances that modify mood and behavior.

C Illustrates how, when, and where certain mood and behavior modifying substances are used for dietary, ceremonial, social, pain relieving, and other reasons.

D Discusses why certain mood and behavior modifying substances are used rather commonly and others only under special circumstances.

CONCEPT 10

FOOD SELECTION AND EATING PATTERNS ARE DETERMINED BY PHYSICAL, SOCIAL, MENTAL, ECONOMIC, AND CULTURAL FACTORS.

A Distinguishes among a wide range of foods.

B States reasons for eating a variety of foods.

C Is aware of factors that detract from or enhance eating certain foods.

D Identifies ways that types of foods and patterns of eating may be related to different cultures.

A Describes food nutrients and their functions as they relate to health.

B Develops acceptable criteria for food selection and patterns for eating.

C Cites examples of social and emotional influences on nutritional behavior.

D Relates different eating patterns to circumstances of living.

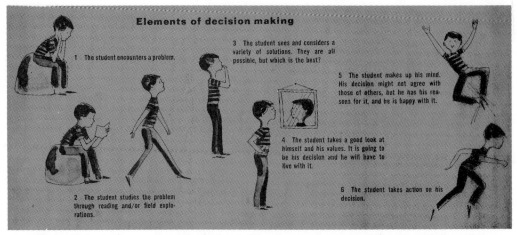

Figure 7–1 Action-centered throughout. (Courtesy *Instructor* and Theodore Kaltsounis.)

fore, is made effective by greatly improving existing courses of study, by following guides to child development, and by using source units or course of study units. The last factor, the unit, is by far the most effective curriculum item. For example, in the health curriculum a very wide variety of learning and materials is organized into areas of experience, or in broad fields, or within single subjects, from which selections may be made. Health may be taught in the broad field of social studies or science, or it may be taught as a separate subject, or both. (It is most effective when taught as a separate subject.) Physical, mental, emotional, and social health embraces so much in the realm of human welfare and behavior that the scope of the health curriculum cannot easily be contained. There are limits, however, to the number and kind of topics that children should be introduced to at any one grade level. And there are obvious limits to the amount of emphasis or concentration afforded a particular topic at a certain grade level.

Determination of Sequence. Sequence is defined in most elementary schools today, but it is not fixed with a rigid order of required topics for each school year. The trend is away from the fixed sequence to the more flexible one.

It cannot be stressed too emphatically that the need for a planned course of instruction is essential for effective health teaching in the elementary school. The chief problem which faces most teachers is not what to teach in the major topical areas, but *how far one should go in the area at specific grade levels*. Solving this would help eliminate or minimize unnecessary repetition. Unfortunately, in many schools today health teaching is simply a "do-gooder" activity. The teacher, feeling sympathetic to the need for health instruction, decides to do "her bit" for the cause. She frequently teaches a little about the teeth, foods, and how to keep clean. This she does, all too often with no knowledge of what her pupils have already received in the way of knowledge from the year before or what they will be getting in the year ahead. Both scope and sequence are foreign terms in such a haphazard setup. A business run in this manner would go bankrupt in six months.

The only sound way to insure proper scope and sequence in health teaching is to set up the essential topical areas of instruction, under which are listed the pupil objectives that should be achieved at each grade level. Until this is done in every elementary school, health teaching will be at best only a "busy work" activity. An excellent way for the new teacher to appreciate the sequential development of health topics is to carefully examine curriculum guides and courses of study. This may be accomplished in a curriculum library of a teacher preparation institution. In this fashion, progressions within an area are observed along with appropriate content, materials and teaching ideas.

Time Allotment and Scheduling

Health instruction has to become a part of the total elementary school program by being scheduled; any program takes time to carry out. How much time should be spent on the health activities? Should a health curriculum, because of its wide scope, justify a rather large part of the school day? Is it conceivable that some teachers, extremely interested in a topic, might spend 30 to 40 per cent of a week's time on it? Who is to say whether this is right or wrong? Of course the classroom teacher must have a fair sense of value and use good judgment when allotting time to health instruction. Time ratios vary because of pupil factors relating to interests, experiences and maturity; environmental factors involving facilities and materials; and the over-all curriculum plans of the particular school.

Many schools have a planned health curriculum which represents the results of long term study and research. This curriculum, coupled with state recommendations, may suggest a time allotment. For example, in New York City 10 per cent of the time allotted to primary grades and 15 per cent in the intermediate grades is to be devoted to science and health teaching. The amount of time spent in any one exposure should be flexible, in keeping with the nature of the lesson, and depending on whether it is taught by an individual or a team. In most schools the teaching is carried on by the regular classroom teacher, as indicated in the requirement for the State of New York. (See Fig. 7–2.) However, assigning suitable time for health teaching is still a problem. In the Massachusetts study, for instance, a high percentage of teachers recognized this lack of time as their first problem.

Although primary graders have a short span of attention, they do not learn too effectively in very short periods day after day. Periods should be of sufficient length to have meaning, perhaps 15 minutes to half an hour. Several authorities prefer a set daily period for direct health teaching.

Daily classroom programs should also be planned so that different types of activity are scheduled for alternate periods; for example, active work following quiet work, such as project construction following reading, or physical education following arithmetic. There is little reason why classroom topics cannot be shifted around from week to week. Children like variety and innovations and respond very well to them. A health topic may be taught in the middle of the morning one day and just before lunch another day.

HEALTH TEACHING IN THE KINDERGARTEN

The health curriculum for kindergarten children may be quite informal. It is integrated with all other areas of instruc-

---

HEALTH EDUCATION IN THE ELEMENTARY SCHOOLS

2. *Health education in the elementary schools.* The elementary school curriculum shall include health education for all pupils. In the kindergarten and primary grades, the health teaching shall be largely done by guiding the children in developing desirable health behavior, attitudes and knowledge through their everyday experiences in a healthful environment. This guidance shall include systematic practice of health habits as needed. In addition to continued health guidance, provision shall be made in the school program of grades 4, 5 and 6 for planned units of teaching which shall include health instruction through which pupils may become increasingly self-reliant in solving their own health problems and those of the group. Health education in the elementary school grades shall be carried on by the regular classroom teachers.

Figure 7–2 Regulations pertaining to health education, State of New York.

tion. Health topics are taught "as though you taught them not." The children are physically active, extremely individualistic, very imitative, dramatic, and imaginative. What they use in the way of material is largely manipulative and experimental. What they understand is generally developed through active participation and first-hand experience. Fantasy and reality appear to be the same to many children. The time-space concept is slow to develop.

Kindergarten boys and girls show interest in a number of items related to health. They are:

Gaining confidence in themselves as persons.

Developing better motor coordination.

Speaking and acting spontaneously.

Assuming some responsibilities.

Learning to clean up and put things away.

Becoming observant of sights and sounds.

Becoming aware of the natural environment.

Gaining a number of specific health interests, such as:

Acting quickly and orderly in fire drills.

Practicing safe ways of going to and from school.

Visiting the school physician.

Carrying a clean handkerchief and covering the cough or sneeze.

Eating midmorning food and having a warm noon meal.

Resting between periods.

Having a relaxed atmosphere for classroom work and playground recreation.

Having proper toilet habits and practicing cleanliness.

Eating the right foods and caring for the teeth.

The observing kindergarten teacher will find numerous opportunities for health instructions every hour of the day. There will be times when it seems desirable to create situations which will appear to the pupils quite natural and unplanned. Daily health experiences in a healthful environment do much to build lasting impressions. Moreover, the kindergarten is a period of culturalization for children who have been neglected, "spoiled," or overprotected at home. It is a place for socialization, for getting to know people of one's age and what they are like.

The over-all kindergarten curriculum in health varies somewhat the country over. Generally, what happens is pretty much up to the individual teacher. Some of the kindergarten teaching opportunities common to most school situations today are as follows:

1. Health examinations and tests, including examination of teeth by dental hygiene teacher.

    a. Opportunity to make friends with the physician, nurse, and dental hygiene teachers and other members of the school health services staff.

    b. Opportunity to learn that everyone should have periodic health examinations by physician and dentist to help in keeping well.

2. Early morning checking time.

    a. Opportunity to inspect children, to recognize achievements and to care for health needs.

3. Weighing and measuring.

    a. Opportunity to arouse interest in growing and gaining and in doing things which will help children grow their best.

4. Mid-session lunch, noon lunch, real and play parties, preparation and tasting of real foods.

    a. Opportunity for practicing washing hands before touching food; sitting down to eat, relaxing, eating slowly and enjoying lunchtime, eating and liking certain foods; taking small bites, chewing food thoroughly and enjoying its flavor; touching only one's own food; washing and preparing food so that it is clean; discarding food which has been dropped to the floor or ground; table manners.

5. Playground activities.

    a. Opportunity to arouse interest

in activities in the sunshine and open air.

b. Opportunity for fun, getting along happily with playmates, promoting physical development, increasing appetite and enjoyment of food, and maintaining or improving posture.

6. Rest periods.
   a. Opportunity to improve ability to relax and rest.

7. Cleanliness and health protection.
   a. Opportunity to learn desirable practices related to cleanliness of body and clothing, food and eating, use of handkerchief, protection of self and others when ill.
   b. Opportunity to learn to use toilet, handwashing, and drinking facilities properly.

8. Reading and other close eye work.
   a. Opportunity for learning proper position of books and other materials and adjustments of lights and shades.

9. Cooperation in keeping air in classroom fresh.
   a. Opportunity to help regulate air conditions by notifying custodian or by other appropriate means; to enjoy the feeling of a well-ventilated room; to become aware of the teacher's attention to the thermometer and air conditions.

10. Seating.
    a. Opportunity to learn to select seats, desks, and tables so that the child may work and play in comfort and to change position to meet changing needs.

11. Clothing.
    a. Opportunity to learn to put on and take off outdoor clothing and to care for it properly.

12. The total program.
    a. Opportunity to enjoy and be reasonably successful in work and play, to get along happily with children and adults, to become increasingly self-reliant in caring for own needs and in helping others.

b. Opportunity to participate fully in the daily program with decreasing need for adult guidance to the end that the child's own safety and the safety of others will be an important outcome of the program.

Research indicates that normal children of kindergarten age, though young in years, are quite receptive to ideas and are capable of learning many presumably difficult things. Because of the interest span and time factor, selecting what to teach is a necessary consideration. Many studies indicate that information on foods and safety is important. Other research indicates a need for emphasis in health instruction to be greatest in the following health areas:

Rest and sleep (correct bedtime and habit of taking a nap during the day)

Grooming (habit of hanging up clothes)

Growth and development (habit of sitting quietly and listening when others speak)

Prevention and control of disease (acceptance of immunization shots and habits of keeping hands out of mouth, and covering mouth and nose when coughing and sneezing)

The new teacher, with the help of the children, will find it wise to build a series of teaching units covering the several areas of emphasis at the kindergarten level. These may be in skeleton form so that they can easily be amended during the period of use or kept flexible from year to year with appropriate modification.

Kindergarten Health Charts

One of the most effective health teaching items for the kindergarten age child is a series of 36 full-color charts (17 inches × 20 inches size).[13] Each chart presents a basic health concept in pictures—a

---

[13]Gallagher, J. Roswell, Spencer, Mary E., and Willgoose, Carl E. *Health Charts for Kindergarten (How About You?)*. Boston: Ginn and Co., 1965. A *Teachers' Manual*, offering detailed suggestions for presenting the pictures, is included with the charts.

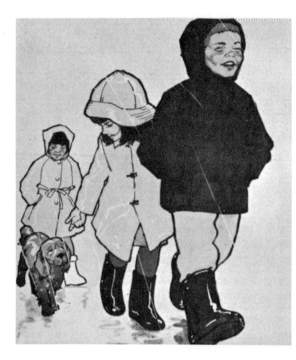

Figure 7–3 Kindergarten health chart. (With the permission of Ginn and Co., Boston, Mass. 02217.)

method of learning most appealing and effective with youngsters of this age level. People, young and old, are portrayed in familiar situations stressing fundamental health and safety practices *with which children can identify.*

Teachers show these large charts (with spiral binding and easel-back for convenient viewing) to their class in order to provoke discussion relative to personal health practices. Figure 7–3 is a greatly reduced picture of chart No. 11 entitled *Warm and Dry?* In this particular illustration the teacher might begin the lesson by showing the chart and asking: "How do you know that it is a rainy, cold day? Do you think the children in the picture are wet or cold? Why not? Do you think the dog is cold? He certainly is wet. Why do you think this picture is called *Warm and Dry?*"

HEALTH TEACHING IN THE PRIMARY GRADES

The health curriculum for the first three grades is one in which the pupil is not held responsible for a great amount of specific health knowledge. Children may engage in a large number of experiences, but informality continues as it did in the kindergarten. The approach is one of definite exploration of the important health practices. There will be opportunities for integration of the health instructional program with social studies, science, and physical education.

Since growth is a continuous process, there will be varying degrees of maturity, capacities, and interests among primary grade pupils. Where first graders are beginning to differentiate between fancy and reality, third graders will have pretty much established this differentiation. As children mature during the primary years they gain in ability to present their own ideas and problems orally and in writing. They gradually begin to appreciate cause and effect relationships, project their feelings more and more toward others, become less individualistic and possessive, and are more cognizant of adult opinion. Growth is slow and steady; they continue to tire less as they approach eight years of age, and show an increase in physical strength and dexterity.

Primary children show interest in a

number of items related to health. They are:

Beginning to show some muscle growth

Advancing to a state of full visual fusion

Watching the first permanent teeth appear

Accepting greater responsibility for personal safety and appearance

Talking about nourishing food, going to bed early, playing out of doors and brushing teeth

Choosing lunch foods wisely

Practicing good sportsmanship

Aware of defective sight and hearing

Concerned with minor cuts and bruises

Curious about disease prevention

Beginning to develop some group responsibility, and are adjusting quite well to school.

The primary grade curriculum in health is designed to help children meet a number of health problems of the moment. This is presented not in great detail, but in the manner of an orientation so that a firm foundation may be laid for the more advanced curriculum content in the intermediate grades. The big teaching task is to arouse curiosity, promote questions and lead pupils to give expression to their thinking.

The teaching areas common to most primary school situations may be seen by reviewing current courses of study. Opinions of health curriculum specialists are also valuable. In the Massachusetts health education study it was found that the popular primary level topics were accident prevention, cleanliness and grooming, dental health, and rest and sleep.[14] Two additional examples of content areas follow:

---

[14]Massachusetts Department of Education. *Health Education in Massachusetts Public Schools: A Summary Report*. Boston: Department of Education, 182 Tremont Street. August 1971, p. 20.

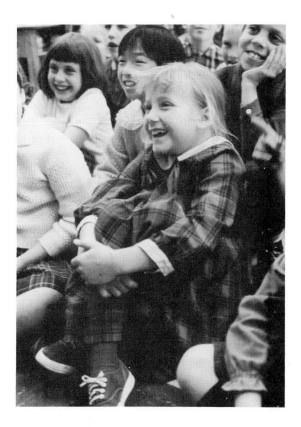

Figure 7–4 A "surprise" activity stimulates everyone. (Courtesy National Education Association and Joe Di Dio.)

ANDERSON[15]

Physical Health
    Personal and school cleanliness
    Rest and sleep
    Eating practices
    Posture
    Play practices
    Dental health
    Lighting
    Common cold
    Safety to and from school
    Schoolroom safety
    Playground safety
    Home safety
    Body growth
Mental Health
    Sharing
    Working together
    Kindness
    Being friendly
    Orderliness
    Depending on ourselves
    Attaining goals
Community Health
    Home life
    Sources of water and milk
    Sunshine and health

TURNER, SELLERY, SMITH[16]
    Cleanliness
    Hands and nails
    Teeth
    Nose and mouth
    Hair
    Elimination
    Clothing
    Food habits
    Table manners
    Play and exercise
    Sleep
    Communicable disease control
    Sanitation
    Harmful substances
    Growth and health
    Mental and emotional health
    Safety

---

[15]Anderson, C. L. *School Health Practice,* 4th ed., St. Louis: C. V. Mosby Co., 1971.
    [16]Turner, C. E., Sellery, C. Morley, and Smith, Sara Louise. *School Health and Health Education,* 6th ed. St. Louis: C. V. Mosby Co., 1970.

HEALTH TEACHING IN THE INTERMEDIATE GRADES

The health curriculum for the fourth, fifth, and sixth grade pupils is one that builds on what has already been taught in the first three grades. The teacher approaches the health topics more objectively. There is greater depth in subject matter and a little more formality than in the primary grades. *The sole reason for this change is that the pupils are ready for more detail.* Now their curiosity is aroused and they ask searching questions having more to do with the exception rather than the rule. They want to know, for example, why some man or woman of their acquaintance who never uses a toothbrush and eats haphazardly has such fine white teeth.

This is the age when the questions asked are often a real challenge to the teacher. It is a period in the growth of the nine, ten, and 11 year olds when there is a magnetic "awakening" to all that goes on around them. There is an adventurous spirit demonstrated by a willingness to try anything once, to look here and there, to explore eagerly. There is a heightened interest in science and machines—how bugs walk, what germs look like under the microscope, how the skeletal muscles hold up the body, and the effect a trip to the craters of the moon has on man in a rocket. Here is a time when dreamers begin to look ahead and imaginative minds are literally "on fire." Health stories of adventure, mystery, travel, science, sports, animal life, and nature go over big.

In addition to placing greater emphasis on the fundamental topics of the primary grade curriculum, there is a need for special instruction in alcohol and narcotics. By the fifth and sixth grade period a number of pupils, boys in particular, have a desire to try a cigarette or taste alcoholic beverages. Both of these items are readily available in many homes today. This is the age when the "gang" develops, and boys and girls begin to conform to the wishes of the group. The ten or eleven year old shows an increase in self-direction and responsibility. The "wise guy" has a cocky walk and the rounded shoulders of the "man about town." He is seen all too often a block from school flicking the ashes from his cigarette as he heads for home. He is ready for a realistic picture of smoking directly from a classroom discussion.

Sex antagonisms grow and become acute by the sixth grade. Boys are interested in boys; girls in girls. Both profit from instruction pertaining to family relationships. Although sex education really begins at home, little is said about it in many cases. It should be integrated with the total health education program at all grade levels. It should not be singled out for separate or undue emphasis. In back of the 11 year old pupil's sex antagonism is a smoldering interest in the subject. This is evidenced by the previously referred to Connecticut report, *Teach Us What We Want To Know.* It should be taught without apology by showing its nobility in terms of creative drive and family happiness.

Arriving at a list of major health topics for the intermediate grades can be ac-complished by viewing the listings of local schools and state education departments. Reports of professional organizations and independent research studies are sometimes helpful. A notable state that has developed and updated health curriculum guidelines and courses of study is New York. It shares top honors with Pennsylvania, Oregon, Washington and California. The New York curriculum was thoroughly researched and set up for grade levels in five strands (see Fig. 7-5): physical health, sociological health problems, mental health, environmental and community health, and education for survival. An examination of the strands indicates where the major subtopics fall. It may be seen that when there is planning for a full program there is opportunity for wide coverage of health problems and concerns. This does not occur countrywide. For instance, in the previously mentioned report, *Health Education in Massachusetts Public Schools*, it was pointed out that there were real omissions in the elementary grades in such areas as sex education and family living, venereal diseases, foot care, alcohol education, and non-com-

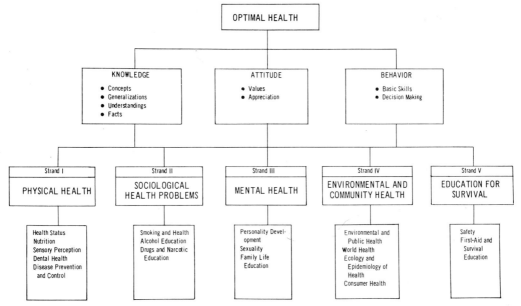

Figure 7-5 The five strands for health teaching. (Courtesy New York State Education Department.)

municable diseases. It was concluded that the updating of present health education programs had not kept pace with revisions in other subject matter areas. Moreover, there was too much emphasis on cleanliness and grooming from kindergarten through grade eight, with too much repetition relative to dental health, sleep and rest. It was also found that topics such as smoking, alcohol, drugs and family living were being held off until grade eight instead of being started by grade five at the latest. The Massachusetts guide is set up by areas somewhat like New York, while the Kansas breakdown is more traditional:

MASSACHUSETTS DEPARTMENT
OF EDUCATION

Area I *Physical Health*
  Body Structure and Function
  Cleanliness and Appearance
  Dental Health
  Fitness and Body Dynamics
  Nutrition
  Diseases and Disorders
  Sensory Perception
  Sleep, Rest, Relaxation
Area II *Mental and Social Health*
  Drugs, Alcohol and Tobacco
  Emotional Development
  Sexuality and Family Life
Area III *Consumer and Environmental Health*
  Ecology
  Health Careers
  Community and World Health
  Consumer Health
Area IV *Safe Living*
  First Aid and Emergencies
  Safety and Accident Prevention

KANSAS STATE DEPARTMENT
OF PUBLIC INSTRUCTION[17]

Nutrition
Disease control
Dental health

Alcohol, tobacco, narcotic drugs
Personal hygiene
Family living
Safety
First aid
Mental health
Community health

THE GRADUATED PROGRAM OF MAJOR HEALTH TOPICS

In view of recent curriculum research, it seems that the most appropriate health instruction curriculum for elementary school children is one that is spelled out in much more detail than the usual programs of the past. This means that teachers must get together and carefully plan for both scope and sequence in health teaching. Precisely, the major health topics or health areas for each grade level have to be established, along with a *graduated* list of knowledges and understandings (or concepts) to be achieved by pupils. This is not an easy task; it requires the combined deliberations of several top teachers frequently under the leadership of the elementary curriculum specialist and the health education coordinator for the school system.

In order to insure a graduated program under each major health topic, *all of the desirable knowledges, understandings, and behaviors should be recorded for all six elementary grades.* This extensive list is then reviewed and arranged in such a manner as to place the easier-to-learn items first and the difficult-to-learn items last. It is then carefully divided into six divisions according to grade level with the more detailed knowledges and understandings falling at the fourth, fifth, and six grades. This kind of order prevents important topics from being omitted and other topics from being taught at an inappropriate time.

The *major health topics* for the elementary school as determined for this text, are as follows: (P-Primary Grades; I-Intermediate Grades)

  1. Personal cleanliness and appearance (P, I)

[17]Division of Instructional Services. *Health Education K-12, Guide for Curriculum Development.* Kansas State Department of Public Instruction, 1967, pp. 13–23.

2. Physical activity, sleep, rest, and relaxation (P, I)

3. Nutrition and growth (P, I)

4. Dental health (P, I)

5. Body structure and operation (P, I)

6. Prevention and control of disease (P, I)

7. Safety and first aid (P, I)

8. Mental health (P, I)

9. Sex and family living education (P, I)

10. Environmental health (P, I)

11. Tobacco, alcohol, and drugs (I)

12. Consumer health (I)

Notice that the topics of Tobacco, alcohol, and drugs (No. 11) and Consumer health (No. 12) are introduced at the intermediate level.

By way of example, the graduated material is outlined for the dental health topic for each of the six grades. It is a brief selection of behavioral objectives to which other related behaviors may be added. Note that there is some overlapping, yet there is progression toward more difficult material. (See chart on the following page.)

It should be pointed out that planning for the first six grades must be done in terms of future junior and senior high school programming. In the above dental health example it is obvious that more technical knowledge and understanding is not called for here, but with this foundation the student is prepared for more detailed study in grades seven or eight. Moreover, a detailed structuring of knowledges, understandings, or concepts should be included in the finished curriculum guide or course of study.

ORGANIZING MAJOR HEALTH TOPICS

How does one organize the major health topics in the instructional program from grades one to six? Is each topic referred to each year? Is there a danger of too much repetition on a yearly basis? Is there merit in a cycle plan in which certain topics are omitted or simply reviewed every other year?

Certainly it has been the custom to have a considerable spread of information through the grades rather than a concentration at certain grade levels. Each major health topic has been taught at each grade level rather than being omitted at any grade level. Sometimes this insures healthy repetition and frequently acquaints the pupil with something that may have been missed the year before, especially in schools that do not follow a planned health instruction curriculum.

It is common knowledge that it is extremely difficult to keep from repeating too often what is said in the second grade to the children in the third grade. Health teaching may be more effective when there is a concentration of instruction on certain health topics on an every-other-year basis instead of spreading a limited amount through each of six or eight grades. Where the *total* elementary school health instruction program has been carefully planned there may be real value in such a cycle plan.

In the Brookline, Massachusetts schools health programs are maximized at certain key grade levels—kindergarten, four, five, and eight. Although other grades are partially ignored there appears to be a "spin off" and spread effect from one grade to another. Also, the feeling is that it is better to do an outstanding job at key developmental points in a child's life than to offer a number of shallow programs every year over the years.[18]

The cycle chosen may vary slightly for each major health topic. Almost all topics should be introduced in the first grade. It may be wise to introduce "nutrition and growth" to first and second grades, skip the third and continue in four and six. The same thing may be true in "safety." Obviously, there is much safety teaching to accomplish right away in the first three grades. Here, one might skip the fifth grade and proceed to the

---

[18]Aubrey, Roger F. "Health Education: Neglected Child of the Schools," *Journal of School Health*, 42:285–288, May 1972.

DENTAL HEALTH

STUDENT BEHAVIORAL OBJECTIVES
Grade One

Brushes teeth in proper fashion
Describes loss of first teeth and appearance of first 6-year molar

Grade Two

Uses toothpaste or powder correctly
Practices proper care and brushing of first teeth and can explain why
Distinguishes between proper care and improper care of toothbrush
Describes and shows how raw foods help keep teeth clean
Relates how sweets affect teeth
Expresses himself clearly on the value of regular dental care

Grade Three

Demonstrates ways the teeth may be cleaned without brushing
Identifies foods that build strong teeth
Relates in detail what the dentist does for children
Improves his appearance through cleaning own teeth and appreciates the reason
  why
Analyzes the several causes of toothache

Grade Four

Presents a clear description of the structure of the tooth
Identifies the several harmful effects of decayed teeth
Plays and works so as not to injure the teeth
Evaluates the importance of teeth for talking and digestion
Examines his own teeth for cavities and appearance

Grade Five

Describes tooth structure and relates it to function
Identifies malocclusion and tries to have something done about it
Distinguishes good dental health practices from poor practices
Is familiar with dental office instruments and their use
Makes a point to interest others in orthodontia when it appears to be necessary

Grade Six

Figures when himself and other sixth graders are apt to have a full set of second
  teeth
Appraises dentifrice advertisements in newspapers and other media
Assists the dental hygiene teacher or other health services personnel with younger
  children
Describes how decayed teeth may cause illness and a disturbance in other bodily
  processes.

(Turn to the Appendix for a graduated list of suggested student behavioral objectives for *each* of the major health topics, grades one to six. This may be employed
as a guide in building a course of study.)

Summary of Topics by Grades

	1	2	3	4	5	6
Nutrition and growth	x	x	R*	x	R	x
Personal cleanliness and appearance	x	R	x	R	x	R
Dental health	x	x	R	x	R	x
Accidents and safety	x	x	x	x	R	x
Mental health	x	R	x	R	x	R
Sex and family living education	x	R	x	R	x	R
Body structure and function	x	x	x	x	x	x
Disease control	x	R	x	R	x	R
Environmental health	x	x	R	x	R	x
Physical activity, sleep, rest, relaxation	x	x	x	x	R	x
Tobacco, alcohol, and drugs	•				x	x
Consumer health			x	R	x	R

*R = Review year (brief treatment of topic).

sixth. There is so much to cover in "body structure and function" that the topic might be spread through all six grades. In the planning stage, a chart would be constructed to reflect the organization.

This cycle plan seeks to get away from needless repetition—repetition that all too often is deadly, because it smothers curiosity and kills the interest of normally intelligent boys and girls. Frequently children are bored with lessons on such subjects as brushing the teeth, or standing tall, or something similar; they see nothing new, fresh, and stimulating. Much of this may be prevented when the major health topics are thoroughly covered on the "on" year and very simply reviewed on the "off" year.

UNIT TEACHING IN HEALTH

One of the most popular and often misused terms in education circles today is the "unit." Teachers loosely use the word, *unit*, to refer to a topic, an outline, a block of subject matter, a project, and even a chapter in a textbook. They divide and subdivide units at random and according to their own particular system of classification of instructional materials.

Most writers agree that a unit, whether for the teacher or the student, represents an organization of activities and information designed to develop useful understandings, appreciations and practices which will contribute favorably to educational goals. Ragan and Shepherd say:

"When this method is used, learning takes place through a great variety of activities; activities are unified around a central theme, problem or purpose . . .; and the teacher serves as a leader rather than as a taskmaster."[19]

If a health unit stays within these definitions, one can hardly question its value. It begins with the health needs and interests of children who, with the help of the teacher, create and arrange an environment out of which will grow the purpose and enthusiasm for the work to be undertaken. Health units cut across subject-matter lines, thereby providing for integration. They furnish "grassroot" or first-hand experiences, and satisfy a number of innate drives to be active, to create, to dramatize, to communicate, and to construct. Lifelike opportunities in which the pupil may build something, experiment, read, share, interview, and express his ideas in various media are important parts of the units. The health unit centers in the

[19]Ragan, William B., and Shepherd, Gene D. *Modern Elementary Curriculum*, New York: Holt, Rinehart, and Winston, Inc., 1971, p. 190.

present but stimulates an interest in future living. Early in its framework it encourages pupil discovery. Meaning is given to factual material when a unit requires problem-solving. Democratic group living is encouraged as desirable social habits are developed while children work on committees and in groups. Moreover, unit teaching stimulates critical thinking. It is rich in opportunities for children with varying degrees of ability and capacity to work along with others toward the success of the unit.

The Teacher's Resource Unit

A resource unit is simply a collection of suggested learning activities and materials organized around some central theme or given topic to be used by the teacher in preplanning. Often a resource unit in health is the product of a committee of teachers pooling their best ideas and then assigning to one teacher the responsibility of organizing the materials and to another the final writing. School nurses, dental hygienists, and even physicians may sit in and help with the unit. These units need not be complex or involved. They may be developed locally or at the state level. In either case they are not units of instruction but are chiefly collections of ideas and materials which may be helpful to an individual teacher in planning her work for the class.

It is worth repeating that the resource unit, no matter how complete, is not a teaching unit; it is strictly an aid to help the teacher and her students in planning a teaching unit. It usually is organized with a title and grade level designation, an introductory statement, a statement of proposed objectives, a content guide, suggested pupil activities, a list of teaching aids — books, pamphlets, music records, and films, and suggested evaluation procedures.[20]

Resource units in health may be built for a separate health course. Sometimes they are built to fit a broadfields or core curriculum. They contribute to the core of a curriculum built around social living or science. This is sometimes thought of as a unit where there is a fusion of subject matter as part of the *integrating* experience which the unit provides. Certainly integration is desirable in health teaching. Children do not put knowledge in categories and classify it the way scholars do; life situations seldom fall within these artificial boundaries. The specialist in health education can be very helpful here in assisting core teachers. A number of classroom teachers will want to turn to the health educator for professional help in setting up units complete with problems to be studied, bibliographies for both pupils and teachers, and suggestions for school and community activities.

The Health Teaching Unit

The essential difference between a teacher's resource unit and a teaching unit involves purposes. The purpose of a resource unit is to give the teacher a well fortified background in a particular area of study. In the teaching unit the organization is in terms of a given class. It is not nearly as broad and inclusive as the resource unit, it includes only those activities, materials, and evaluation techniques that will actually be used. Thus it is quite realistic and practical both in terms of time available and the nature of the learner. Where a number of stories, films, and suggested activities appear in the resource unit, in the teaching unit the second grade teacher might read only one story, carry out two projects, and show one film.

Some planning of a teaching unit has to be done by the teacher in advance of meeting the class. Then the pupils are given a chance to select activities. They may examine or be given a choice of activities that appear in the resource unit. Those that seem to arouse enthusiasm may be selected for the teaching unit. This unit is then ready to implement.

---

[20]Klausmeier, Herbert J., and Dresden, Katherine. *Teaching in the Elementary School*, 2nd ed. New York: Harper & Brothers, 1962. Chapter 5.

Needless to say, when pupils share in the planning of their own work in health they have greater retention of what they learn. Activities tend to be vital and are more apt to promote new health habits and appreciations. This is modern education at its best.

There is a difference in emphasis in health teaching between the primary and intermediate grades. It influences the building of the teaching unit. Health education in the primary grades is centered on helping children to live healthfully at home and at school. Much health is taught incidentally, indirectly, and informally in an effort to put across elementary health concepts and simple health practices. It would be very easy, therefore, for the teacher to "overorganize" the teaching unit in the kindergarten and first three grades. A few "tried and proven" ideas or activities may well make up the major part of the unit. Obviously, during the planning stages of a unit, children come up with suggestions that are both excellent and impracticable. Through proper manipulation of the planning session the teacher guides the boys and girls into agreeing on the better suggestions. Evidence abounds in the primary grades to show that young, creative, and dramatic minds have imaginations that at times run wild. Gently curbing this wonderful quality, without at the same time reducing enthusiasm, is what makes teaching an art as well as a challenging profession.

Health teaching in the intermediate grades tends to be more specific, more formal, and generally planned in relation to broad areas of experience. Teaching units, therefore, are often constructed as subunits or integrated units of the broader field. Although they should not attempt to cover too much material in any one health area, nevertheless, it is difficult sometimes to strictly limit them. This is because health, in its fullest meaning, relates to physical, mental, emotional and social welfare. Practically everything that affects man may in some large or small way be connected to health teaching.

Organization of Health Teaching Units

There are a number of ways to organize the teaching unit. Basically it needs some kind of introduction followed by objectives, a main body of activities, source materials, and finally some reference to evaluation.

Teaching units are generally organized along specific lines. This crystalizes the thinking of teachers and pupils. Klausmeier and Dresden use the same form that was employed in the resource unit. Various writers and educational groups have their differences and similarities in unit arrangements, but the similarities seem to outweigh the differences.

As a rule, the following outline is satisfactory for the development of teaching units for the major health topics:
1. Title
2. Introductory statement
3. Concepts and behavorial objectives
4. Outline of Content (Primary Level) (Intermediate Level)
5. Suggested learning activities
6. Resource aids and materials
7. Evaluation techniques
8. Student and teacher references

An example of an especially detailed presentation dealing with a major health topic is taken from the guide of the New York State Education Department.[21] The strands and topics have already been mentioned. (See Fig. 7–5.)

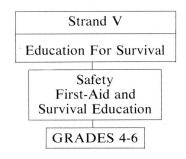

---

[21]The State Education Department Strand V *Education For Survival (First Aid and Survival Education)*, Grades 4-6, Albany, New York: The State Education Department, 1971.

Outline of Content	Major Understandings and Fundamental Concepts	Suggested Teaching Aids and Learning Activities	Supplementary Information for Teachers
I. Introduction to First Aid	First aid involves immediate temporary care and not treatment.	What is first aid? What is the difference between first aid and treatment?	
A. Definition	First aid is the immediate and temporary care given to an injured or sick person until the services of a physician can be obtained.		
B. Values of first aid training	Having knowledge of first aid will give the student a feeling of some competency to care for himself and others and will serve to make him aware of preventable safety problems.		The pupil can care for his own injuries and the injuries of others. He is helped to improve his safety consciousness which aids in the prevention of accidents. First aid can be extremely valuable during catastrophes such as wars, floods, hurricanes, earthquakes, and tornadoes.
C. General procedures to follow in first aid emergencies	The first aider should function in a logical and systematized way rather than in a state of panic and disorganization.	Describe several accident situations and discuss with pupils the general first aid procedures that should be followed in each case.	Factors that should be considered include: determining the victim's injuries; determining what injuries should be dealt with first; getting the victim's name and address; carrying out the determined procedures; securing necessary help; protecting victim from further harm; psychological reassurance for the victim; dealing with external factors of weather, traffic, crowds, etc.
	Learn the meaning of panic.	Example: A man has just been hit by a car. He is lying in the street and a large crowd is beginning to form around him. As a first aider, what would you do to help this man?	
		Point out that securing necessary help is vital. Call for professional help as soon as possible.	The following bibliographical sources may be checked for further information: Cole, pp. 1–16, and Henderson, pp. 34–56
		Show McGraw-Hill film *Your Responsibilities In First Aid.* An introductory film also may be shown, such as the American Red Cross films, *Checking For Injuries* and the *How and Why of First Aid.*	
		Discuss the consequences that might occur if it were proven that a first aider did something that further injured the victim.	It is best to summon medical help immediately and keep the victim comfortable.
		Panic can be worse or as bad as an injury. Keep yourself and the injured person calm. Encourage others to do the same. Discuss possible injurious results of panic. Act out in simple skits.	A first aider might find himself in a lawsuit if he negligently and carelessly administered first aid which resulted in injuries or aggravation of the original injury.
		If an injured person is found unconscious keep him lying on his side so	See bibliography: Gold and Gold: "First Aid and Legal Responsibility."

Table continued.

Outline of Content	Major Understandings and Fundamental Concepts	Suggested Teaching Aids and Learning Activities	Supplementary Information for Teachers
		that his tongue does not fall back in his mouth to choke him.	
D. First aid kits and materials	First aid kits *should* be available in situations where accidents are likely to occur. Very often the first aider must improvise with available materials.	Have several kits available to show to pupils. Show and discuss the contents of each kit. Have pupils report on first aid supplies they have in their homes. Have the pupils make first aid kits for the home, car, and one for camping trips. Wooden boxes 8″ × 5″ × 2″ may be constructed to house these kits. Make a list of possible kit items and discuss this list with your school's nurse teacher. Discuss materials that might be available when there is no first aid kit for supplies.	Contents of kits usually include adhesive compresses, bandage compresses, plain gauze pads, gauze roller bandages, eye dressing packets, plain absorbent cotton, triangular bandages, tweezers, and scissors, antiseptic soap, aspirin, elastic bandage 3″ wide, and safety pins.
II. Wounds and the Control of Minor Bleeding		It is vital to keep wounds clean. Wash with soap and water if possible.	First aid for wounds varies according to the nature and possible results of each.

(This is only the first part of the guide—pages 1–3, out of 39 pages.)

SIGNIFICANT HEALTH CURRICULUM TRENDS

If there is any one over-all trend in health curriculum planning it is to teach health through a variety of experiences in a broad and flexible program. There are other trends:

1. The health curriculum is not limited to the activity and four walls of the classroom. It moves about the building. Primary grade children discuss playground accidents out where they might occur. Sixth graders visit the local sanitation department; they talk with restaurant owners about food handling and dishwashing practices. The health curriculum is practical.

2. There is increasing emphasis on the manner in which principles and objectives influence the curriculum.

3. The health curriculum is being revised continually by classroom teachers working together with health services personnel, supervisors, and parents. Health needs change, and teachers are becoming more flexible in their teaching. They are more alert to the values of cooperative planning for health.

4. Health in the school is integrated with health in the community through the curriculum and teaching methods. Elementary teachers are learning more about their community health programs and agencies that can enrich their own health instruction.

5. Provision is being made in more schools for formal, direct teaching of health in the elementary curriculum.

6. Health curriculum aids, such as bulletins, courses of study, and the state syllabus, are considered only as suggested guides for the teacher. The teacher must be sufficiently oriented to

the modern elementary school purposes and instructional methods to be able to choose wisely those activities best adapted to the health learning situation in her classroom.

7. Because of the impact of advertising and quackery, a sharper evaluation is being made of health services and products.

8. The school nurse is more than ever an important member of the school health teaching team.

9. Sex and Family Living Education is being introduced in more elementary school health education programs.

10. There is slowly emerging a unified approach to health teaching in which all major health topics are properly considered instead of singling out one or two urgent topics (such as drugs and smoking) for special attention. There are fewer "one shot" assembly programs as token gestures of a health education program.

As indicated in a national committee report, elementary schools desperately need a school health coordinator, a designated, interested, and well-qualified faculty member who is responsible for the efficient operation of the health education program.

Team Teaching

A number of approaches to defining the functions of the elementary school teacher are being tried. One of these which has had an early success in Davidson County, Tennessee, and Lexington, Massachusetts, is *team teaching*. Here, an instructional team—free from the record-keeping clerical duties, teaches children in large or small groups or individually according to the nature of the subject matter. This arrangement, for example, makes it possible for all sections of an entire third grade to assemble for one type of lesson such as a superb film, a special lecture, or a speech by an outstanding resource person. Classroom teachers especially interested and talented in a phase of health may handle certain parts of the instructional program while others are free to develop new teaching materials or work with individual pupils.

The health curriculum lends itself to this kind of teaching. Although the large group will meet, often to introduce a unit of work, it is the medium group in which the bulk of the teaching is regularly done, so that teachers can have a continuing relationship with the same children over a period of time. The small group is especially valuable for carrying out vital discussions of health problems of interest to the age group. Also, there is ample room for individual tutoring within the school. Finally, to use the words of Mallan and Hersh, there should be "no GODs in the classroom" when this kind of teacher-student activity occurs. In fact, the "Giver Of Directions" should be a thing of the past.[22]

In one large school in a suburb of Rochester, New York, all of the fourth grades studied a unit on digestion under team teachers. Working in small groups, each student posed questions that were placed on a large chart in the classroom and were subsequently answered. The team teachers found the approach challenging because children of various levels of ability could be reached. Moreover, the children enjoyed the format and greater flexibility that allowed for a more individualized instruction. The more able students acquired a sizable amount of information, as evidenced by their sophisticated reports and high test scores. However, as Polos suggests, there is no magic in team teaching, but in the light of many experiments it is effective in improving instruction.[23]

The Self-Contained Classroom

About three-fourths of all schools group students according to grade level in self-contained classrooms. The teacher gets to know the students well and has a chance to employ flexible grouping within the classroom. A well-prepared teacher can teach health effec-

---

[22]See *No G.O.D.'s In The Classroom* by John T. Mallan and Richard Hersh, Philadelphia: W. B. Saunders Company, 1972.

[23]Polos, Nicholas C. *The Dynamics of Team Teaching*. Dubuque, Iowa: William C. Brown Co., 1965.

tively this way. In several places there is a health specialist, along with the music, art, and physical education specialists, who comes into the classroom to give a lesson.

Non-graded Classes

A number of large school systems are currently using a non-graded sequence in at least some elementary schools. In this arrangement grade levels are removed from some or all classes, and the children who would normally be in these classes are placed in the non-graded sequence. This occurs mostly in the primary grades. Each pupil works according to his ability — beginning the new school year where he left off the year before.

Those who favor this organization point out that the pressure is off the pupils, and material is better understood. There is also an opportunity for more continuity in learning experiences. One of the limitations of non-graded plans is the burden on the teacher to follow individual pupil progress. Another limitation has to do with parents who need much help to understand and work with the plan.

Because of the built-in flexibility, the non-graded class seems to be a good place to try new ideas that may make health education more dynamic. Micro-unit work is an example. This is a technique of weaving (integrating) health education content into a topic the students are already studying. For example, disease rates can be integrated with arithmetic, and nutrition can be worked into the social studies unit dealing with far-away cultures in other lands. The micro-unit has been very well received in the Novato, California elementary schools. Four units: "The Waves Rolled and the Ship Creaked — Health Conditions on the Mayflower"; "Puritan Land of Plenty — Food and Medicine in Colonial America"; "Sugar and Spice and the F.D.A."; and "Into the Valley of Death — The State of Medicine at Valley Forge" were highly successful.[24]

---

[24]Feldstein, M., and Swabb, L. "The Use of the Micro-Unit in Health Education," *Journal of School Health,* 42:105–107, February 1972.

Alternative Schools

In an effort to get away from the stultifying climate of so many public schools, close to 1000 "alternative" schools have been born. Some last a week or two and others have been operating much longer. Founders of such schools, influenced greatly by the writings of Kozol, Holt, Glasser and others, seek an education for children that is unregimented; alive with flexible teachers; and a fertile climate for learning because of sympathetic administrators. Teaching groups are small, and what is taught appears unconventional only because it doesn't take the usual subject matter form. When health conditions and practices are referred to it is usually done in an integrated fashion with other kinds of information.

Alternative schools get started easier in the ghetto community than elsewhere, for the simple reason that student failure is clearly visible over prolonged periods and the frustrated parent seeks options — options which provide a quality education. Numerous educators feel that the well-managed public school should provide these options — and in each school building at every educational level. In short, alternative ways to educate should be available everywhere in public education — programmed learning, Montessori classrooms, community-oriented projects, non-graded sections, multi-cultural arrangments, etc., to supplement and compliment traditional models.

Compensatory Education

The health problems of the disadvantaged are such that education for them should be different — not so much in terms of subject content, but in terms of teaching emphasis. In their writings Gentry, Jones and others make it clear that because there are disadvantaged and culturally handicapped children a variety of misdirected programs have been created to get at the problem — based primarily on the proposition that ghetto children need "compensatory," "special," "catch-up," or "head start" programs.[25] The authors claim that the assumption that compensatory education will clear up the difficulties is a myth. The assumption leads to *lowered expectations* and thereby results in lower educational successes. Children of the blacks and other minority groups and the poor are shortchanged because less is expected of them as "disadvantaged" people. What is really needed is a teaching approach that is as vigorous as it would be with so-called normal children, and void of defeatist attitudes. There would be no need for compensatory types of education, says Shane, if a *curriculum continuum* was introduced into school systems — "an unbroken flow of experiences planned with and for the individual learner" throughout his total school years.[26] All health and other learning experiences would be personalized and individualized, and middle class values would not be brought somewhat abruptly to lower class children and youth.

Decentralization of Schools

When this occurs in the larger city school systems it permits parents and local agencies in new districts to directly affect the total educational program. From a health education viewpoint there is an opportunity to devise programs which meet local health and safety environmental conditions and child needs. If health problems are critical — such as drug abuse or poor nutrition among Hispanic children — a district can increase its distribution of funds spent for prevention. From the New York City experience there is reason to hope that as local groups take a greater interest in the schools the positive relationship between decentralization and successful education will be verified.

Differentiated Staffing

Instead of having groups of children assigned to a teacher in a traditional way, a "differentiated staff" is formed where there might be 160 children in a class with two senior teachers, two staff teachers, and four teaching assistants or aides. It is a team teaching effort which attempts to accommodate the many learning styles of children with different instructional approaches. The teacher becomes an "instructional manager" and resource person, and not a "giver of directions." From a health curriculum viewpoint there is hardly a limit to what might be planned for pupils of various backgrounds and needs. Differentiated staffing anticipates the introduction of new personnel into the instructional process. Resource people from the health professions and health-related areas of the community are worked into programs in a meaningful way. Currently, there is little to report relative to the successes of differentiated staffing in advancing understandings and practices relative to health education. Cooper offers some ideas and potential values to be obtained, but for the most part this kind of organization for teaching is yet to be proved.[27]

Other Aspects of the Health Curriculum

The Emphasis on Physical Activity

The role of exercise in the health of the individual has long been recognized. In recent years it has become a very popular school activity due primarily to the age of automation, the era of the overfed, overprotected and underactive child. Thus teachers of health should seek to cooperate with physical education instructors so that the vigorous physical activity in the gymnasium or on the playground may be related to such items as weight, diet, fatigue, personal cleanli-

[25]Gentry, Altron, Jones, Byrd, et al. *Urban Education: The Hope Factor*. Philadelphia: W. B. Saunders Company, 1972, pp. 12–14.

[26]Shane, Harold G. "A Curriculum Continuum: Possible Trends in the 70's," in *Curriculum: Quest for Relevance* (William VanTil, editor). Boston: Houghton-Mifflin, 1971, p. 211.

[27]Cooper, James A. *Differentiated Staffing.* Philadelphia: W. B. Saunders Company, 1972.

ness, and general well-being as taught in the classroom.

Where there are no special physical education teachers it will be necessary for classroom teachers to teach the games, dances, stunts, and exercises themselves. Carefully planned activities are effective in raising individual pupil physical fitness. This has been ably demonstrated by the President's Council on Physical Fitness and Sports. Where ongoing programs exist failures on tests of physical fitness are around 25 per cent or less, but where there has been no previous program of physical education the test failure rate runs around 45 to 55 per cent. Professional leadership in physical education, therefore, is helpful in building a better health program in the elementary school.

THE SCHOOL LUNCH PROGRAM

In many schools today a special, and somewhat formal effort is made to improve the nutritional status of children, while at the same time increasing their knowledge and appreciation of foods, through the school lunch program.

In 1946 Congress enacted the National School Lunch Program as a "measure for national security, to safeguard the health and well being of the nation's children, and to encourage the domestic consumption of nutritious agricultural commodities and other foods." The program was amended in late 1970 to put more emphasis on school feeding of children of the identified poor. This program is carried on today on a nonprofit basis without physical segregation or other discriminations by the school against any child because of his inability to pay the full cost or any part of the cost of the meals.

A school plan with such worthy objectives as these certainly cannot go unnoticed as a means of further implementing the health instruction program. One cannot dismiss the educational implications of an activity that serves over two billion lunches to millions of children. Surveys,

however, indicate that school personnel are not capitalizing on the opportunities inherent in the school lunch situation and little is said about the school lunch as a learning laboratory.

The school lunch offers a place to teach diet and food practices in their natural setting, making the lunch program an educational operation rather than a business function. Here, boys and girls may learn to be self-sufficient, to make decisions, and to spend their money wisely. There are meals to plan and serve, sanitation to be considered, and numerous chances to promote climates favorable to appetite, to growth, and to mental-emotional health. There are few total school activities so conducive to a practical, down-to-earth kind of teaching as that afforded by the school lunch operation. This is a real-life situation where the teacher can find in a single lunchroom an assortment of eating patterns—from the plate lunch to the à la carte lunch; from the home lunch supplemented with school lunch items to the all too typical lunch with the weak combination of a jelly sandwich and a piece of cake.

Beginning in the primary grade classroom with the study of foods, the teacher encourages her class to share their thoughts relative to school lunch menu planning. The planning, especially in the third grade and above, may begin with a school survey of current dietary practices or a study of the components of a well-balanced lunch as a part of the total daily diet. Other ideas include the following:

Discussions may be directed toward overcoming food dislikes. Foods left on the trays may provide a basis for such a study.

New foods may be accompanied by a class discussion on the values of the foods and ways of acquiring a taste for them.

Assisting with the serving of lunches gives pupils a first-hand opportunity to learn about proper sanitary practices.

Help in the preparation of food and cleaning up the lunchroom after the meal may be arranged. Where this is done, pupils should be rotated so that all have an equal chance.

Survey the school lunch facilities and consider ways of implementing their findings.

Observe the social graces. Take turns as hosts and hostesses. This is a social hour for pupils and teachers. It is pleasant and enjoyable—a tonic to learning.

Where proper studies have been conducted, the school lunch has proved to be an effective medium for developing good eating practices—a fact that has been sustained throughout the school year. However, the nutritional status of children on school feeding programs does not always improve. This was found to be true in the Paige study.[28] This lack of success was attributed to high rates of absenteeism among nutritionally disadvantaged children, incomplete consumption of lunch, and poor nutritional reinforcement at home.

Perhaps the biggest difficulty in the school lunch program has been with the children who bring lunches from home. Many schools and homes have cooperated to improve the homepacked lunch. In Petaluma, California, for example, the school health council and local PTA got together, established the nature of the problem through a city-wide survey, cooperatively prepared a *Guide to Home-Packed School Lunches*, and took steps to revise the health curriculum to integrate this nutrition work into the classroom situation.[29]

In Long Beach, New York, a very complete booklet entitled *For Your Children at Lunchtime* was developed by the PTA for parents. The school health council and classroom teachers assisted.

[28]Paige, David M. "The School Feeding Program: An Underachiever," *Journal of School Health*, 42:392–395, September 1972.

[29]Manning, W. R., and Olsen, L. R. "Home and School Cooperate to Enrich the Home-Packed School Lunch," *Journal of School Health*, 32:87–89, February 1962.

QUESTIONS FOR DISCUSSION

1. Bloom, Hastings and Madaus have written at length on the structuring of objectives in education so that adequate evaluations can be made after learning activities have taken place (see *Selected References*). How might this kind of information be used wisely in planning a new elementary school health curriculum?

2. What is the relationship between health knowledge and health attitudes? How does this relationship affect the planning of unit activities? Give an example to illustrate this.

3. Because of its high drop-out rate, teaching has been called a profession of low commitment. Many people undergo training for teaching, but few make a career of it. Cooper feels that this may be due to personal disappointment with the first teaching experiences (see Cooper in *Selected References*). Differentiated staffing may have an answer to this concern. What are your comments?

4. As a humanist Joseph Wood Krutch felt that the school curriculum should provide more opportunities for social intercourse that would foster mental health. Comment on how this can be planned for in the local elementary school.

5. From what you have been able to observe, what are some of the needed improvements in elementary school health programs?

6. List several ways of achieving both scope and sequence in planning a health education curriculum. Also list the references on curriculum development that you consulted.

SUGGESTED ACTIVITIES

1. John Goodlad points out that "health has never been a clearly defined study in our schools." Ask two or three elementary classroom teachers how they feel about this statement. Is it generally true of generally false? And what is the reasoning behind the answer?

2. Recently curriculum changes have been more widespread and intensive than at any time in the history of American schools. One should ask if the curriculum changes are really significant. Do children learn better in the new programs than they did in the old? Suggest several means of finding out how valuable certain curriculum changes are in a school.

3. Through small committee action, survey several school lunch programs at the elementary level to ascertain where the educational influences come in. Relate this to the findings of David Paige as reported in the article referred to in this chapter.

4. Read some of the material that has been written about the advantages of differentiated staffing. From the point of view of health instruction does it seem to be more or less practical to teach by this method or the method frequently employed in the self-contained classroom unit? Support your answer with appropriate references to the literature on the topic.

5. Formulate your own list of concepts suitable for a grade of your choice which pertains to one of the major health topics. Examine several curriculum guides before putting your list in final form.

6. Select one of the following topics and prepare a resource unit for use in a primary grade of your choice:
   a. Safety
   b. Dental health
   c. Sleep, rest, and relaxation
   d. Communicable disease control

7. Visit the college library and look over a number of curriculum guides in health education. List some of the ways they differ and some of the ways in which they are similar.

SELECTED REFERENCES

Bair, Medill, and Woodward, Richard G. *Team Teaching in Action.* New York: Harcourt, Brace & World, 1966.

Bloom, Benjamin S., Hastings, J. Thomas, and Madaus, George F. *Handbook on Formative and Summative Evaluation of Student Learning.* New York: McGraw-Hill Book Company, 1971.

Bruner, Jerome. *Toward a Theory of Instruction.* Cambridge, Mass.: Belknap Press of Harvard University, 1966.

Cooper, James A. *Differentiated Staffing.* Philadelphia: W. B. Saunders Co., 1972.

Darrow, Helen F. "Conceptual Learning." *Childhood Education,* 287–288, February 1965.

Ebel, R. L. "Behavioral Objectives: A Close Look." *Phi Delta Kappan, 52*:171–173, November 1970.

Fast, Charles G. "Comprehensive School Health Education." *School Health Review, 3*:34–35, September–October 1972.

Goodlad, John I. *School Curriculum and the Individual.* New York: Blaisdell Publishing Company, 1967.

Hillson, Maurie. *Change and Innovation in Elementary School Organization.* New York: Holt, Rinehart, & Winston, Inc., 1971.

Kilander, H. Frederick. *School Health Education.* 2nd ed. New York: The Macmillan Company, 1968, Chapters 12 and 16.

King, Arthur R. J., and Brownell, John A. *The Curriculum and the Disciplines of Knowledge.* New York: John Wiley & Sons, 1967.

Krutch, Joseph Wood. "A Humanist's Approach." *Phi Delta Kappan, 52*:376–378, March 1970.

Lehman, Edna S., Schumacher, Corrine, and Vitek, Mildred. "The Conceptual Approach to Health Education." *Journal of Health, Physical Education, and Recreation, 38*:32–35, February 1967.

MacDonald, J. B. and Wolfson, B. J. "A Case Against Behavioral Objectives." *Elementary School Journal,* December 1970, pp 119–128.

Means, Richard K. "The School Health Education Study: A Pattern in Curriculum Development." *Journal of School Health, 36*:1–11, January 1966.

Nagel, Charles. "A Behavioral Objectives Approach to Health Instruction." *Journal of School Health, 60*:255–258, May 1970.

Oberteuffer, Delbert, Harrelson, Orvis A., and Pollack, Marion B. *School Health Education,* 5th ed. New York: Harper and Row, 1972, Chapters 2 and 4.

Phenix, Phillip H. *Realms of Meaning.* New York: McGraw-Hill Book Company, 1964.

Plesent, Emanuel. "Kindergarten Through Twelfth Grade Curriculum in Three Weeks." *Journal of School Health, 38*:113–115, February 1968.

Purpel, David E. and Belanger, Maurice. *Curriculum and the Cultural Revolution.* Berkeley, Calif.: McCutchan Publishing Corporation, 1972.

Ragan, William B. and Shepherd, Gene D. *Modern Elementary Curriculum.* New York: Holt, Rinehart & Winston, 1971, Chapters 6 and 14.

Sliepcevich, Elena M. "School Health Education Study: Appraisal of a Conceptual Approach to Curriculum Development." *Journal of School Health, 36*:145–153, April 1966.

Van Til, William. *Curriculum: Quest for Relevance.* Boston: Houghton Mifflin Co., 1971.

Willgoose, Carl E. "Saving the Curriculum in Health Education." *Journal of School Health, 42*:108–112, March 1973.

Woodruff, Asahel D. "The Use of Concepts in Teaching and Learning." *Journal of Teacher Education, 20*:81–99, March 1964.

IMPLEMENTING THE HEALTH CURRICULUM

8

*We can start releasing the nation's self-educational energies . . .
by building new learning environments and offering enough of
a variety of learning experiences to do justice to the diversity
of American learners.*[1]

—Paul Ylvisaker

There is no clearer way to call attention to the need for a diversity of student experiences than that which has been stated above by the dean of the Harvard School of Education. It is a straightforward pronouncement relative to the implementation of educational programs, and applies as much to health teaching as it does to social studies or language arts. Acknowledged here is the fact that *there is an educational need to nourish the dissimilarities, variations, and pluralism of modern life.* To think otherwise is to invite further restrictions on individual growth, and emphasize conformity and discipline—both of which retreat from creative individualism that is required to survive in a multidimensional society.

IMPLEMENTATION—THE BIG WORD

If indeed the educational need *is* to offer "a variety of experiences" in order to prepare youth for the diversified culture, then the process of implementation takes on greater meaning.

Coming from the Latin *implere,* the word implementation means to fill up or finish. It is associated with such words as fulfill, accomplish, carry out, and complete. It relates to getting somewhere by putting plans into action through the careful selection of learning activities, the variety of student experiences which get at things to think about and try, together with pertinent resources and aids. The work implementation is an all-encompassing term which ultimately gets at the roots of the curriculum by answering the old question of "*how* to do" in education. It is a term which makes methodology practical; and in this chapter it is spelled out by a wide variety of school-community tested learning activities designed to challenge the diversity of learners by providing something that should capture the imagination.*

The view that the program of health activities at any grade level should be a

---

[1]Ylvisaker, Paul V. "Beyond '72: Strategies for Schools," *Saturday Review, 55*:33–35, November 11, 1972.

---

*Chapter 9 will provide a more thorough discussion of methodology, in terms of both student behaviors and teaching techniques.

broad and varied one can be supported—not only on the basis of a pluralistic society—but on the firm understanding that children differ widely in their personal interests, and need to be able to make choices in a school setting. In such fashion sooner or later everyone will discover something that he likes very much. That which is liked is apt to be more successful when undertaken.

As teachers and health coordinators work together to prepare interesting content for a major health topic, they have to keep in mind that the selection of learning activities to be engaged in has to be carefully chosen from an ever-growing list of ideas and activities embracing a great many facts and concepts. With such a wide variety of possibilities and a limited amount of teaching time, *selection* becomes the essence of planning. The learning activities selected must be so succinct and reasonably complete that they will serve to generate the kinds of student concepts that relate to total instructional content instead of isolated views and bits and pieces of information.

Although a number of research studies have been carried on relative to pupil interests, major health problems, the nature of the elementary school health curriculum, the major topics for elementary school study, and the particular knowledges and understandings for each grade, very little has been done regarding specific *teaching activities* in the major topical area of instruction. This has resulted in a conglomeration of activities and experiences under a particular topic, with or without reference to properly stated outcomes. Needless to say, every activity employed to teach a health topic, whether it be an experiment, a story play, a poster drawing, or an independent project, should contribute to the predetermined objectives, and be subject to periodic reappraisal.

SUGGESTED ACTIVITIES FOR MAJOR HEALTH TOPICS

A number of special health topics for elementary schoolchildren follow below. These topics are the ones that make up the health curriculum and were set forth in some detail in Chapter 7. In order to do justice to current courses of study and at the same time be complete, a total of 12 categories or topics are covered. They are (1) Personal Cleanliness and Appearance; (2) Physical Activity, Sleep, Rest, and Relaxation; (3) Nutrition and Growth; (4) Dental Health; (5) Body Structure and Operation; (6) Prevention and Control of Disease; (7) Safety and First Aid; (8) Mental Health; (9) Sex and Family Living Education; (10) Environmental Health; (11) Tobacco, Alcohol, and Drugs; and (12) Consumer Health. These topics have been set up separately as follows: *Comments* relative to instruction; *Behavioral objectives* for primary level and intermediate level students; *Suggested activities* for each elementary school level. The *Behavioral objectives* are samples of what might be developed at the local level. They are reasonably appropriate for the grade level. They tend to be more realistic in any community when developed by teachers themselves. The same can be said in part for the *Suggested activities*. The teacher should find them useful when considering how far to go with any one particular guide. Although primary grade children are quite different from intermediate graders as a group, there will be times when there is considerable overlapping of interest between children of different grades. More specifically, a precocious third grade child may be ready for a suggested experience or project suitable for the typical fifth grade class.

Another reason for presenting a wide range of activities under each topic is that in many parts of the United States there are schools administratively set up in such a way that one teacher may teach one or more grades in one classroom. It is not uncommon in some areas to find combined grades, such as second and third or fourth and fifth. In some places there are non-graded schools where the teacher has a class made up of several grades. In such a situation a great amount of attention is given to individual pupil differences, and boys and girls make progress in their subjects more or less at their own rate of development and often without the pressure to complete a specified quantity of work in any one year.

The activities suggested for the primary and intermediate grades are not all-inclusive nor are they offered as ideals or "musts" in any way. They are simply a collection of appropriate experiences for a particular category of health instruction. No teacher will carry out all of the suggestions, but she may use those most applicable to her particular grade. Practically all of the activities have been tried in one school or another and found to be worthwhile in promoting a greater understanding of health. Many of them are suitable for initiating a unit of study. When employed with appropriate questions, they contribute to the discovery method of instruction. Obviously, depending on local circumstances or local teachers, some of the activities are better than others in their tendency to change behavior and promote acceptable health practices and attitudes.

In using this suggested material, *keep these points in mind*: (1) the effectiveness of the activities will be increased after a review of the chapters on methods and materials; (2) evaluation techniques (Chapter 12) will help measure the worth of the activities selected; and (3) sources of materials to accompany these activities (films, filmstrips, charts, posters, pamphlets, and stories for children) should be used. These are listed in detail in Chapter 11.

1. PERSONAL CLEANLINESS AND APPEARANCE

> **Behavioral Objectives* (Primary Level)**
>
> Explains why cleanliness and grooming are important to personal health and appearance.

---

*For a finer breakdown of behavioral objectives grade by grade see the Appendix. All of these are attainable pupil objectives which lend themselves to appraisal by the teacher.

> Demonstrates ability to wash the hands when necessary, use toilet facilities properly, brush teeth, keep clean, use the handkerchief, care for the clothing, comb the hair.
>
> Dresses appropriately for the climate and weather.

> **Behavioral Objectives (Intermediate Level)**
>
> Relates why clothing needs to be changed frequently, and in keeping with weather conditions.
>
> Distinguishes proper from improper practices of cleanliness related to food and eating.
>
> Explains the structure and function of the skin and the elimination of wastes through the skin.
>
> Describes the relationship between appearance and daily living, social success, and self-respect.
>
> Analyzes the several ways to assume personal responsibility for the maintenance of good health.

Comments

The child entering school is faced with the somewhat new idea of being responsible, more than ever before, for his personal cleanliness and appearance. As he progresses through the grades he grows in understanding the reason why cleanliness and grooming are important to personal health and appearance. He becomes aware of how cleanliness helps to prevent the spread of disease and how it makes him more acceptable to his classmates.

Although standards of cleanliness vary, most homes are equipped with the basic facilities for helping children keep clean. When children, through no fault of their own, fail to meet accepted standards of cleanliness or appearance, care should be taken not to humiliate them unintentionally.

In the intermediate grades cleanliness may be related to the prevention and control of disease. (Merely keeping clean for esthetic reasons will no longer hold attention.) After learning the characteristics of bacteria and their relationship to disease, the practice of keeping clean becomes more closely related to a real desire to preserve health. Cleanliness then becomes a social asset.

With the active aid of the students, cleanliness and neatness in the classroom can be achieved. With a little encouragement children take pride in the condition of their books, desks, and materials. The alert teacher recognizes that it is only a step from such individual accomplishments to the development of pride in the group. Such things as work tables, floors, blackboards, bulletin boards, the coat room, the toilet room, and lockers can become objects of group concern and of group action in keeping them clean and presentable. The NEA-AMA Joint Committee on School Health Problems clearly points out that "when a child feels that a desk is *his* desk and when children feel the classroom and everything in it is *their* classroom, they will act and react differently from times of stubbornness when they feel they must do certain things simply because they are told. Class lessons in cleanliness become important because of their personal application."[2]

*Suggested Activities**

Primary Level

1. Show the 7-minute film, *Health: The Dirt-Witch Cleans Up* (Encyclopedia Britannica Educational Corp.), which encourages younger children to enjoy bathing and developing regular routines of washing hands, faces, bodies, and hair. Then discuss differences between a bath and a shower. Ask: How do you *feel* after a bath?

2. Take turns dusting the room, books, bookcases, and arranging shelves and clothing racks.

3. Draw pictures illustrating taking a bath, washing clothes, ironing shirts, and cleaning fingernails. A first grade child can draw a meaningful picture of himself washing his face in the bathroom at home without much difficulty. Have several children illustrate their own story of cleanliness by holding their pictures up for all to see.

4. Discuss the different ways people take baths (full tub, wash tub, shower, sponge, or steam baths). Read the poem "After a Bath" by Aileen Fisher.

5. Visit the school nurse for a personal inspection. This may be quite rewarding, especially if done with a little advance planning.

6. Have the students demonstrate to the class the proper method of:
   a. Washing and drying hands
   b. Combing the hair and cleaning the hairbrush
   c. Covering coughs and sneezes
   d. Blowing the nose properly
   e. Drinking from a drinking fountain

7. Have a child bring his pet cat or dog to school and show the class how he brushes it and keeps it neat.

8. Appoint all class members as "Health Detectives." Before the weekend begins ask everyone to keep his eyes open on Saturday and Sunday and note what he can see involving the cleanliness and appearance of people, animals, buildings, roads, walks, lawns, and gardens. On Monday permit everyone to tell what he saw. This may be made more interesting by having the group make little cardboard badges which may be worn right away on Friday afternoon:

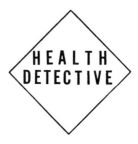

[2]National Education Association—American Medical Association. *Health Education*, 5th ed. Washington, D.C.: National Education Association, 1961.

*For an extensive listing of teaching aids and sources to be used with these and the following major health topic activities, see Chapter 11.

9. Talk about personal experiences such as falling in the mud, walking through mud puddles, or getting covered with paint. When is getting dirty fun? When is it unpleasant? Have you ever felt embarrassed or out of place because you were dirty?

10. Give each child a coat hanger for his clothes. Give each child a large number cut from a calendar. Play a game with numbers until each child can tell his own. Then he can paste it over the hook where he hangs his clothes.

11. Appoint a committee to prepare an exhibit of different types of clothes for different occasions. Work clothes, rubbers, raincoats, riding clothes, snowsuits, bathing suits are all designed for special purposes. Appoint another committee to collect various types of hats which express native customs, i.e., felt hat, cap, turban, straw hat, fez, fur hat, hood (applicable for third grade).

12. Create a classroom store and engage in buying and selling experiences which will help to provide a better understanding of the kinds of clothing best suited to health needs and appearance.

13. Talk about the protective covering of animals, fish, birds: the fur of the bear, fox, squirrel, raccoon; the feathers of the wild duck; the shells of clams and oysters; the bark of the trees.

14. Invite the school custodian to class to talk about how the school is kept safe and clean.

15. Construct a Health Check Wheel.

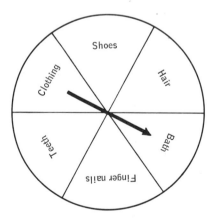

Use a wheel 20 inches in diameter. Use a brad to fasten an arrow to the middle of the wheel. Use pictures of health practices made by pupils or illustrations from magazines. Ask a pupil to spin the arrow to select a health practice to be checked for the day.

Intermediate Level

1. Raise questions about being careful in the use of certain cleaning solutions. Some products are harsh to the skin or highly flammable; some may damage the floor or furniture if spilled. List the cleaning solutions your mother keeps at home. Are any dangerous if used in the wrong way?

2. Discuss ways and means of making the classroom more attractive.

3. Examine the skin on the back of the hand with a magnifying glass. See the creases and folds when the hand is relaxed. See also the dirt which will disappear after washing (good for a fifth or sixth grade class). Have the class note the pores and tiny hairs. Discuss perspiration and body odors. Note oil and hair glands and tell what they do for the skin and one's appearance.

4. Have the class bring in pictures from magazines depicting how the skin works. Pictures, such as a man shivering from the cold or sweating from the noonday sun, or of a little boy burning his finger over the hot stove, are good examples. Magazine advertisements for beauty aids may also be discussed. Do the aids do everything the ads claim they do?

5. Discuss injuries to the skin which may affect health and personal appearance. Talk about cuts, bruises, blisters, burns, and splinters. Show the class or have the nurse demonstrate how to treat a blister and remove a splinter of wood from a finger.

6. Prepare an article for the school paper on some topic of cleanliness.

7. Experiment with the wearing of wet clothes by taking a piece of dry cloth and a piece of wet cloth and placing both on the skin. Ask the class which feels cooler? Which takes more heat from the body? What conclusion should be

drawn? Proceed from there to study types of seasonal clothing. Refer also to clothing used in tribal areas and other sections of the globe.

8. Discuss germs and how they cause disease when the hands, tableware, and family utensils are not clean. Use the microscope to see the germs. Point out that germs are both helpful and harmful, that washing with water may remove a few, but only careful washing with soap and hot water will remove enough of the germs to protect our health.

9. Show how "hidden dirt" stays on the skin, even when a pupil thinks he is clean, by rubbing the back of the hand with a small piece of cloth dipped in alcohol. Let the class see the cloth before and after rubbing the skin.

10. Find out how Jenner, Pasteur, Koch, Reed, and others have benefited humanity.

11. Visit the school cafeteria to inspect and observe the methods used to maintain sanitary conditions. The same approach may be made at a park, picnic area, or public beach to note hygienic conditions.

12. Show the relationship of posture to personal appearance.

13. Plan, find out, report on, make, draw, collect, write, discuss, and sing about cleanliness and neatness. Notice that the words above suggest activity—*doing something* with the topic.

2. PHYSICAL ACTIVITY, SLEEP, REST, AND RELAXATION

Behavioral Objectives (Primary Level)

Explains how one balances exercise, play, work, sleep, and relaxation to provide for optimum achievement in physical and mental well-being.

Describes the need for play and large muscle activity, daily relaxation periods, and a wide variety of leisure time activities.

Identifies reasons why sound sleep in quiet surroundings is healthful, and why quiet activities before bedtime or mealtime are beneficial.

Behavioral Objectives (Intermediate Level)

Demonstrates how exercise builds and maintains health.

Explains the importance of outdoor play and recreational activities.

Analyzes the real value of sleep and rest, and how to rest and relax.

Personally observes regular hours of retiring and rising together with other requirements for sleep and rest.

Employs hygienic practices when engaging in physical activity at school and in the community.

Comments

Boys and girls at all age levels should reach the end of the day free from undue fatigue and irritability. They should rest a while before eating and engage in pleasant and quiet activities before going to bed. They should arise in the morning rested and ready for schoolwork or play. What could be more simple? Yet, getting this knowledge across to all elementary school pupils and having them modify their living practices accordingly is indeed a difficult task.

Health teaching on this topic relates to a number of significant variables. Children themselves vary in their sleep requirements. Those from four to eight years of age need a total of 12 or 13 hours of sleep. For 11 year olds, 10 hours is generally sufficient. By age 12 or 13, nine hours is usually enough. But the quantity of sleep is not nearly as important as the quality. The quality is affected by numerous home and community stimuli. In every neighborhood there are items such as street noises, factory noises, industrial odors, barking dogs, older children at play, and other factors which have a negative effect on the quality of the night's sleep.

Parents must have an understanding of sleep and rest needs, of wholesome physical activities, of signs of fatigue, and many more conditions conducive to adequate growth. When parents fail to guide their children properly at home, the efforts of the classroom teacher may seem quite meager. Late evening programs, movies, television shows, radio, and after dinner visits tend to cut into the optimum sleep requirements for growing children. Over a period of time pupil behavior is affected. Children in such instances become more fatigued, lose their keen appetites, drop in scholarship, and frequently demonstrate a less social behavior. Fatigue in children is sometimes a sign of anemia caused by insufficient iron in the blood. This can usually be corrected by better nutrition and prescribed medication.

Although children are more discriminating than they used to be in what they choose to watch on television, there are still many who spend hours per week sitting and watching. There are, of course, many excellent offerings on television, but numerous children stay up too late watching.

There is an excellent opportunity for the teacher to work with the home, to see that all pupils receive their due share of vigorous growth-stimulating physical exercise, relaxation, and sleep each day. Probably more bacterial and virus diseases get a foothold in the human organism because of chronic fatigue than from any other hygienic shortcoming. Children need school activities which will point up the fact that satisfying school work, outdoor play, rest, sunshine, proper food, and happy associations at school and in the home neighborhood help them to secure a restful night's sleep.

Today, more than ever in the past, considerable attention must be given by the teacher to the role of physical exercise in the maintenance of organic health.

Physical fitness is the prerequisite to everything else. It is the wherewithal that permits movement; it is in a very real sense the capacity for activity — any and all activity. Tyler says that the muscles are the "organs of the will." Since the muscular fitness items of strength and endurance (which relate to organic health and mental-social health as well) cannot be stored, it is necessary that daily attention be directed to vigorous physical exercise. Although most students appear quite active, a knowledge of the benefits of exercise needs to be

stressed academically in the classroom, as well as directly on the playgrounds and gymnasiums. There are numerous boys and girls today who are under their normal strength and well below a minimum level of muscular fitness. Their physical efficiency is too low for them to live fully and function with a full display of energy. The quiet, chore-free activities of a somewhat sedentary adult population have reached the schoolchildren. Even those pupils a few blocks from school ride the bus; others sit and watch much of the time; still others are tense and emotionally on edge due in part to the rapid pace and stresses of modern civilization. With overeating and underactivity it becomes clear that education for health is more important than ever. Suitable activities which are carried on in a pleasant atmosphere, free from the pressure and rapid pace of modern society, can be most profitable.

The role of the classroom teacher is to demonstrate clearly to her particular grade that exercise, nutrition, and rest build a quality of physical fitness that is a forerunner for all other activities. This means that the classroom teacher is a physical education teacher and as such is a teacher of health. The value of physical skills cannot be overemphasized, for fitness in later life is related to skills acquired during the early years. Emerson, in his *Essay on Education*, refers to "educated eyes in uneducated bodies." In so doing he makes a strong point in favor of physical efficiency and skills.[3] Thus each instructor of youth, particularly at the elementary level, teaches the mimetics and story plays, the games, the rhythms and dances, and the recreational skills that contribute to growth and understanding at the moment.

A large percentage of classroom teachers carry on their own programs of physical education. It is the minority that have the services of the trained specialist to teach activities. It is important, there-

---

[3] ". . . let us have men whose manhood is only the continuation of their boyhood, natural characters still; such are able for fertile and heroic action; and not that sad spectacle with which we are too often familiar, educated eyes in uneducated bodies."

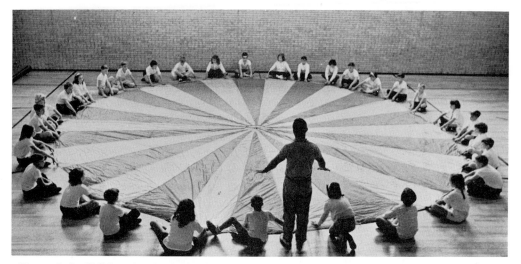

Figure 8–1 Children in physical education class prepare to jump to feet and raise parachute vigorously overhead. (Courtesy Baldwinsville Schools, Baldwinsville, N.Y.)

fore, that each teacher be well acquainted not only with the behavior characteristics of the age group, but also with the appropriate activities for each grade level, season, and facility. The program must be a broad and varied one so that all children have a number of experiences and find something that they are interested in. It is the concomitant learnings associated with these games and dances that foster social efficiency, cultural appreciations, and moral ethical values. This becomes emphasized when one considers that activity—play, games, stunts, rhythms, and dance—is to the child as work is to the man. It is serious, special, and full of meaning—the child's way of life. Through it he learns about himself, the people and the things around him.

In this connection, a word about movement exploration is appropriate. This is a relatively new direction in elementary physical education. It is taught by problem-solving methods, affording all children the opportunity to perform as individuals—being creative as they discover new ways of handling their bodies and objects. The teacher sets the problem. She may ask, "Can you jump *over* the beanbag?" "Now, can you jump over it again and *land* without making any noise?" Or she might say, "Show me how *high* you can bounce the ball. Can you make your body *low* and bounce the ball?" Original responses are encouraged throughout movement exploration activity. This builds concepts of level change, direction, force, speed, timing, and space relationships needed in mind-body understandings. Not only does it contribute to joy in activity, physical fitness and motor development, but it measurably improves listening habits, creativity, and confidence in ability to adapt to the immediate environment.[4]

There is a fantasy of motion associated with creative dance that younger children thoroughly enjoy. Music, rhythm, communication, line and form may all be tied to the dance activity. Children express themselves as they move and sway the way they feel.

Suggested Activities

Primary Level

1. Talk about the relationship of physical activity to "feeling good." Show how overactivity relates to fatigue, sleep, and relaxation.

---

[4]See "Movement Education: Play With a Purpose" by Elsie Werra in *Instructor, 80*:84–85, October 1970. See also "Creative Dancing" by Monica Pendergast in *Instructor, 81*:62–63, March 1971.

2. Have the class tell about the games and dances they enjoy playing most. Play one or two favorite games in the classroom as an illustration of something "we like" to do, or do the same thing on the school playground.

3. Put the following poem on the blackboard in big letters.[5]

WE ARE PLANNING OUR DAY

WE PLAN OUR WORK
WE PLAN OUR PLAY
TO MAKE A HAPPY
BUSY DAY.

Have the class plan the work, play, and rest periods for the day. Point out the balance between these three items. Ask the class to tell why they think this kind of planning may make them happy.

4. Teach some exercise which will strengthen abdominal and back muscles and contribute to good posture and body mechanics. Play games to release tensions built up in concentrated activities. Engage in fundamental rhythms such as walking, marching, skipping, hopping, sliding, twirling, and jumping to music (applicable to kindergarten and first grade). Use the balance beam. (Even a homemade $2'' \times 4'' \times 12'$ piece of wood with side supports can be used.)

---

[5]Reprinted through the courtesy of the Metropolitan Life Insurance Company.

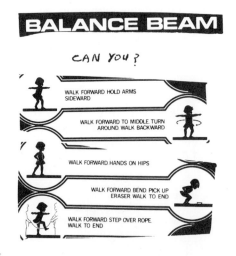

5. Have fun acting out mimetics such as story plays that are full of actions. Dramatize such things as going to a fire, swimming along the shore, rowing a boat on a fishing party, tree branches bending before the force of the wind.

6. Have a quiet period. Speak to the class: "Stand up very slowly. Sit down very slowly. Go somewhere on your feet—now go a different way. Go somewhere on your hands and feet—now find a different way to go—go faster. Move somewhere on any part of your body. Find a space and make yourself small, very small, as tiny as you can. Now stretch every bit of your body way out. Squeeze up very tight. Stretch again and relax."

7. Bring a kitten to class. After the class has been under way awhile, tell everyone to look at the kitty. See how many children have pets. Have them tell how their animal friends rest or sleep. Ask where birds go to sleep.

8. Make a clock out of cardboard. Place the pointer at a reasonable bedtime. For first graders set it at 7 P.M. Inquire as to when the various children go to bed.

9. Bring a globe of the world to class. Explain daytime and nighttime by pulling the shades to darken the room and holding a flashlight over the globe to represent the sunshine. Notice in what countries people are sleeping when it is daytime in America.

10. Talk about the nice feeling of going to bed. Let the pupils suggest how nice the sheets feel and the softness of the bed (first grade).

11. Check on the number of children having baby brothers or sisters. Have the children answer questions on how long the babies sleep, what awakens them, and why they need more sleep than older children (first grade).

12. Have someone demonstrate a cartwheel. Let everyone try a few. Then do cartwheels along a line; along a set of hoops on the floor; along a line and picking up an object in the process; over an object such as a rope; with a run, etc.

13. Take the opportunity to capitalize on the daily rest period in school. Listen

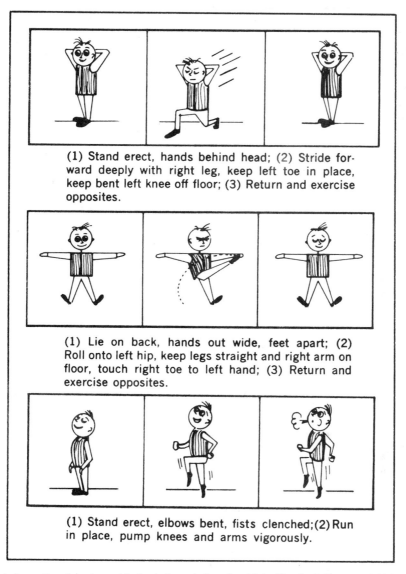

(1) Stand erect, hands behind head; (2) Stride forward deeply with right leg, keep left toe in place, keep bent left knee off floor; (3) Return and exercise opposites.

(1) Lie on back, hands out wide, feet apart; (2) Roll onto left hip, keep legs straight and right arm on floor, touch right toe to left hand; (3) Return and exercise opposites.

(1) Stand erect, elbows bent, fists clenched;(2) Run in place, pump knees and arms vigorously.

(Adapted from the American Medical Association booklet, *Physical Fitness,* A.M.A., Chicago, Illinois, 1966.)

to soft music before the rest period (kindergarten to second grade). Examples: *Lullabies For Sleepy Heads,* Dorothy Olsen (RCA Victor), *The Swan* from *Carnival of the Animals* by Saint-Saens.

14. Construct a model bedroom on a large table. Use doll furniture and doll people. Show a comfortable room with clean bedclothing, opened window, and other optimum physical factors. Put a clock on the wall set for bedtime. Vary

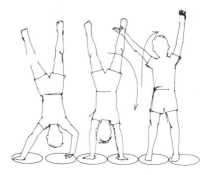

the model according to the known socio-economic level of the students.

15. Display activity posters during the teaching period. For example, the 22″ × 28″ colorful poster *Keep Physically Fit*, available free of charge from School Services Division, Florida Department of Citrus, Lakeland, Florida.

16. Make pictures or posters suggesting activities conducive to play, sleep, or relaxation.

17. Prepare a wall board with pictures brought to class depicting sleep, work, play, and relaxation (second and third grade).

18. Plan a program of action with children and parents. In one community a letter sent home was quite effective.

Intermediate Level

1. Formulate a well-balanced daily schedule that makes ample provision for each of the functions of exercise, relaxation, and sleep which affect the growth and development of the human body.

2. Discuss the values of muscular work as a health measure. Point out that a muscle in good tone is firm and ready to act; muscle tone is the foundation for further development of strength and skill; sufficient strength and endurance reduce fatigue and permit a child or adult to keep going longer; agility, flexibility, speed, and precision are improved; increased heart action results in a more efficient heart with more blood being pumped together with fewer beats per minute; oxygen is better distributed to tissues; all organic functions in the body are improved; and general health is advanced (fifth or sixth grade).

3. Use a wall chart to show how the muscular system works and how its use puts demands on the other body systems; the demands in turn tend to keep the other systems organically and functionally healthy.

4. List on the board a number of physical activities that may be engaged in around the home. Number these activities according to the degree of vigor required. Do the same for occupations in the community and for sports and games in the school physical education program.

5. Display pictures of prominent athletes or pictures of athletes in action.

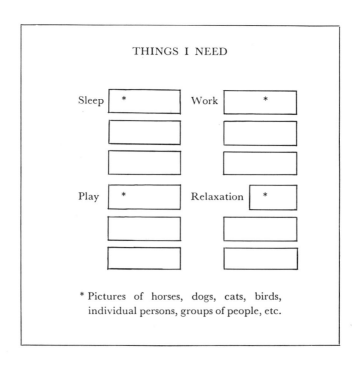

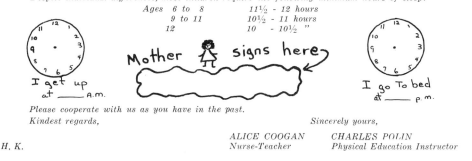

EAST SCHOOL

Dear Parents,   Long Beach, N. Y.

    Are you willing to give your children a longer sleeping hour?

    For many years we, at East School, have been interested in your child's good health. We know you, too, are concerned. With this in mind, we feel it is necessary that you help us with a serious problem that has come to our attention. We have observed the students and find that a great many of them are tired and sleepy. After further investigation, we learned that too many children go to sleep at a rather late hour. This, combined with a late wake-up time, results in fatigue, as well as neglected toilet habits and insufficient time for a nutritious breakfast. The children are, therefore, poorly prepared for a day's work and play, and are at a low level of efficiency.

    We can overcome this undesirable situation by insisting that the children retire at a reasonable hour, receive the proper number of hours of sleep, and awake at 7 a.m. They are then prepared for school, and have a nourishing breakfast and are ready for a full day's work.

    Despite individual differences, most children require the following minimum hours of sleep:

Ages 6 to 8	*11½ - 12 hours*
9 to 11	*10½ - 11 hours*
12	*10 - 10½ "*

    Please cooperate with us as you have in the past.

Kindest regards,   *Sincerely yours,*

                                         ALICE COOGAN   *CHARLES POLIN*

H. K.   *Nurse-Teacher*   *Physical Education Instructor*

Magazines such as *Sports Illustrated* abound in excellent pictures of swimmers, golfers, tennis players, baseball batters, football carriers, and ice skating champions.

6. Plan a hiking, camping, or bicycling trip. Make the trip if possible.

7. Practice relaxing. Have the class stand by their desks with both arms extended above the head. On command, relax only the hand by allowing the wrist to "break." Then relax to the elbow joint, and then the rest of the arm. Repeat by relaxing the whole arm on command. Point out how difficult this seems at first (fifth and sixth grades).

8. Discuss the meaning of recreation. Ask the children what their parents do for recreation. Suggest and list on the board several reasons that play is not a waste of time.

9. Prepare a hobby exhibit. Show pictures of the hobbies of prominent people. Suggest to the class that they illustrate some of the hobbies of their older brothers and sisters and their parents.

10. Encourage informal discussions of why we tire, how rest affects posture, work, and play, and why anxiety, fear, anger, and eating before bedtime may affect sleep.

11. Keep individual records of the number of hours sleep each night for one whole week with notations on "How I felt in the morning." Discuss the records at the end of the week. Bring into the discussion the advantages of sleeping alone, the kinds of mattresses slept on, restlessness in sleep, and sleep practices (sixth grade). (See ill. on following page.)

12. Count pulse rates before and after a period of exercise. Note also the respiratory rate, its increase and return to normal. This may be made quite interesting. Have the children stand by their desks and count their own pulse beats for 30 seconds. Multiply by two and record on a piece of paper. Then run quietly in place for one minute and quickly take the pulse rate again for 30 seconds. Record in the proper place on the paper. Sit down and rest. Take the pulse two minutes later and record.

Find out who had the greatest rise in pulse rate. How many came close to returning to their original pulse rate? Discuss what has happened in the body, with particular reference to physical con-

MY SLEEP RECORD

Day	Hours Slept	How I felt in the morning
Monday		
Tuesday		
Wednesday		
Thursday		
Friday		
Saturday		
Sunday		

dition and fatigue. Plot individual line graphs (see example below).

13. Interview the school nurse regarding the relationship of excessive fatigue, inadequate sleep, and activity to the common cold.

14. Invite the physical education teacher into class to talk about athletes he has known. Encourage questions from the class relative to the eating, sleeping, and resting practices of athletes.

15. Appoint a comittee of three to find out about the Harvard Step Test of Physical Fitness for elementary age pupils. Give the test and check individual student scores.[6]

16. Run an indoor track meet when the class needs a "restless" break. (See box at top of facing page.)

---

[6] Adequate instructions may be found in Carl E. Willgoose, *Evaluation in Health Education and Physical Education*. New York: McGraw-Hill Book Company, 1961, pp. 117–118.

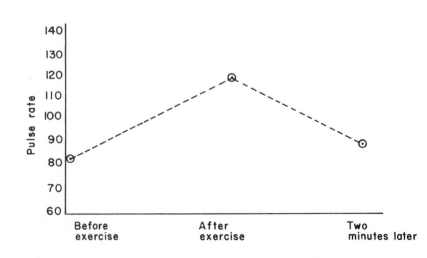

The Hundred-Inch Dash: Draw a starting line and a finish line one hundred inches apart. Starting with their feet together, contestants move forward by touching the heel of one foot to the toe of the other foot.

The One-Minute Mile: Time each person for one minute as he runs in place, lifting feet at least twelve inches. Every time the contestant's right foot hits the floor, it counts as one. The child with the highest count within a minute is the winner.

The Paper-Bag Put: Grab a paper bag and crush it into a ball. You now have an indoor shot that can't damage anything. See who can throw it the farthest, using proper shot-putting form.

The Javelin Throw: Save a few straws from lunchtime—they make harmless javelins! Let kids experiment with different ways of throwing them.

3. NUTRITION AND GROWTH

Behavioral Objectives (Primary Level)

Explains that a variety of food is needed by the body for growth and energy.

Investigates a variety of nutritious foods, good eating habits, and customary social behavior at mealtime.

Relates how energy is necessary for work and play, and that some foods provide more energy than others. Outlines how appetite can be improved by careful planning of work, play, and rest.

Portrays how being tired, sick, and unhappy is often related to poor nutrition.

Describes a happy, pleasant mealtime.

Behavioral Objectives (Intermediate Level)

Interprets the concept that a well-balanced daily nutrition includes food from each of the four basic food groups.

Structures a well-balanced diet which helps to achieve success in work and play, and shows how it relates to one's emotional outlook.

Selects foods that contain various nutrients, minerals, and vitamins which have something to do with prevention of disease, personal vigor, and enthusiasm.

Interprets the concept that the body is composed of cells which need wholesome food for proper growth and development.

Investigates how foods are used in other parts of the world and how food is handled, preserved, and stored.

Demonstrates ability to be able to personally choose suitable meals when he must select his own. Investigates common food fads, misconceptions, and superstitions.

Cooperates with others (including parents) in meal planning.

Comments

The White House Conference on Food, Nutrition and Health called for ". . . a dynamic nutrition education program that begins in early childhood and continues through the early elementary and secondary schools." This was the cry as 1970 began. It hasn't changed; and the burden is on the teacher. Unfortunately, most teachers have little real preparation for the assignment.[7]

In a Los Angeles study to determine the effectiveness of a nutrition education program, 1,720 second grade pupils were divided into three groups for instruction: (1) those whose teachers were trained by nutrition educators and were given teaching materials; (2) those whose teachers were not trained, but were supplied with materials; and (3) a control group whose teachers were supplied with nutrition objectives only.[8] Pretest-

---

[7]Sinacore, John S. and Gail Harrison, "The Place of Nutrition in the Health Education Curriculum," *American Journal of Public Health*, 61:2282, November 1971.

[8]Lovett, R., E. Barker and B. Marcus, "The Effect of a Nutrition Education Program at the Second Grade Level," *Journal of Nutrition Education*, 2:80–88, Fall 1970.

ing was done for nutrition knowledge and its application in the selection of meals. Post-tests were given after the instruction was finished. The students in group one who had the trained teacher increased 360 per cent in knowledge and 150 per cent in ability to select balanced meals. No significant improvement was noted in the other two groups. It is clear from this study that elementary teachers can indeed help children if they broaden their general education with some work in nutrition. At present, little nutrition education will occur in the grades unless classroom teachers do it themselves.

Over the decades nutritional deficiency diseases such as rickets and scurvy have been reduced, and the diet of the schoolchild has been improved despite parental indifference and poverty. Yet there are major difficulties regarding nutrition to be overcome. One of these has to do with an adequate breakfast. For some time research studies have indicated that about 25 per cent of the daily nutritional needs should be supplied at breakfast. How many chil-

dren, even in affluent communities, meet this requirement? (See Fig. 8–2.) A great number do not. In a 1971 study of 80,000 Massachusetts public school children it was discovered that 24 per cent of all children came to school without an adequate breakfast. Even more startling, 13 per cent ate no breakfast; younger children did better than older children, and boys did better than girls. Moreover, lunch meals were not all good either.

There are several studies, such as the one by the School of Medicine of the University of Washington, which show that a large number of boys and girls are significantly overweight. The studies indicate that girls frequently lead a soft existence—underactive, overeating, passive, and very dependent on parents. Also, Mayer's studies at Harvard University of obese girls indicates that they are far less active than girls of normal weight.

Moderately severe and prolonged undernutrition in children can produce alterations in brain activity which may

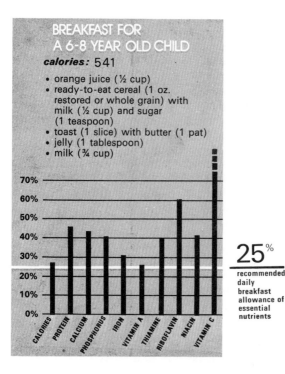

Figure 8–2 Breakfast for the primary grade school pupil. (Courtesy Cereal Institute, Inc.)

never be corrected.[9] Through improvement in diet, the child may catch up to his peers in physical size, but limitation of nutrient intake during the early years occurs during the period that normally produces some 90 per cent of normal brain structure. In addition, recent research indicates that malnutrition delays puberty and slows the development of mental ability. This is frequently expressed through a lack of mental vigor and reduced ability to concentrate.

It is not easy to tell when a child is malnourished. It may help, however, to check the characteristic deviations in appearance and behavior listed in Chapter 5. A familiarity with these signs will not only be beneficial in terms of individual cases of malnutrition, but will also suggest items for study in the food instruction program.

There are certain essentials one must bear in mind for effective nutrition teaching. This should never become a fixed or stereotyped area of instruction. The teacher needs a knowledge of nutrition coupled with an appreciation of home-school-community relationships. To check herself on her own methods she may ask such questions as these.[10]

1. Do I relate classroom experiences and other activities to the daily food practices of children?

2. Do I make clear to the children the habits that are desirable for them to establish?

3. Do I provide parents with information and solicit their suggestions so that I may expect full cooperation from them in habit formation?

4. Am I guided by the needs of children and the community in selecting learning situations?

Most nutrition educators point out that nutrition teaching to be most successful should begin early in the grades.

This is the time when the school supplements the home, and here, perhaps more than ever again, there is mutual interest of parent and teacher. In this respect, a set of reasonably attainable primary and intermediate level behavioral objectives have been arranged by the National Dairy Council (New England branch) and may be obtained from 1084 Commonwealth Avenue, Boston, Mass.

In the primary grades there is a breadth of teaching possibilities built around growing big and strong, farm and market visits, growing vegetables in the classroom or school garden, preparing foods, tasting foods, enjoying foods, and the sociability of the occasion. The list of possible teaching units in nutrition is lengthy indeed. One can fire the imagination of the enthusiastic child with such headings as, "Getting Ready for Our Picnic," "The Animal Way," "Off to the Farm," "To Market with Mother," or "Making Butter the Hard Way." Moreover, the list of available top-rate films on nutrition is extensive; many are excellent. (See Chapter 11.)

The nutrition area is rich in teaching materials available from commercial organizations. The Cereal Institute, for example, has several kits which include colorful cartoon filmstrips, records, and duplicating masters for activity sheets. In *Alexander's Breakfast Secret* (Alexander is a talking dog) there is music and sounds of the morning to go along with a number of activities. The same organization makes the booklet, *Breakfast Cereals — Part of Modern Life*, available for intermediate grade level children. Here again a transparency master is free of charge along with duplicating masters for student worksheets. The Florida Citrus Commission also makes duplicating masters available to teachers at no charge. These help call attention to vitamin products. (See current addresses of companies referred to in Chapter 11.) The posters and charts of the National Livestock and Meat Board are the most realistic made. Meats and other foods as depicted look real enough to eat right off the paper. Their *Primary Grade Nutrition Education Kit*, for which there is a

[9]Coursin, D. B., "Effects of Undernutrition on Central Nervous System Function," *Nutrition Review*, March 1965. See also Philip L. White, "Nutrition and Genetic Potential," *Journal of School Health*, 36:341–345, September 1966.

[10]Martin, Ethel A. *Roberts' Nutrition Work with Children*. Chicago: University of Chicago Press, 1972.

$2.00 charge, services 30 children with three pieces of material pertaining to "food power."

Other organizations worth singling out that supply teachers with nutrition education materials are National Dairy Council—the organization most prolific in dispensing teaching aids, with everything from posters and leaflets to white rats for animal feeding experiments; H. J. Heinz Company with *Facts About Foods;* American Institute of Baking with many colorful pamphlets and *The Wonder of You*—an informative 12-page manual for the teacher and intermediate pupils; General Mills, Inc. with *Nutrition Guide* developed to help the new teacher; Pet, Inc. with the carefully detailed *Meal Planning Guide;* and Sunkist Growers and their filmstrips, posters, and big orange booklet for the teacher, *Build a Better You With Fresh Citrus.* A noncommercial manual designed for the elementary teacher, grades kindergarten through six, is *Focus on Nutrition.* It may be obtained from the Massachusetts Dept. of Education, 182 Tremont St., Boston, at a small cost. It is a complete curriculum guide

loaded with fine ideas on how to make the subject of human nutrition alive and vital to younger children.

In the intermediate grades the proper food and living practices which were started in the primary grades continue to grow, but with more answers and meaningful experiences provided. Children now learn more specifically what foods will do for them with a minimum of emphasis placed on technical names.

Simple, outstanding functions should be selected for emphasis. Such an example might be growth and energy. Too many functions demand more time than the average teacher can spare. Time can be used wisely by combining nutrition and social studies activities involving the lives of people in other lands. In addition there should be a chance to exercise judgment involving real nutrition problems—problems which lend themselves to class exploration and reasonable conclusions.

Suggested Activities

Primary Level

1. Show the *Guide to Good Eating* and stress the need for food each day from the four basic groups (third grade). The *Guide to Good Eating* (in color) is made available by the National Dairy Council (See Fig. 8–4.)

2. Keep a record of height and weight. Interest in growth, especially through the individual pupil's readily visible characteristics, is generally high. Particularly useful charts which may be hung on the school wall for groups of children to use may be obtained from Travelers Insurance Company, Hartford, Connecticut (second grade activity).

3. Establish the EE and FF club. Copy the daily lunch menu on the board. Children read this and compare the food items with a food chart also on the board. Everyone goes to the cafeteria knowing what they are eating and *why*. On return, the pupils report themselves as EE (eat everything) or FF (fussy feeder). Then they discuss why they think they acted the way they did (first and second grades).

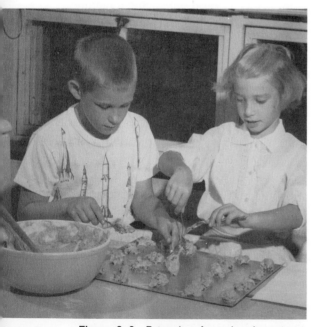

Figure 8–3 Preparing for a lunch party at school. (Courtesy American Institute of Baking.)

A Guide To Good Eating
USE DAILY...

Most people are motivated to follow a food guide more closely when they understand why certain foods are em-phasized. On the next pages you will find ideas that may help you explain the importance of each food group.

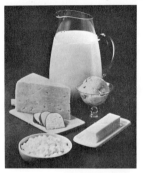

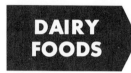

DAIRY FOODS

3 TO 4 GLASSES—CHILDREN
4 OR MORE GLASSES—TEEN-AGERS
2 OR MORE GLASSES—ADULTS

CHEESE, ICE CREAM AND OTHER MILK-MADE FOODS CAN SUPPLY PART OF THE MILK

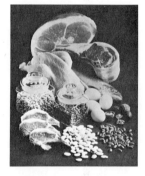

2 OR MORE SERVINGS
MEATS, FISH, POULTRY, EGGS, OR CHEESE—WITH DRY BEANS, PEAS, NUTS AS ALTERNATES

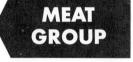

MEAT GROUP

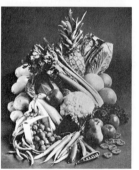

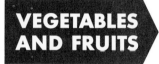

VEGETABLES AND FRUITS

4 OR MORE SERVINGS
INCLUDE DARK GREEN OR YELLOW VEGETABLES; CITRUS FRUIT OR TOMATOES

4 OR MORE SERVINGS
ENRICHED OR WHOLE GRAIN ADDED MILK IMPROVES NUTRITIONAL VALUES

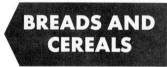

BREADS AND CEREALS

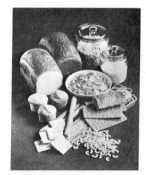

This is the foundation for a good diet. Use more of these and other foods as needed for growth, for activity, and for desirable weight.

The nutritional statements made in this guide have been reviewed by the Council on Foods and Nutrition of the American Medical Association and found consistent with current authoritative medical opinion.

Figure 8–4 A daily reminder. (Courtesy National Dairy Council.)

4. Prepare a flannelboard presentation about foods (first grade). *Ollie and the Orange* and *Smile, Ralph, Smile* are excellent stories with complete teacher instructions which may be obtained free from Sunkist Growers, Inc. in Los Angeles, California.* The same company puts out the filmstrip, *Vitamin C Makes the Difference*—an interesting narrative on vitamins and disease.

5. Visit the local milk bottling plant or bakery to see how foods are preserved through sanitary and other processes. Arrange for samples of the product ahead of time. Be certain, also, that the class knows what to look for.

6. Study color in foods. Begin by asking the class to bring in colored pictures of foods. In the fall of the year a blue hubbard squash cut down the middle is brilliant. So is a pumpkin, a sweet potato, a box of freshly picked cranberries, a handful of sweet apples.

7. Ask the class where their food came from. Some foods come from seeds, others from fruits, leaves, stems, roots, and animals. The class may bring in special foods to illustrate this point.

8. Display several animal bones and human teeth. The children may have samples of first teeth at home and are usually happy to bring them to school. Then discuss the makeup of bones. Calcium and phosphorus are obtained from a number of items which the teacher may take, one at a time, from a large basket on a table at the front of the class: milk, celery, hard cheese, eggs, almond nuts, dried beans, turnip tops, and broccoli, peanut butter, and a piece of lean meat (liver, kidney, heart). See also the excellent wall chart, "For the Calcium You Need," Evaporated Milk Corporation (free) and the *Nutrition Guide*, available free from General Mills, Inc., Minneapolis, Minnesota.

9. Make clay and cardboard food models which can be used in building combinations for meals. Models already made in appetizing colors may be obtained from the National Dairy Council. Make place mats and place cards for the table. Discuss and arrange flowers for the table (first grade).

10. Make paper cups by folding clean sheets of paper. Enjoy drinking water from them.

11. Visit a farmer in the chicken yard or in the fields raising grain. See turkeys at Thanksgiving time. Have one brought to class in a cage if the class cannot visit a farm. Notice how foods like milk, butter, cheese, and bread are kept safe from dirt and flies.

12. Play grocery store; pool the knowledge of the class for an efficient operation. Use real canned goods and solid vegetables such as potatoes, onions, and carrots.

OUR CHILDREN suggest

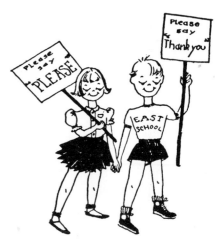

13. Show the colorful, 75-frame filmstrip, *The Power of Food*, and have each class member tell what he learned when the showing is completed. (Available for $2.00 from National Livestock and Meat Board, Chicago, Illinois. Much of this relates to bodies and growth.)

14. Prepare and taste fruit and milk drinks. Milk may be flavored with honey, chocolate syrup, peanut butter, or bananas.

---

*All addresses of companies referred to may be found in Chapter 11.

15. Look over various food advertisements brought to class. Post the better ones so that they may be seen. Discuss accuracy. Talk about food values, truths, and half truths (third grade).

16. Prepare a cookbook made chiefly of pictures instead of words. Each pupil will collect all kinds of colored pictures of foods. Past issues of popular magazines may be cut up at home or in class. These pictures are then pasted on sheets of paper in groups, and the sheets may be combined into one small booklet.

17. Conduct an experiment in which two tomato plants are used—both plants to be given sunlight, air, and water, but one to be planted in poor soil and the other in good soil.

18. Use the clock when talking about regular meal habits, sleeping, work, and play.

19. Make large posters showing the body engine in action, such as hopping, running, dancing, skating, swimming, playing games. Other posters depicting active children, and relating to food and rest, are available from General Mills, Inc., Minneapolis, Minnesota.

20. Ask about appetite. What makes a person eat well? Draw rough sketches of two kinds of eaters and display in classroom.

21. Make butter in class; then spread it on crackers to eat as a midmorning snack. (Obtain instruction leaflets for all class members from the National Dairy Council.)

22. On different days prepare and serve raw vegetables: cauliflower, carrots, turnips, lettuce, celery, spinach, broccoli, cabbage, tomatoes. Serve a small bit of the vegetable which is broken and washed by the children.

23. In discussing breakfast foods, make a display or "store front" of empty cereal boxes brought from homes of the children.

24. Using a large map of the United States, find and mark the places from which meat comes. Locate the sources of the different kinds of fish.

25. Keep a weekly record of the basic four groups eaten every day. (Use chart distributed by Maltex Company, Burlington, Vt.)

26. Hold a mother-children breakfast at school.

27. Use a committee of interested mothers and children to do planning. Follow up with a breakfast discussion. How about the 25 per cent rule and breakfast appetite?

28. Have a "Crazy Milk Day" in the classroom. Help the children make butter to eat on crackers, buttermilk, cottage cheese, yogurt, and cream cheese. Call attention to cheese with some "Did You Know?" posters:

DID YOU KNOW?

. . . that in Switzerland, when a baby is born, a wheel of Saanen cheese is marked with his name? On all the holiest occasions of his mortality his private cheese is served. When he dies the mourners consume the last of this ceremonial Wheel of Life.

. . . that the holes in Swiss cheese form themselves naturally through the chemical changes that take place during aging?

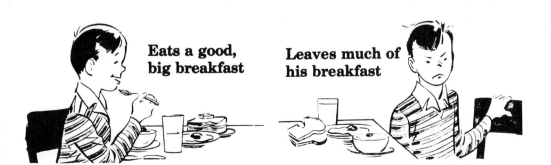

Eats a good, big breakfast

Leaves much of his breakfast

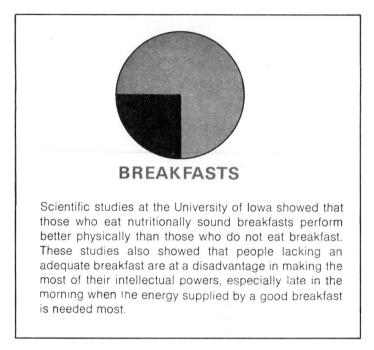

BREAKFASTS

Scientific studies at the University of Iowa showed that those who eat nutritionally sound breakfasts perform better physically than those who do not eat breakfast. These studies also showed that people lacking an adequate breakfast are at a disadvantage in making the most of their intellectual powers, especially late in the morning when the energy supplied by a good breakfast is needed most.

29. Coloring books, *Jane and Jimmy Learn About Fresh Fruits and Vegetables*, are available with *Tips for Teaching* from United Fresh Fruit and Vegetables Association. Coloring familiar foods is still a first grade activity that holds interest.

Intermediate Level

1. Discuss the statement, "It's smart to eat a good breakfast." How much breakfast should one eat, and what kind? The Iowa breakfast studies and a number of others show that 25 to 30 per cent of the day's nourishment should be provided by breakfast. The bacon and eggs type of breakfast can be equaled by one consisting of milk, cereal, toast, and butter. Present-day cereals have a far greater food value than most people realize. A single serving of Cream of Wheat, for example, contains as much iron as a serving of liver. And many cereals are rich in high vitamin wheat germ.

2. Prepare several breakfast menus. Divide the class into "Try Out" committees. Each committee will try out two or three menus, considering such things as ease of preparation, taste, cost, food values, and personal preferences (sixth grade). Further discussion might center around the factors involved in establishing personal preferences.

3. Study food dishes from other lands. Consider the nationalities represented by pupils in the classroom. Possibly an Italian dinner, Greek lunch, or Brazilian breakfast could actually be served in the school with or without parental assistance. In the dairy areas of Brazil, for instance, a breakfast would consist of a hard roll *(pãozinho)*, butter *(manteiga)*, mineiro cheese *(queijo mineiro)*, and warm milk flavored with coffee. A Chinese meal complete with chopsticks, plate, and spoon affords quite an experience. See *It's Always Breakfast Time Somewhere* (National Dairy Council) for suggestions and facts of particular interest to middle grade children.

4. Have the class raise questions on nutrition. Then post a question with its appropriate answer on the bulletin board.

5. Request the local or county agent to visit the class to explain some of the problems of local agriculture and animal husbandry. Before he arrives, have the class prepare a list of questions that they

---

Can't Danish pastry or doughnuts be considered an adequate breakfast for some people?

It may be "breakfast," but it probably won't get you through the morning. If you eat two Danish pastries, with two pats of butter, you've consumed some 400 calories, but only five grams of protein. This negligible amount of protein in a high calorie breakfast may provide a quick pickup, but can result in symptoms of hypoglycemia (low blood sugar) in two or three hours. As a result, you'll feel tired, despite the fact that you've eaten "breakfast." Ounce for ounce, doughnuts have even less protein than Danish pastries. Two plain doughnuts (250 calories) provide three grams of protein; two raised doughnuts (also 250 calories), four grams. Nutritionally speaking, neither Danish nor doughnuts adds up to a good breakfast.

---

would like to have him answer (fifth and sixth grades).

6. Request the state agricultural college or county agent to send some samples of various types of soil for actual use in the classroom. Fertilizing additives may be used to stimulate plant growth and to demonstrate why the farmer must employ crop rotation to insure the return of certain elements to the soil after a crop has been harvested. One New England school has for years demonstrated the necessity for proper fertilizers by having an experimental garden in the classroom. Seed quality may also be demonstrated this way.

7. Correlate such factors as rainfall, temperature, altitude, and frost dates with the food belts for corn, wheat, cotton, or dairy products.

8. Look over a simple diagram of the digestive and elimination tract. Answer questions on digestion, appetite, hunger, assimilation, and the elimination of waste. Most children enjoy talking about appetite — good and bad.

9. Investigate the "romance" of food. Milk in Holland is churned into butter. Lobsters in Maine are a state export item of considerable significance. Chile con carne from Mexico can be discussed first and tasted afterwards; Heinz, Libby, Campbell, and others pack it in cans. Massachusetts is the "land of the cod." Why? (A helpful booklet on the story of fresh fruits and vegetables may be obtained free from United Fresh Fruit and Vegetable Association.)

10. Secure several recordings of music and experiment with each while the class eats. How do marches compare with soft string music as a background for eating?

11. What is meant by a pleasant, cheerful atmosphere at meal time? Post the following poem just before lunch period.

When supper's almost ready

We rest a little while

And think of something funny

That will make the family smile.

---

12. Grind some dried corn kernels in class. This may relate well to a study of Indian life. (See Fig. 8–5.)

13. Conduct an animal feeding experiment with white rats, hamsters, or baby chicks.[11] This is especially good for a fourth grade class. Two 65-gram rats, weighed each Monday over an eight week period, may yield startling results. In an Indiana classroom one rat was fed the regular school luncheon diet and grew to 180 grams. The other rat was fed only hard candy, vanilla wafers, unenriched bread, jelly, and soft drinks; he wasted away to 55 grams. (For more on this see Chapter 9.)

---

[11] Local National Dairy Council offices are generally able to meet requests for these experimental animals (free). See also *White Rat of Hawkins Halls*, a story of a white rat experiment, Evaporated Milk Association.

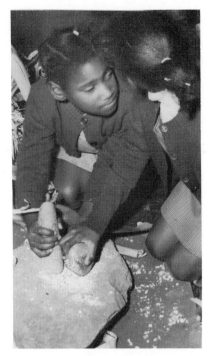

Figure 8–5 Discovering foods by grinding corn the Indian way. (Courtesy *Instructor* magazine.)

14. Investigate food fads, dieting, and calories. Build calorie charts for typical quantities of common foods. List foods consumed during previous three days and calculate calorie intake. Excellent calorie lists which may be obtained in quantity free of charge are contained in the booklets below.

> *Breakfast Source Book*. Cereal Institute, Inc.
> *Your Guideline to Nutrients* and *The Wonder of You*. American Institute of Baking
> *Choose Your Calories Wisely*. Kellogg Co.

Compare differences within the class. Compare daily activities of the various pupils at home and at school, and relate to food intake.

15. Become calorie conscious for a time. Post a chart for all to see. (See Fig. 8–6.) Relate calories to daily activities (6th grade). Estimate the number of calories used to perform an activity: (1) Multiply body weight by number of calories used per pound per hour. (2) Multiply this figure by the fraction of an hour actually spent on the activity.

Activity	Calories Per Pound Per Hour
Dressing and undressing	0.7
Eating meals and snacks	0.2
Sitting in classes	0.4
Dancing	2.0
Laboratory work	0.5
Walking	1.1
Walking rapidly	1.8
Running	3.7
Piano playing	0.9
Typewriting	1.0
Housework	1.2
Carpentry	2.0
Swimming	4.1
Writing	0.4
Ping-pong	2.5
Sleep	0.1

EXAMPLE

If you weigh 80 lbs. and play ping-pong for 15 minutes you will be working at the rate of 200 calories per hour. Thus, in 15 minutes you will use about 50 calories. (Would a tablespoon of peanut butter provide enough energy?)

16. Collect food superstitions and discuss these in terms of scientific knowledge.

Day	Breakfast	No. of Cal.	Lunch	No. of Cal.	Dinner	No. of Cal.	Snacks	No. of Cal.	Total Calories For Day
1									
2									
3									

_____Total Calories

HOW WE IN THE UNITED STATES GET OUR CALORIES

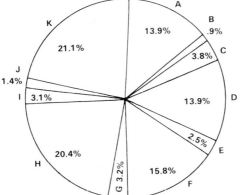

A. Meat, poultry, and fish

B. Leafy, green, and yellow vegetables

C. Other vegetables and fruit

D. Dairy products, excluding butter

E. Eggs

F. Sugar and syrups

G. Dry beans and peas, nuts, soya flour, and cocoa

H. Fats and oils, including pork, fat cuts, and butter

I. Potatoes and sweet potatoes

J. Citrus fruit and tomatoes

K. Flour and cereal products

A 13.9%
B .9%
C 3.8%
D 13.9%
E 2.5%
F 15.8%
G 3.2%
H 20.4%
I 3.1%
J 1.4%
K 21.1%

about 200 CALORIES

Cake, plain . . . . . 3x2x1 ½ inches
Doughnut, cake type . . . . 1 ½
Ice cream . . . . ¾ cup
Meat, except pork . . . . 2 oz.
Peanut butter . . . . 2 tablespoons
Potato chips . . . . 20 medium
Sherbet . . . . ¾ cup

Cake, frosted layer . . . . 2-inch wedge
Chocolate candy bar . . One 2-2 ½ oz. bar
Cookies, plain and assorted . . . 3
Frankfurter and bun 1
French fried potatoes . . 16 pieces
Ham . . . . 3 oz.

about 300 CALORIES

Hamburger and bun 1
Milk shake with ice cream . . . . ½ serving
Peanuts, roasted . . . . ⅓ cup
Pie, 9-inch diameter . . . . . ⅐ pie
Spaghetti, with meat sauce . . . . ¾ cup

Figure 8–6   Calories do count. They come from many sources.

17. Work with the terms "enriched," "restored," and "fortified." Flour and bread were first enriched in 1941. The law requires the enrichment of flour and bread in most states. The American Bakers Association reports that 80 to 90 per cent of all commercial bread is currently enriched. Bring food packages to class.

18. Ask pupils to help you prepare *be-*

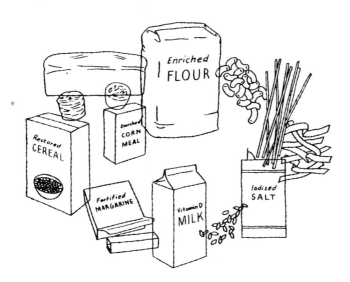

havioral objectives that can be measured at a later date. A sixth grader might suggest the following:

    a. Identify the information required on a food package label in front of the class.

    b. Give an example of the difference between factual and misleading sales presentation for a given food item.

19. Show intermediate level filmstrips, *Project A.M.*, which shows how food scientists relate to one's daily nutrition. Available from Cereal Institute, Inc.; a Spanish version is also available.

20. Place a number of up-to-date colorful booklets on a side table for independent study use. Most can be obtained free from companies. Five examples:

Food for Growing Boys and Girls — Kellogg Company

Vitamin Supplements and Their Correct Use — American Medical Association

Citrus Fruit and Nutrition — Florida Citrus Commission

Build a Better You — Sunkist Growers

Meal Planning Guide — Pet, Inc.

21. Cook dried fruit. Make a fruit salad. Make chopped vegetable sandwiches using dark bread. Serve in class following a discussion of the food values involved. Arrange a centerpiece of vegetables for a classroom table.

22. Take husks from oats and have the children roll them with a rolling pin to make rolled oats. Discuss how oats are rolled in the factory.

23. Conduct an experiment using chickens to show the need for green, leafy, or yellow vegetables. Give one chicken feed without vitamin A. Give the other the same diet, but add one of the many sources of vitamin A.

24. Construct and post on the bulletin board a diet for some special people: the Olympic athlete, the Arctic explorer, the astronaut.

25. Sketch a diagram of the digestive tract; indicate by arrows what takes place along the way and label it "Digestion In Action." For an excellent $8\frac{1}{2}'' \times 10\frac{1}{2}''$ chart see American Institute of Baking booklet, *The Wonder of You* (free), p. 6.

26. Interview officials of the local health department regarding food protection practices.

27. Read and report about some of the harmful effects of overweight and underweight (sixth grade, independent study).

28. Under committee leadership, conduct an "experimental kitchen"; prepare and try out nutritious snacks, sandwich spreads, and drinks. Example:

Hot Spiced Cider

Heat apple cider with lemon slices and lemon peel. Spice with cinnamon sticks, cloves, and allspice.

29. Ask the school nurse to explain red cell blood count. Have pupils study foods which provide iron and protein needed to maintain a normal red cell blood count (fifth grade). Note that certain cereals now contain 100 per cent of daily iron requirement.

30. Construct a mobile of the foods in an adequate breakfast. Prior to this, examine carefully the labels on breakfast cereal packages.

31. Try some food experiments. For ideas see Ethel Austin Martin, *Nutrition Education in Action*. New York: Holt, Rinehart, and Winston, 1966.

4. DENTAL HEALTH

Behavioral Objectives (Primary Level)

Demonstrates how to brush the teeth using the toothbrush.

Explains without apprehension what the dentist does, something about his equipment and where he is located.

Rinses the mouth with water after eating when at all possible. Investigates how raw foods help clean the teeth.

Distinguishes clean teeth from dirty teeth.

Behavioral Objectives (Intermediate Level)

Explains clearly that dental health is a significant part of one's total health.

Compares crooked teeth with straightened teeth in terms of appearance and efficiency.

Describes the causes of toothache and the need for immediate treatment. Explains how diseases in the body may be related to diseased teeth.

Evaluates dentifrices through reading and discussions with dentists.

Illustrates how water fluoridation functions to reduce tooth decay.

Depicts practices that may injure the teeth.

Comments

The American mouth is a disaster area!

About 97 per cent of all the children in the United States are affected with dental caries, and half of them under 15 never have been to a dentist. Moreover, a large number have broken front teeth. This accident most frequently occurs in the eight to 11 year age group and is particularly serious inasmuch as the treatment is very difficult.

The makeup of a thorough dental program consists of dental information for the general public, including educational material for civic groups, a patient education program in the dentists' offices, and a dental health program for schools. These three means of improving dental health have a strong bearing on classroom activity. Every child who learns that the dentist is his friend and why he is becomes a walking dental health educator when he enters his home at the end of the school day. Parents often "move" under the pressure of their children's candid remarks. Procrastination and even indifference are sometimes put aside when the child urges his parents to take him to the dentist "because the teacher says so." Literature distributed in the schools in the afternoon sometimes finds its mark in the family kitchen or across the dinner table that evening.

As a result of a two-year pilot program in the San Antonio schools, sponsored by the U.S. Public Health Service, it is now considered feasible to train children in effective personal dental care prac-

tices in the elementary classrooms.[12] knowledging that mouth care program in the home and dental office have not proved effective, it was decided to train the teacher as a dental health educator. Through a series of workshops 36 teachers were trained in small groups; and then they taught 1100 elementary grade children the proper practices. In ten weeks time 88 per cent of the students showed improvement in gum tissue health and reduction in plaque scores. Brief classroom exercises took place to integrate dental health concepts with pupil training in tooth cleaning techniques. This study developed a package curriculum which could be transported to any elementary school in the country. Films, models and guides for teachers and parents were developed and used. Prepackaged toothbrushing kits containing brushes, dental floss, disclosing wafers, mirrors and models for a 16-week program were assembled.

Several commercial organizations make teaching kits available that are used in numerous school health programs. Colgate-Palmolive Company has a program for students in grades K-4 which includes a filmstrip and record, "The Mouth I Live In," a disclosing tablet for checking teeth cleanliness (excellent for home use), and teacher's guide. This kit is made up to serve 35 students. A similar kit, together with step-by-step instructions to the third grade teacher, is available from the Procter and Gamble Company. A class toothbrushing chart for posting is used along with a dental health quiz. First-rate, large, colorful posters can be obtained from the company at no cost. Dental health posters for classroom display are also available from Florida Citrus Commission (free).

Most state health departments, as well as the American Dental Association and the numerous companies that make dentifrices, are very willing to make available for the teacher's use a variety of

[12]Masters, Donald H. "The Classroom Teacher . . . Effective Dental Health Educator," *Journal of School Health*, 42:257–261, May 1972.

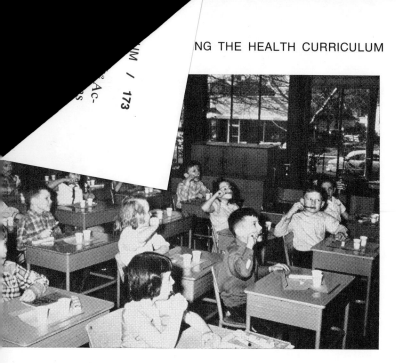

Figure 8-7 The toothbrushing drill—a pleasant experience.

teaching aids, brochures, and suggested learning experiences. The majority of these are good when used in the right way. It must be remembered that some elementary schoolchildren have heard about tooth decay and have drawn pictures about teeth for several years. Yet tooth decay is present today as much as it ever was. One might ask what is wrong with the effort. For one thing, the effort has been a weak one. For another, when it has been made it has not been made *vital*. There has been too much talk and not enough action. Experiences have not been lifelike. There has been little imagination employed. In one Missouri kindergarten the children were "fired up" because the teacher fostered role-playing and acting in a play, "Superbrush and the Molars." The children put it on closed circuit television to an audience of parents and fellow students. It was an exciting new experience with noticeable carry-over.[13]

Suggested Activities

Primary Level

1. Ask the class to tell what they know about teeth. How the teeth chew

food, how they help in talking, and how they look.

2. Show the primary grade film *Health: Toothache of the Clown* (Encyclopedia Britannica Educational Corporation)—the story about a circus clown who is not happy because he is suffering from a toothache. An excellent teaching script is available for the teacher using the film. The same organization puts out a 9 full-color 8mm loop film dealing with oral health, grades K-6.

3. Talk about toothbrushes. Are some better than others? Have a few samples of new and well worn brushes on hand to look over. Discuss proper care of the brush.

4. Teach about teeth in an incidental way, especially when a child loses a baby tooth or has just returned from a trip to the dentist.

5. Bring animal and human teeth to class. The local meat market may have teeth and the local dentist will be happy to lend teeth. Bring a live cat and dog to class so that the teeth of pets may be seen. Or show pictures of the teeth of different animals.

6. Demonstrate and practice proper toothbrushing. Recent studies, reported by the American Dental Association, show that a total of one hour of instruction (in four sessions) usually is ade-

[13]Wyper, Marian. "Introducing Kindergartners to Dental Health," *Journal of School Health, 42:* 97, February 1972.

quate. Drills may be executed by the whole group right in the classroom. This is easy when below-cost toothbrushing kits are available. A free publication with full instructions for a toothbrushing drill is available from the American Dental Association entitled, *You Can Teach Toothbrushing*. The Division of Dental Hygiene, Ohio Department of Health, distributes (free) an excellent booklet, *School Toothbrushing Program*. Post brushing diagrams shown below.

7. Discuss reasons for considering the dentist as a friend. Write the statements formulated by the class on the board. These may be copied later on a ditto sheet for each pupil to carry home. This may, on occasion, alert the parents to take their child to the dentist right away instead of waiting until there is toothache or other complaint.

8. Have each child look into a well-lighted mirror to see if his mouth is clean and to see what the dentist did or can do for him.

9. Demonstrate decay in an apple. Start with two sound apples. Break the skin of one and place both on the window ledge for daily observation. After a few days observe what has occurred. Compare this to tooth decay when a "break" in the tooth occurs.

10. Illustrate ways to protect teeth, such as using the drinking fountain correctly and being careful when playing ball. Ask if anyone knows someone who has broken a tooth.

11. Demonstrate how acid can dissolve calcium in tooth enamel. Place a whole hard-cooked egg in a bowl of vinegar (acetic acid) for about 24 hours. As vinegar decalcifies the shell it becomes soft. Before the experiment, try pushing the egg through the top of a milk bottle; after decalcification the egg can be pushed into the bottle easily.

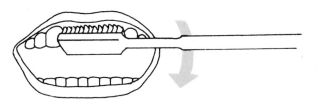

DOWN FROM THE TOP inside and out . . . starting on the gums

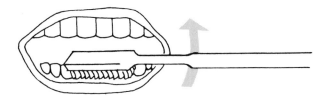

UP FROM THE BOTTOM inside and out . . . starting on the gums

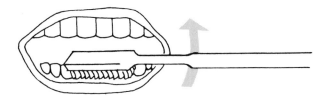

ACROSS THE TOPS (chewing surfaces)

12. Mimeograph a chart such as the accompanying one on 8 inch × 11 inch paper: (*see below*)

Post the charts in class. Every time the pupil brushes his teeth—breakfast (B), lunch (L), or dinner (D)—he may color the proper square. He may use different colors (first grade).

13. Practice (play telephone) making appointments to see a dentist. The student playing the dentist should ask proper questions about whether there is an emergency toothache, accident, or need for regular checkup.

14. Have all classmembers take the "Tablet-test." Procter and Gamble distributes free two little tablets containing a harmless coloring agent. Colgate also supplies these disclosing tablets. The pupils first brush their teeth the way they always do. They then chew one tablet, letting it dissolve in the mouth. They swish the solution around in the mouth, then rinse the mouth. When they look in a mirror the children will see red areas here and there indicating harmful, decay-producing deposits that were missed in brushing. Rebrushing, of course, will remove the stains. Also, along with the tablets, each pupil gets a set of seven rules with brushing instructions—drawings entitled, "Handy Guide to Good Toothbrushing" (third grade).

15. Post a list telling how much sugar there is in some common foods. Then discuss factors influencing wide use of sugar (third grade).

16. Keep a daily record of toothbrushing in the home.

BRUSH UP ON YOUR BRUSHING

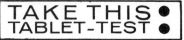

TAKE THIS ●
TABLET-TEST ●

17. Encourage parents to supervise the brushing of teeth at home. Consider sending an information letter to the parents.

Intermediate Level

1. Examine the wall chart showing a sound tooth. Refer early to three factors associated with tooth decay: nutrition, brushing, and individual differences (hardness of teeth and hereditary strengths or weaknesses). This last factor is important. There will always be people, exceptional cases, who eat poorly and appear to have good teeth. Children see them and often draw erroneous conclusions. Thus these exceptions, together with other examples of variation, need discussion in the classroom.

2. Have a student committee visit a local dentist and report back to the class with their findings regarding tooth decay, extractions, dental tools, filling materials, and anesthetics.

3. Make tooth powder. Have the class members mix one part of salt to three parts of baking soda. Put a few drops of wintergreen extract into this to

	Sunday	Monday	Tuesday	Wednesday
B				
L				
D				

give it a pleasant smell. Let it dry, then try it out. Everyone may comment. Perhaps the group will want more wintergreen added to a new batch of powder, or another flavor may be desired.

4. Show pictures of crooked teeth, diseased teeth, and bright, clean, sound teeth. Learn the parts of the teeth. Investigate the functions of the joints and heart for the purpose of associating disease in these areas with infected teeth. Show how decayed teeth are bathed by the blood stream so that one's total efficiency may be reduced through poor teeth.

5. Teach dental health in connection with a study of foods and nutrition. Emphasize experiences dealing with bone building foods.

6. Formulate and record by way of tape recorder a list of reasons why teeth are important and how teeth should be cared for. Play back the tape and appraise it in terms of its effectiveness in changing behavior. Encourage suggestions for shortening the recording and making it appealing. Compare it to radio and television advertisements for dentifrices and foods.

7. Collect toothbrush and dentifrice advertisements; study the claims made. Gather information to determine whether the claims are reasonable and accurate.

8. Prepare, as a group, such snacks as apple slices, dried fruit, celery, carrot sticks, and nuts that can be eaten between meals. Talk about how satisfying they are to the appetite and the values of each kind of snack. Note how celery and carrot sticks help keep the teeth clean (fourth grade).

9. Have a dentist or dental hygienist come to class. Have a panel of students on hand to ask questions. From such an interview the class should find that the dentist does at least the following important things: he makes a complete health inventory and dental history; he cleans and scales the teeth; he x-rays every tooth, locating the cavities no matter how small; he detects abnormal conditions of the gums or mouth; and he gives a full explanation of his treatment plan,

number of visits, and proposed fees. Print on the board:

ASK YOUR DENTIST WHY

10. Stress the relationship of good grooming, appearance, and pleasant breath to success both in school and in the community. For upper grade pupils this approach may hold more interest and shape more attitudes than the approach through foods, disease, and body physiology.

11. Show the Johnson and Johnson film, *Take Time for Your Teeth.* Have each pupil list the essential points when the showing is over.

12. Using small pocket mirrors, one for each row of pupils, have each child look at his own teeth and try to answer the questions, "How do our teeth work?" "What work do the different shaped teeth do?" "Do my teeth meet evenly when I close my mouth?"

13. Make wax impressions of the teeth. Use household preserving wax, 2 inches × 2 inches and 1/4 inch thick (molds may be made in class to this size from heavy aluminum foil). For further hints on this project secure a copy of the free booklet, *The Way to Smile,* from Procter and Gamble Co.

14. Find out how much sugar is in many of the popular foods. There is more than a casual relationship between excessive sugar consumption and dental decay. Most children hear about this at an early age, but they do little about it because of other more impressive factors. Discuss these other factors; the pupils will know what they are.

There is a substantial amount of sugar in most popular foods. For example:

		sugar	
Coca-Cola	6 oz. bottle	$4\frac{1}{3}$	tsp.
root beer	10 oz. bottle	$4\frac{1}{2}$	tsp.
candy bar	1–5 oz.	5–10	tsp.
angel food cake	4 oz. piece	7	tsp.
ice cream sundae	1	7	tsp.
cherry pie	1 slice	10	tsp.

15. Make and display a diorama of a dentist's office. Use pipecleaner figures.

16. Post this sign at the front of the classroom:

PAUL REVERE MADE FALSE TEETH FOR GEORGE WASHINGTON AND ADVERTISED HIS PRACTICE IN THE *BOSTON GAZETTE* IN 1786! WHAT ELSE CAN YOU FIND ABOUT THE EARLY PRACTICE OF DENTISTRY?

(See the book by Esther Forbes, *Paul Revere and the World He Lived In.* Boston: Houghton-Mifflin Co.)

17. Include dental words in spelling lessons. Fourth and fifth grade pupils should be able to spell words such as:

erupt	enamel	fluoride
cuspid	pulp	abscess
bicuspid	decay	malocclusion
calcium	tartar	orthodontist
molar	bacteria	
permanent	Novocain	

18. Do not overlook the opportunity to point out that water fluoridation is a classic example of the public health approach to dental disease control (sixth grade). Over three decades of brilliant research have shown that the community may reduce the dental caries attack by over 60 per cent by fluoridating the water supply.

19. Distribute a 10-inch piece of dental floss to each pupil. Have class practice using the floss to clean the area between the teeth. A leaflet suitable for grade four or above may be obtained (free) from Johnson & Johnson. It is entitled *How to Use Dental Floss.*

20. Examine "before" and "after" plaster of paris molds of sets of teeth showing malocclusion and orthodontia results. Local dentists are usually helpful with the loan of materials. Have class relate malocclusion to a number of mouth problems. How may halitosis occur here? Will mouthwashes overcome effects of crooked teeth and an unclean mouth?

5. BODY STRUCTURE AND OPERATION

Behavioral Objectives (Primary Level)

Describes the basic bone and muscle structure of the body and compares it with the framework of other structures such as automobiles and buildings.

Shows where vital organs of the body are located and what they do.

Identifies elements in health examination and tests of seeing and hearing.

Demonstrates proper posture in sitting, standing, and walking.

Relates key ways in which to protect the eyes and ears from injury.

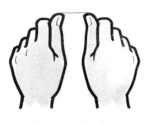

For upper teeth

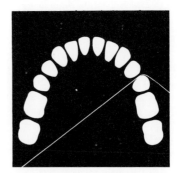

MOVE FLOSS GENTLY BACK AND FORTH BETWEEN TEETH

(Courtesy of Johnson & Johnson leaflet: *How to Use Dental Floss.*)

Behavioral Objectives (Intermediate Level)

Explains how sound body structure is a prerequisite to proper functioning.

Investigates and describes how exercise and recreation tend to relax tensions caused by strong emotions and overambitious living.

Identifies the structure of cells, tissues, organs, and systems.

Portrays what is meant by normal growth.

Chooses scientific terms to describe the body and its functions.

Interprets the close relationship existing between systems of circulation, respiration, digestion, and elimination.

Applies an understanding of the special senses to the care of eyes, ears, and mouth.

Comments

According to Abraham Maslow, one of the characteristics of a healthy, self-actualizing person (his term for maturity reaching toward the fulfillment of the individual) is that he has an understanding and appreciation of his body which lead to less actual body consciousness and greater use of the body *as an extension of his whole personality.*[14] If this is true, then educators for years have been missing an opportunity to influence human effectiveness through a study of the physical self.

A study of the body structure and its function is a fundamental one. It is a biological topic that should be carried on as soon as the class is ready for it.

Primary graders require very little reference to body function. Short general answers to questions of "why" usually suffice, but the upper grade pupils very often want a detailed reason. This is the time to bring in elementary anatomy and physiology — not in a cut and dried approach, but with familiar examples and choice references to personal well-being and appearance. In fact, in many cases boys and girls are impressed more with how they look to others and feel on special occasions than they are with the circulation of blood or the physiology behind good sight and hearing.

Children of all ages tend to be interested in their posture and their general body mechanics if the topic is presented in terms of personal growth and well-being. Measuring growth in the classroom by checking height against the wall and weight on the scales seldom fails to ferret out a number of excellent questions, especially in grades one to three. Here the teacher has an opportunity to demonstrate good standing posture, to discuss ligaments, tendons, and muscles that maintain this posture, and to relate this function to sound nutrition, adequate sleep, and freedom from disease organisms. It may readily be shown that poor eating and fatigue cause many things, that postural attitudes tell much about a person's mental health.

Upper grade children will be especially fascinated by a study of how the foot works, the nature of the longitudinal and metatarsal arches, why the policeman is called a "flatfoot," why sneakers are not advisable for use on hard pavements, the benefits of good shoes and foot exercises, why top rate athletes practice proper foot hygiene, and how overweight can cause pain in the feet. Of course, merely lecturing to a class about the position of the feet in walking or how they should stand or sit will not in itself change the body mechanics of many children. In fact, talking is not enough. In every class one finds a child whose poor posture represents a kind of rebellion against nagging parents and teachers who have overpreached on this topic. Postural changes are brought about when children hear, see, and *feel* what optimum posture is. Bring a mirror to class. Have boys and girls take a side view look at themselves. Have them back up against a flat wall and with their hand feel how much space there is between the hollow of the back and the wall. Let them "stand tall" and walk away from the wall to the mirror so that they can reinforce the way they feel with what they *see.*

---

[14]Maslow, Abraham, *Motivation and Personality.* New York: Harper and Row, 1960, p. 196.

In the case of the tall girl who is seen stooping a bit while talking with a number of friends, it may be that her defect is due strictly to an intense desire to "keep up with the Joneses" by lowering the body to the level of her shorter friends. Such an illustration is rich in instructional ideas. Tall children should know that many a tall person has a kind of upright bearing and grace in movement that is the envy of others.

Included in this particular topic of structure and function is the care of the special senses. Primary grade children need to discuss in detail how to protect their eyes and ears. They should understand the relationship of light and glare to seeing and eye comfort, and they should know how eyeglasses work and how to watch television. Intermediate classes should have a simple understanding of how the eyes and ears work as well as how to take proper care of them. Fifth and sixth graders almost always show in-

terest in a large size model of the eyeball or ear, especially if the parts as shown are immediately related to abnormalities shared by members of the class. For example, nearsightedness (myopia) or farsightedness (hyperopia) are readily explained. A simple eyeball sketch on the blackboard showing a convex or concave lens which is used to correct the particular difficulty will be effective. This is especially true if it is used with actual eyeglasses which the children are permitted to examine. The flexibility of an eyeball can be demonstrated by noting the properties of a hard boiled egg. A Snellen Test chart, employed to measure simple visual acuity or accommodation, can be used in the classroom both as a screening instrument and a teaching device. Some reference should be made, when the special senses are being investigated, to the relationship between safe driving and optimum seeing and hearing. Good eyesight has much to do

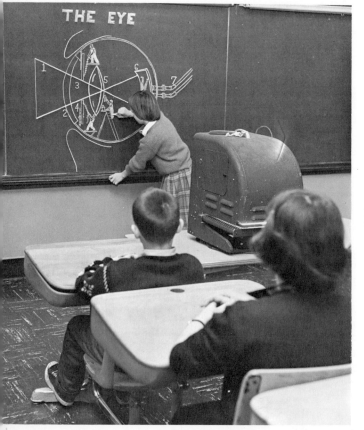

Figure 8–8 Intermediate students are ready for detailed work. (Courtesy Cincinnati Public Schools.)

with personal safety—riding bicycles, crossing streets, and reading roadside signs and markers. The question of how blind and deaf boys and girls behave and how they feel is one that provokes discussion.

Help is available for the teacher who is concerned with the care of the special senses. The primary grade film, *Health: Eye Care Fantasy* (Encyclopedia Britannica Educational Corp.), runs 8 minutes and usually provokes a number of good questions and student observations. Perhaps the finest teaching manual, *Teaching About Vision*, was developed by the American School Health Association and the National Society for the Prevention of Blindness, Inc. especially for classroom teachers. (Price $2.00 from the Society). Lessons are suggested and all scientific words are explained in simple terms. Also, when it comes to the skin as a sense organ, the American Association for Health, Physical Education and Recreation has a very popular intermediate grade level filmstrip, *Every Body's Skin Makes Everybody Kin*; it deals very well with appearance, sensation, and feeling.

The body structure and its operation simply cannot be taught in terms of systems, processes, and mechanics to elementary school children. It has to be taught quite personally with pertinent questions being answered as they are raised by the class. Good teaching motivates the questions the teacher knows to be important. Most children want to know sooner or later what they look like with the skin off and why their bodies function as they do. They want to know how the heart beats and what it sounds like, why they perspire in summer, how the arms move, and a hundred other such practical questions. Without the teacher's moralizing, the class can be shown that the body, in the words of the poet, is the "temple of the soul" and the "organ of the will." It is, by simple statement, an amazing machine with intricacies so numerous that man has not yet figured out all of its actions. Finally, and this is significant, children will not treat the body as a fine instrument until they learn to appreciate it for what it is. With this in mind, the first and second grade children in Kansas City, Missouri were exposed to an award-winning television program (Telecourse) over KCSD-TV. There were twenty 15-minute lessons taught by a former director of the 21-Inch Classroom. A brief description of a few lessons follows; note how attractive they appear:

LESSON NOTES

Are You a Machine?

Content: Introduces "Mr. Machine," a walking, squawking, mechanical man who cannot hear, learn, or understand. Shows how much more wonderful the child is than any machine ever invented. Identifies, with the aid of an anatomical model, important organs inside the human body.

What's Your Fuel?

Content: The lesson is planned to help children understand that their bodies need fuel for energy. A toy steam engine leads off this lesson. Children review what they know of how food is changed to fuel—how it is mashed, moistened, and swallowed. Diagrams and models show where the food goes in the process of digestion.

Take a Deep Breath

Content: Tell the children they are going to learn about something that is more important to them than eating and drinking. It is something that they have been doing from the moment they were born. It is something they can stop doing, but for a short time only. Allow them to guess and then watch the program to find out.

My, How You've Grown

Content: Pupils learn that their bodies are made of little blocks called cells. The story of how they came to be called that is told with the help of honeycomb and a plant stem. The lesson closes with the guest appearance of a charming baby boy who will one day be a man. Thus do the children see living proof of the constant wonderful changes taking place in the development of a human being.

Your Birthday Suit

Content: Describes the skin as an organ that wraps the child completely, protects his body germs, removes liquid wastes, and helps keep his body at an even temperature. Tells the story of skin growth, explaining what each layer does for the body. Answers questions like: "Why are some skins brown and some white?" "What are freckles?" and "What are goose bumps?"

Suggested Activities

Primary Level

1. Post baby photographs around the classroom. A set that shows development through the years is most valuable. Pictures of babies, children, and young people may be cut from magazines and brought to class by the pupils. These can be graduated in such a way as to depict the story of a steady growth.

2. Bring pictures of machines to class and discuss similarity to body functions. Feel arm and finger bones and shoulder and hip joints and see how they move. Choose a pupil to bend, twist, and straighten his backbone to show that the spine is made up of many little bones (second grade).

3. Measure each child for height and weight at intervals. Tie this activity in with body growth. Refer to the growth of the hair, fingernails, and toenails. An excellent "How Tall" wall chart for measuring height is put out by the Travelers Insurance Co., Hartford, Connecticut (free). It is hung on a wall or door, 2½ above the floor. The names of the children may be written in at the head of the height column. Each time a measurement is made, add the date near the height mark. Seven charts will service a class of 28 pupils.

4. Using this growth measuring activity show the relationship of height to standing posture; stress standing tall without affecting a braced type of posture. Illustrate this by dropping a string plumb line from the ceiling of the classroom. The line should run approximately through the tip of the ear, the center of the shoulder, the hip joint, the knees, and the outside ankle bone. Let each class member try this. (A window pole held vertically may be substituted for the plumb line.)

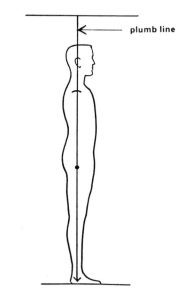

5. Play a game where everyone chooses an animal and mimics its movements by carefully moving about the classroom or recreational area. Then stop and discuss what animals and humans have in common relative to movement.

6. Listen to the beat of a heart. A stethoscope may be borrowed from the

health service department so that each child can hear a heart beat. This is a good project to engage in just before visiting the school physician for a medical examination.

7. Compare the ears with an ordinary telephone receiver. A simple demonstration can be made with an upright telephone. This may be borrowed from a secondary school science department or the local telephone company office. First graders will be amused; third graders will want to see the telephone taken apart.

8. Identify objects by taste, odor, or sound while blindfolded. This can be carried out after the initial demonstration by making a game out of it. In a class of 28 children, four teams of seven children each may, for example, listen to a particular sound. The first child in each group guesses first. The first to give the correct answer scores a point for his team. He then moves to the end of the line. The game continues with different sensory items being introduced. This game motivates the class to want to talk about their smell, taste, and hearing and how these items work with the big sense of sight. Material to have on hand for this game might include a piece of chocolate, a spoiled orange, sour milk, or a musical record.

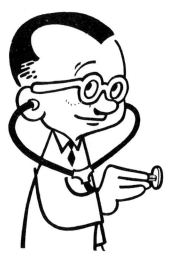

9. Use bellows to demonstrate breathing. Compare a sponge to the lung structure. Look at an x-ray picture of a pair of normal lungs (third grade). A school physician or local health department will usually be able to supply a no longer needed negative for classroom use and storage. Have pupils breathe in deeply, holding their hands on their sides to feel the ribs.

10. Talk about reading books which are printed in a type which is easy to read and sitting in a comfortable position while reading in order not to get tired. Examine some fine print with a reading glass or ordinary magnifying glass.

11. Check sight in class by using the Snellen chart. Use it more as an object lesson than a screening device. Have children talk about their own seeing problems and what they should consider doing to correct the difficulty. (See reference to Snellen chart in Chapter 3.)

12. Let the class hear high and low vibrations to show that certain sounds are more readily heard and recognized. Use whistles, pipes, or a flute to compare with the sound of a tuba, cello string, or low note on a saxophone. One of the many records on the individual instruments of the orchestra may prove helpful here.

13. Teach special senses safety. Point out that only a clean handkerchief should be used near the eyes, that one should refrain from pointing objects such as scissors, pencils, or sticks at anyone, that nothing should be put in the ear.

14. Show why it is necessary to play carefully so that the ears and eyes will not be injured. Point out that running while carrying sharp objects or glass is not a good practice. Warn pupils about shouting into ears. Make pictures of objects that may injure the eyes and ears, such as pencils, scissors, paper clips, snowballs, BB guns, slingshots, or rubber bands. Have children talk about their pictures to the class.

15. Distribute bookmarks so that each class member has one. These are available free from the American Optometric Association. (See next page.)

16. Find out what to do in case of earaches. Bring the school nurse into the classroom to help.

17. Collect pictures of different kinds

EYES

WERE

MADE

FOR

SEEING

APPROXIMATELY

80%

OF LEARNING
DEPENDS ON

VISION

of eyes from magazines and newspapers. Put together a large mural-sized montage of the pictures. Be sure to get pictures of fish, birds, animals, insects, as well as humans.

18. Make a list of pleasant sounds and unpleasant sounds. Relate these sounds to richness in living.

Intermediate Level

1. Discuss growth. Of what does it consist? Look over body diagrams or wall charts (Dennoyer-Gebhart wall charts of body systems are available in many schools). Refer briefly to the relationship of the various areas of the body, i.e., circulation to respiration, digestion to elimination. This should be brief and merely introductory in nature.

2. Make a bulletin board display showing three levels of growth: the first grader, the fifth grader, and the ninth grader. Together with the class fill in the appearances (growth signs) and skills (social, intellectual, and motor) usually seen at each level of growth. This may cause much thought and reflection by the pupils as they think in terms of older and younger people of their acquaintance (fourth and fifth grade project).

3. Listen to the heartbeat with a stethoscope. Study a simple diagram of the heart. Have one pupil jump up and down for 30 seconds. Then notice the increased heart action by listening again with the stethoscope. Notice also the increase in breathing. Show how the lungs perform the function of securing oxygen for the blood.

4. Locate and feel the pulse beat; relate this to the heart beat. Point out that other arteries near the surface of the body may serve as a pulse. Note the notch along the side of the chin, the artery under the upper arm, in the groin, and near the ear on the side of the head. Check these pressure points and indicate briefly how severe bleeding may be controlled by causing pressure over these points.

5. Post an open map on the wall alongside a diagram of the body showing the road or path followed by the blood stream. Point out such items as:

   a. Blood, bathing an infected

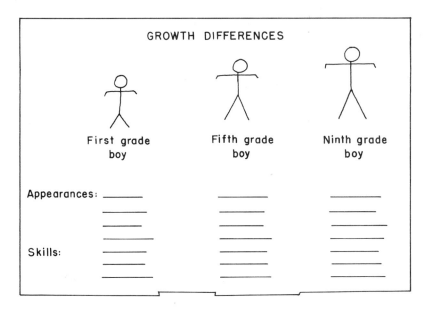

GROWTH DIFFERENCES

First grade
boy

Fifth grade
boy

Ninth grade
boy

Appearances: _____

Skills:

tooth area, can carry germs to the lining of the heart, to another organ, or to a joint.

b. The force and rate of the heart beat has a bearing on the efficiency of the system.

c. Vigorous physical exercise calls for more oxygenated blood to be supplied to the muscles.

d. An effective brain depends as much on the blood and oxygen supply as on the muscles.

6. Show the effect of fatigue, food, rest, disease, emotions, and exercise on the pulse beat. Let the class add to this by telling their experiences. Answer the "why" questions in terms of elementary physiology.

7. Illustrate, through experiment, the relationship of physical fitness (strength and endurance) to heart efficiency. Set up a simple exercise test which is related to the rise and fall of the pulse rate.

8. Discuss the relationship of body posture to body function. Let the class point out that poor nutrition, inadequate sight or hearing, and personal feelings have a bearing on posture.

9. Illustrate the connection between poor standing and sitting posture and general fatigue. Have two pupils stand at the front of the classroom with their left

arms extended horizontally to the side. Continue with the lesson, and about five minutes later ask the two pupils where they are tired. They will mention the extended arm together with the opposite side of the body. Point out that they have expended considerable energy while in "poor posture" by trying to keep from falling away from the line of gravity. Illustrate this further by using kindergarten building blocks. (See next page.)

Show that there is less strain in the building block molecules when they come close to approximating the line of gravity B than there is in figure C, and that there is more stress and strain in the materials of the blocks in C. This is similar to the stress and strain in boy A who is attempting to stay on the gravitational or "fall" line. Then have several pupils walk across the classroom, illustrating a number of pronounced postural defects such as a head forward position, rounded shoulders, a high shoulder, and a hollow back curve. Relate these conditions to A and C and fatigue.

10. Discuss the mechanics of walking, sitting, and sleeping. Show the relationship of poor sleeping posture, mattresses, and beds to chronic fatigue and irritability. Further discuss the social benefits of correct posture. Practice sitting down and getting up from a chair.

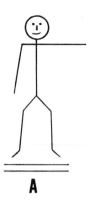

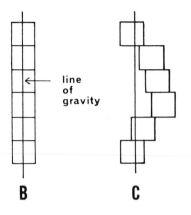

A   **B**   **C**

Demonstrate the proper way of moving a chair to seat a girl or lady.

11. Display some animal bones, which may be obtained from a meat market. Show longitudinal and cross sections.

12. Choose a girl to respond to the role of *Jane*, and another for the role of *Sue*.

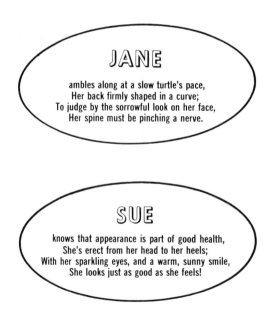

JANE

ambles along at a slow turtle's pace,
Her back firmly shaped in a curve;
To judge by the sorrowful look on her face,
Her spine must be pinching a nerve.

SUE

knows that appearance is part of good health,
She's erect from her head to her heels;
With her sparkling eyes, and a warm, sunny smile,
She looks just as good as she feels!

13. Organize a posture contest. This might resolve itself into a full elementary school assembly program. Some preparation should precede this event. Fourth, fifth, and sixth grade posture contest entrants may be checked at each of seven stations:

   a. Sitting (at a desk)
   b. Walking (across the platform)
   c. Exercises (for coordination and flexibility)
   d. Posture screen (by school nurse)
   e. Plumb line test
   f. Foot and leg alignment (by the nurse)
   g. Roaming judgment (by a judge who judges posture at all times in between the stations)

Score on the basis of 70 points for a perfect score. Many good activities and experiences may be derived from such a contest.

14. Talk about good foot health. Secure an animal's foot or the bones of a leg and foot from the local meat market. Show a cow's knee joint. Have a leg and foot of chicken on hand to show how muscles and ligaments are associated in the human foot. Explain the longitudinal and metatarsal arches and the relationship of their functional efficiency to gait, shoes, and posture.

15. Measure a footprint angle with the protractor (fifth grade activity). Supply each child with a piece of brown paper, a ruler, pencil, and protractor. Have each child step on a damp towel and then stand on the brown paper. Do the same for each foot. Before the paper dries, draw lines A-B and C-D. Measure the angle formed by these lines:

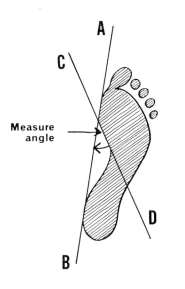

C

A

Measure
angle

D

B

of the human eye. Assign parts of the eye for several pupils to define. An encyclopedia, health tests, and eye booklets may be laid out on a side table for independent use. Compare the eye to a camera. Discuss the rods and cones of the retina and their relationship to good nutrition, disease, and body poisons. The eye of a sheep is especially useful for classroom use.

17. Smear a drop of blood on a glass slide and examine it through a microscope to observe the structure and arrangement of blood cells.

18. Collect and display pictures that depict people from all walks of life taking part in various work and play activities in which good eyesight, good hearing, and a fine sense of balance are necessary. Supplement the display with pictures that show how certain handicaps and inadequacies can be compensated for by the use of such devices as braces, hearing aids, artificial limbs, and eyeglasses.

This is a project that will promote all kinds of foot questions. What is a good arch? What is a flat foot? Why should policemen sometimes do foot exercises while standing on the corner? Are sneakers and moccasins harmful to the feet? How should the heels wear down on the shoes? How should we walk? Is pigeon-toed walking harmful or helpful?

16. Make a large, simple diagram or picture that shows the component parts

19. Tell stories to illustrate how the emotions affect the body. Show how stress items such as fear, anger, jealousy, hate, and worry increase the pulse rate and make people tense. Read a particularly exciting and suspense-filled story or show a movie along these lines. Stop the

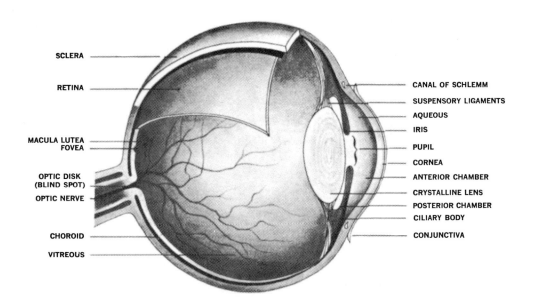

SCLERA

RETINA

MACULA LUTEA
FOVEA

OPTIC DISK
(BLIND SPOT)

OPTIC NERVE

CHOROID

VITREOUS

CANAL OF SCHLEMM

SUSPENSORY LIGAMENTS

AQUEOUS

IRIS

PUPIL

CORNEA

ANTERIOR CHAMBER

CRYSTALLINE LENS

POSTERIOR CHAMBER

CILIARY BODY

CONJUNCTIVA

class at the critical moment to have them notice their heart and respiration rates.

20. Match up everyone with a partner. Blindfold one partner and have the other serve as his guide. One by one each blindfolded pupil should try to explore the classroom, locate his desk, identify other persons and objects in the room, etc. Then have the partners switch places so that everyone will have a turn to be blindfolded.

21. Dramatize the story of Thomas Edison and his hearing problem.

22. Introduce the subject of the heart with a large drawing of a giraffe standing next to a basketball. Have the class try guessing the heart size of a giraffe.

23. Demonstrate the use of an audiometer by the school nurse.

24. Draw and label parts of the respiratory system. Follow this with demonstration of how mouth-to-mouth breathing is administered to a person in need of artificial respiration. Leaflets for class distribution are available from Johnson & Johnson (free).

25. Play a game linking language and thought through sensory awareness activity. Prepare a paper bag, putting in such objects as a smooth stone, a rough stone, a small piece of metal, hard bread, a piece of wax, soap, modeling clay. Blindfold a pupil and let him take an object out of the bag and discuss its texture. To further illustrate sensory awareness create other bags with different materials such as burlap, cotton, silk, velvet—or honey, butter, relish, and detergent powder. A fun activity.

6. PREVENTION AND CONTROL OF DISEASE

Behavioral Objectives (Primary Level)

Describes how children go freely to visit the nurse and other medical personnel.

Explains a few activities carried on by some health workers in the community who protect the health of others.

Relates elementary disease conditions to personal unhappiness.

Drinks properly from a water fountain and does not share glasses and straws.

Describes germs and relates them to sneezes, sore throats, and similar occurrences.

Identifies hospitals as important items in the process of recovery from disease.

Explains the necessity for proper healthful practices concerning himself and others and shows favorable attitudes toward the school physician and nurse and their equipment, thereby overcoming any fear of medical personnel.

Demonstrates several practices which will protect the individual and others from common diseases and illnesses.

HOW LARGE IS THE HEART?

BOY'S HEART	=	A FIST
RABBIT'S HEART	=	AN EGG
DOG'S HEART	=	A TENNIS BALL
GIRAFFE'S HEART	=	A BASKETBALL

Behavioral Objectives (Intermediate Level)

Differentiates between germs that are harmful, others that are harmless, and some that are helpful.

Describes how germs may be spread, and their relationship to common communicable diseases.

Explains how the body defenses react to disease, and that scientists are laboring to obtain more information about disease.

Demonstrates understandings by staying home when ill, keeping immunizations up to date, covering coughs and sneezes, keeping appointments with physicians and dentists, and practicing cleanliness in the preparation, serving, and storage of food.

Identifies the disease prevention value of professional health workers in the community.

Analyzes sources of infection: bacteria, viruses, fungi; people, animals, climate, insects, water, food.

Distinguishes men in science for what they have done to conquer disease.

Comments

Disease prevention and control has more than a slight bearing on the lives of schoolchildren of all ages. Illustrations of this are everywhere, and disease experiences come to every pupil. This fact should do at least one thing for the teacher; it should contribute significantly to the pupil interest level.

Teaching the concept that germs cause disease and that disease can be prevented through the control of germs may seem like uphill work in the elementary grades. Yet children have been successfully taught that micro-organisms are everywhere and can be controlled. But because they are not completely controlled, they cause such things as upper respiratory infections sometimes leading to hearing impairment, pneumonia, colds, and stomach and intestinal upsets. "Strep" germs alone can cause sore throats, tooth decay, and heart damage. Today, some of these germs can "come alive" in the classroom through the use of special slides, films, filmstrips, overhead transparencies and powerful microscopes.

An especially effective film, entitled *Spot Prevention* (color, sound, 13½ minutes), designed to show the chase and capture of the measles "germ," is available for showing to children in kindergarten through second grade. It is distributed by the U.S. Public Health Service, Audiovisual Facility, Atlanta, Georgia 30333. The films, *Germs and the Space Visitor* and *Your Protection Against Disease* (Encyclopedia Britannica), are also good.

As far as the primary grade children are concerned, the prevention and control of disease might well come under the area of personal cleanliness and appearance. Certainly disease control is related to one's personal habits of cleanliness. Children in the first three grades are quite capable of understanding this, especially if the subject is treated lightly and tied in directly with such routine health practices as covering the mouth when coughing, washing the hands before eating and after going to the bathroom, drinking properly from the drinking fountain, keeping away from others when ill, and staying at home when ill.

During the primary grades the teacher is especially concerned with day-to-day signs and symptoms of infectious diseases and defects. She is alert to note deviations from normal health and performance. She has an excellent opportunity to make clear to her pupils that they should remain at home when ill, and not place too great a premium on perfect attendance. Third grade pupils, for example, may be interested in preparing a note to their parents encouraging them to make careful observation of their children before sending them to school. Third graders are also interested in the first stages of the common communicable diseases such as measles and chickenpox, immunization and vaccination, and simple first aid procedures. Upper graders, of course, may want to talk about specific immunization for whooping cough, tetanus, typhoid, and diphtheria, and smallpox vaccinations (see Chapter 5).

As one grows older and must accept additional responsibility, the topic of disease control and its prevention takes on greater meaning. At the intermediate level it offers discussion possibilities greater than the topic of cleanliness and personal appearance. An effort is now made to use scientific knowledge and give decisive answers to "why" certain practices are helpful or harmful. Children show interest in scientific materials. The mystery surrounding bacteria, and why some kinds are difficult to see even with powerful microscopes, and such questions as whether or not bacteria are useful arouse much comment.

It would almost be a mistake to miss an opportunity to present real case studies to a fifth or sixth grade class. Two case studies, such as the following, could be used to initiate a unit and provide immediate kindling of interest and discussion:[15]

CASE 1 — Seventeen persons aboard a ship became ill within 8 hours after eating a noon meal. Nausea, vomiting, cramps, and diarrhea were the symptoms. Macaroni had been cooked prior to the meal, and chopped pimentos, lettuce, boiled eggs, mayonnaise, and mustard were hand-mixed by two mess cooks. One of those cooks had several minor cuts on two fingers. These finger cuts yielded *Staphylococcus aureus*, the same kind of bacteria found in the salad.
PREVENTION. — *Never use your hands to mix foods when clean sanitized utensils can be used! Never work with food when you have infected cuts because the germs causing the infection may be a source of foodborne illness!*

CASE 2 — One hundred and fifty-five persons became ill with severe diarrhea and stomach pains. The suspect meal, roast beef and gravy, had been eaten by 170 persons. This beef and gravy had been prepared the day before and allowed to cool in open trays without refriger-

---

[15] From *You Can Prevent Foodborne Illness.* U.S. Public Health Service, Publication No. 1105, Washington, D.C. 20201.

ation for 22 hours. *Clostridium perfringens* organisms were found in the beef and gravy.
PREVENTION. — *Potentially hazardous (readily perishable) foods should be thoroughly cooked and then either kept hot (140° F. or above), or cold (refrigerated to 45° F. or below) until serving.*

When upper elementary grade schoolchildren review the long and stimulating record of medicine and hygiene practices, there is a good opportunity to impress them with the historical emphasis on disease prevention and control. The control efforts came first, for people were plagued with sicknesses. Even today, in countries like Egypt, some 80 per cent of the population is disease-ridden. Problems of control are of first importance, followed quickly by prevention techniques. The first project is to save the life of the afflicted, then set out to prevent the disease in others. It is suggested, therefore, that intermediate graders take a look back through the pages of history and see what has gone on in the past. Superstitions, magic, and witchcraft in primitive society, the worship of special gods during the early days of Egypt, Greece, and Rome, and the slow transition from alchemy and astrology to the science of chemistry and astronomy are items that challenge the imagination of eager fourth, fifth, and sixth grade pupils.

Studying disease can be very practical in inner city areas where there are predominantly black schoolchildren. A discussion of sickle cell anemia is appropriate from the fourth grade up. Information relative to this genetic disease needs to get around. Moreover, anemic children suffer shortness of breath and tire easily. Unfortunately, too few parents and their children know if they have sickle cells in their bloodstream.

Suggested Activities

Primary Level

1. Consider germs from a general point of view. Ask if all germs are harmful. Talk about helpful little germs that give cheese its wonderful flavor. If possible, emphasize this point by giving each child a little cube of milk cheese to eat on a small cracker. Talk about the yeast that

makes bread rise and the germs helpful in turning apple juice into vinegar. Ask how many children have tasted apple cider. Follow this discussion with some information on harmful germs that make canned fruit spoil and milk and cream turn sour. Continue by relating germs to disease—the common cold and sore throat.

2. Ask someone to tell the class what measles, chickenpox, or some other common communicable disease is like. Why do people feel sick when they have a disease? What are some of the ways to keep germs away from the body? Emphasize cleanliness, injections by the doctor, vaccinations, good food, rest, and sleep.

3. Post on the board an enlarged picture of the common housefly. Or employ an opaque projector to enlarge a real fly a dozen times on the screen. Discuss other disease-carrying insects and rodents. West of Colorado, rats, squirrels, and rabbits spread more disease germs than in the East. Examine a fly under a magnifying glass. Note the hairs. Discuss how flies spread disease.

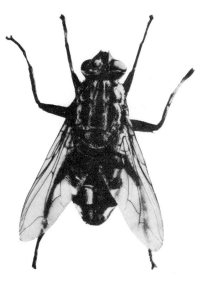

4. Build a simple exhibit of items about the house that help people control disease germs. A number of items, including a garbage can, a trash basket, a refrigerator, a clean toilet bowl, a bath tub, or a garden hose, may be made from cardboard (third grade).

5. For one week keep a record of the people who have been absent, taking notice of the reasons people are not in school. Emphasize improved health, not improved attendance.

6. Call attention occasionally to an opened box of clean paper tissues on the corner of a classroom table.

7. Have class members describe personal cleanliness and its relationship to the transmission of diseases. Call attention as often as needed to the manner in which germs travel among boys and girls:

    a. By coughing and sneezing

    b. By dirty hands and fingers of one person touching those of another

    c. By picking up and eating food that has fallen on the floor or sidewalk

    d. By failing to refuse food that has been bitten into by another person

    e. By sharing individual cups, glasses, and straws

    f. By coming to school with a bad cold

8. Call on a cub scout to describe his part in a cleanliness campaign. Perhaps the class could talk over how to organize a small one.

9. Have the class find how the early American settlers kept clean in such settlements as Jamestown or Plymouth.

10. Make a list of all the housekeeping chores engaged in by the mother to help keep the home clean. Then have each pupil choose a chore and illustrate it in mimetic form, or the chores may be selected by the class members as a topic for a drawing.

11. Engage in pupil-teacher planning of ways to keep the school washroom clean.

12. Demonstrate how to use the soap dispenser and towels.

13. Build a model hospital on a small classroom table. Dress several dolls as the doctor, nurse, and patient. Have a garage where a toy ambulance is ready

and waiting. A total class project can be planned by having the children, voluntarily or by assignment, secure the necessary items.

14. Post on board for a third grade class to see:

COMMON COLD PERPLEXES RESEARCHERS

Why is this so? There is little hope that a vaccine can be developed against the common cold; there are too many viruses that cause a cold (latest count = 113).

15. View the colored movie film, *How to Catch a Cold.* It may be obtained on a free loan basis from Kimberly-Clark Corporation (Kleenex) or Associated Films, Inc. Following the movie discuss the 2000 year old problem, the common cold.

16. Hang an attractive sign from the ceiling which may readily be seen by all pupils (see below).

Point out that colds are related not only to cleanliness, but also to getting overtired, wet, or chilled, balanced diets, sleep and rest, and fresh air and exercise.

17. An independent research project for some children is to find out how nursing started. A student may want to talk to some nurses. The teacher may read the booklet, *Florence Nightingale* (Metropolitan Life Insurance Co., free). Or, the 35 mm filmstrip of the same title and available from the same source may be shown.

18. Hold a clinical thermometer up for all pupils to see. Ask questions. Do you have a thermometer at home? Is it an oral or rectal thermometer? What does it tell? Should we encourage our parents to get a thermometer if they do not already have one?

19. Discover how dishwashing affects the family health. The commonplace food utensil is a potential carrier of many infectious diseases. Discuss hand washing, proper rinsing of dishes, hot water, soap, detergents, drying, and machine washed dishes (third grade). The machine washed dishes are the cleanest, according to the research results available from the American Public Health Association.

20. Create drawings to illustrate ways in which children can avoid infection, supplying appropriate captions for each poster, for example:

    a. "Catch That Sneeze" (a child may be shown coughing or sneezing into a disposable tissue).

    b. "Cut the Apple to Share It" (indicate the danger that can result from several persons taking bites from a single article of food).

    c. "Use Your Own" (show a child drying his face with his own towel or combing his hair with his own comb).

21. Look into the ways in which people live around the globe. They have special ways for living in hot, dry deserts; in hot, wet jungles; and in snow covered lands. Where does the *Zebra*

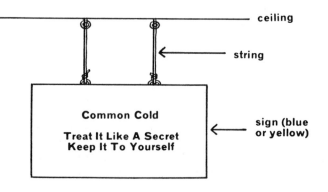

come from? (Africa) Are diseases different there than in USA?

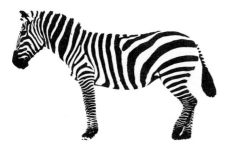

Intermediate Level

1. Prepare immunization record forms for parents to complete and keep at home. An excellent sample form may be obtained from the U.S. Public Health Service, Washington, D.C. 20402. Have pupils enlarge these forms and discuss their meaning.

2. Collect newspaper clippings concerning communicable diseases, community sanitation and cleanliness; and magazine advertisements having to do with health protection, cleanliness, and disease. Post these accounts and compare the number of magazine advertisements with the number of advertisements used for other topics. The soap and beauty ads alone will be quite plentiful.

3. Experiment with bacteria. Show that the germs "like" a warm, moist, and dark atmosphere in order to thrive and multiply.

a. Crush several dried beans. Place half of the beans in each of two containers. Cover with water. Store one of the containers in a warm, dark place and the other one on the classroom sill. After several days note the results.

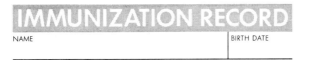

NAME				BIRTH DATE	

ADDRESS

IMMUNIZATION	YEAR SERIES COMPLETED	YEAR BOOSTERS RECEIVED			
		1	2	3	4
D.T.P.					D.T.
POLIO					
SMALLPOX					
MEASLES					
OTHER					

U.S. DEPARTMENT OF HEALTH, EDUCATION, AND WELFARE / Public Health Service

GUIDE FOR FUTURE IMMUNIZATION

THIS IS A GENERAL GUIDE ONLY. See your doctor or health department for your own schedule of immunizations.

D.T.P. Diphtheria, Tetanus (Lockjaw), and Pertussis (Whooping Cough) should be repeated at 18 months and 5 years of age.

D.T.* (Diphtheria-Tetanus), after age 8.

T.* (Tetanus)

SMALLPOX*

> *BOOSTERS ARE RECOMMENDED EVERY 3 TO 5 YEARS!

POLIO See your doctor about boosters.

b. Secure two apples. Peel one and place it in a dark, moist, and warm place; leave the other exposed to the air and sunlight on the teacher's desk. Note the results in a few days.

c. Indicate how the human skin acts as an envelope somewhat like the apple skin to protect the body.

4. Using a magnifying glass, study the molds that have grown on stale bread, fruit, or other material. Point out that there are other bacteria so small that only a microscope can magnify them enough for the human eye to see. Bring a microscope to class. Let each child use it. Talk about Leeuwenhoek's discovery of the microscope.

5. Identify and be able to use correctly such words as:

contagious	bacteria	scientists
disease	dangerous	laboratory
harmless	superstition	infection
sterilize	microscope	immune
pasteurize	health	ferment
quarantine	science	illness

6. Analyze the poem, *Strictly Germproof*, by Arthur Guiterman.

7. Demonstrate the ways in which drinking water differs. Illustrate the passage of water through stones and sand. Have a committee of several persons build a stone and sand model for class use: pour muddy water in at the top of the box; see how much cleaner it is when it comes out at the bottom.

8. Post and encourage comments regarding local rules about dogs and rabies immunization.

9. Inquire about raw milk. What are the dangers in drinking it? What is meant by tuberculin tested cattle? How does this compare with pasteurization in terms of health protection?

10. Read excerpts from the stimulating book by Hans Zinsser, *Rats, Lice, and History*. Here is a man who did a great deal of research and writing on typhus fever and wrote a best-seller. Follow this reading by discussing head lice. What are nits? What are graybacks? How may lice be controlled? Name other small insects and animals responsible for carrying disease.

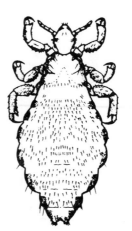

Pediculus humanus or head and body louse

Ye ugly creepin' blastit wonner,
Detested, shunn'd by saunt and
*   sinner!*
How dare ye set your fit upon her,
*   Sae fine a lady?*
Gae somewhere else, and seek your
*   dinner*
*   On some poor body.*

from To a Louse
by Robert Burns

11. Search out illnesses attributed to meats. Point out such things as the following:

a. Meat killed in the woods is not always properly refrigerated in time.

b. To prevent spoilage of meats a farmer sometimes coats it liberally with salt. Notice how salty country hams taste.

c. Look for the federal or state inspection stamp on meat that has been processed under favorable conditions.

d. Many animals are capable of carrying undulant fever and diarrhea to people. Swine spread hookworm, tapeworm, and muscle worms (trichinosis). All animals may spread tuberculosis.

e. The first meat inspections were made by early Egyptians and Israelites. Mohammedan food regulations today are similar to those of years ago. Meat inspections by the Federal Government began in 1890.

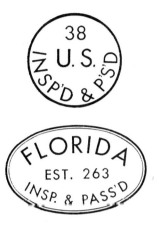

12. If at all possible, visit a meatpacking plant and see what takes place in the way of inspections, cleaning, and refrigeration. Post two large stamps of approval.

13. Assign library research reports on the stories of the lives of such scientists as Koch, Jenner, Pasteur, Reed, and Salk.

14. Ask a restaurant owner or any food handler to come and speak to the class on the rules and regulations for protecting the public from spoiled foods and inadequate sanitary practices.

15. Find the oath of Hippocrates.

1. Have you heard of the *oath of Hippocrates?* (See Encyclopedia.)
2. Is it as useful today as it was for doctors over 2000 years ago?

16. Set up the huge wall-chart on cancer cells. This superb chart is available (free) from Eli Lilly and Company. Investigate the 7 warning signs of cancer shown.

17. Compare normal red cells with sickle red cells. Introduce sickle cell anemia and encourage black children to find out if they have the sickle cell trait or actually have sickle cell anemia. Secure copies of *Where's Herbie?*, a sickle cell anemia story and coloring book, very well done and available from Children's Bureau, U.S. Dept. of Health, Education, and Welfare, 1972. (See Fig. 8–9.)

18. Investigate several dimensions of cancer. Show the American Cancer Society film *From One Cell.* Discuss how

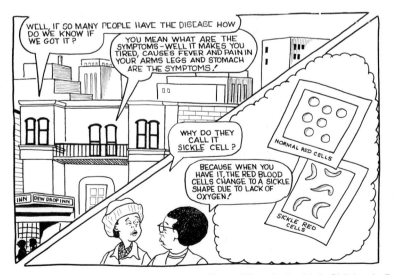

Figure 8–9 Sickle cell anemia needs attention. (From *Where's Herbie?*, Children's Bureau, U.S. Department of Health, Education, and Welfare.)

cancer spreads. Illustrate uncontrolled growth in plants (galls). Plants can be induced to develop cancer-like growths by applying chemicals. Encourage school laboratory or home experimentation: Paint the stems of growing tomato, castor bean, or sunflower plants with diluted tar or with a solution of ammonia in water. Irregular masses will form on the stems.

19. Post the words

MENS SANA
IN CORPORE
SANO

and ask the questions:

What does this mean?*
What are the implications for our lives?

20. Most North Vietnamese make a fetish of cleanliness. Prevention of disease is stressed through sanitation. Public health teams inspect the family outhouse. Families get special red slips if their outhouses are "clean enough to write poetry in." Try this information on a 5th grade class. How do they react?

7. SAFETY AND FIRST AID

> *Behavioral Objectives (Primary Level)*
>
> To understand and be able to practice such items as the following:
> Crosses the street safely.
> Travels the safest route from home to school.
> Demonstrates ability to give name, address, name of school, and name of parents.
> Demonstrates ability to get on and off the bus safely and behave safely when riding on buses, cars, and trains.
> Walks and runs in the right places.
> Shows what to do in cases of illness or injury to self or a companion. Describes how to report accidents and emergencies to an adult.

(*A sound mind in a sound body)

> Uses swings, slides, and other playground equipment properly.
> Recognizes the need for keeping buildings, walks, gymnasiums, and playgrounds safe.
> Demonstrates ability to use and properly store such items as saws, scissors, hoes, rakes, pins, needles, and other school-home equipment.
> Does not accept rides with strangers.
> Accepts responsibility for helping protect younger children.
> Acts properly in case of fire and practices simple rules of fire prevention.
> Chooses safe bicycle practices.
> Explains why he should refrain from teasing pets and playing with strange animals.
> Chooses to practice safety at home as well as at school.

> *Behavioral Objectives (Intermediate Level)*
>
> Crosses streets at intersections, obeying traffic signals, lights, and traffic rules.
> Practices safety in free play situations.
> Demonstrates safety in using a bicycle, the school bus, and all forms of public transportation, tools, electricity, and playground game equipment; and in flying kites where there are no power lines and no danger from automobile traffic.
> Shows skills required to administer first aid for slight injuries, such as sprains, fainting, insect, dog, or snake bites, burns, blisters, nosebleed.
> Describes safety precautions needed while swimming, fishing, boating, canoeing, and water skiing.
> Explains fire prevention in the home and in the community.

Comments

The magnitude of the accident problem today is reflected in the figures of the National Safety Council. According to this source, accidents to children outrank all other causes of death—killing more children between the ages of five and 14 years than cancer, congenital malformations, pneumonia, and polio-myelitis combined.

The need for safety education continues to increase despite the slight decline in child deaths and injuries. Recognizing the enormity of the problem, the U.S. Public Health Service expanded its accident prevention program, making it equal officially with the study of mental illness, cancer, and heart disease. This is understandable in view of the fact that there was a 12 per cent increase in drownings in the last decade; 500 children die each year from poisoning; and out of 800,000 dog bites a year there are thousands of children who haven't learned not to pet strange animals, and not to tease a dog or take away his bone. Also, there are over 50,000 children injured a year in pedestrian accidents. Those children in the first three grades fare poorly as compared with older groups. (See Fig. 8–10.) These figures are not surprising since primary graders are prone to cross streets at the wrong time, pass between parked cars, and dart into the street during their informal play activities.

Certainly the school, where half the accidents to children occur, has a definite responsibility in the area of safety instruction. Teachers must be cognizant that young people usually seek adventure and excitement. This is as it should be, for it is through adventure, challenging experiences, and bold activities that young people grow and develop their personalities. Frequently, however, children become absorbed in their classwork or in their play and forget to exercise precautions essential for their personal protection and the protection of other children around them. It is the little things sometimes that cause the greatest trouble and alert the teacher to a health teaching need. For example, among the non-hospitalized accidents to youngsters, injuries caused by cutting and piercing instruments and those involving bicycles exceed even the accidents due to motor vehicles. Falls in and about the school occur continually. Rabid dogs bite and sometimes disfigure children. Firearms explode at the wrong time. Drownings occur in every community where there is a body of water. Primary grade children become victims of their curiosity when it comes to poisons. The newly formed poison centers in one state alone handled 470 cases of poisoning in a

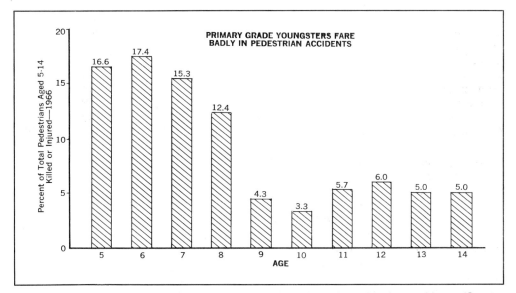

Figure 8–10 Percentage of school children killed or injured in pedestrian accidents. (Courtesy American Automobile Association.)

recent year. There were 48 cases of children drinking kerosene, 40 eating roach tablets, and 92 eating too many aspirins. These are items the school can do something about. In this respect, an excellent teaching guide is available from the Division of Accident Prevention, U.S. Public Health Service. It is entitled *Teaching Poison Prevention in Kindergartens and Primary Grades.*

About a quarter million products designed for use in the home contain toxins, and many of these seem to be attractive to youngsters for chewing, drinking, and eating. Products such as cleaning and polishing agents, detergents, shoe polish, cosmetics, paint, plant and food sprays, and a variety of medicines have all been involved in accidental poisonings. Efforts to decrease the number of home poisonings led to the passage in 1960 of the Hazardous Substance Labeling Act. It requires the labels of household aids and medicines to list poisons, antidotes, and recommendations for use. An important innovation in poisoning treatment procedures is the poison control center, organized by physicians and coordinated by the Department of Health, Education, and Welfare. There are almost 500 such centers in hospitals throughout the nation. Here the poison contents of thousands of trade-name products are cross-indexed. These are primarily information centers. However, neither the law concerning hazardous substances nor the poison control centers can help to decrease the number of poisonings if parents do not do their share.

Teachers have a real role to play. Once a year they should be instrumental in getting the message to all parents of primary grade children that poison hazards can be reduced by:

1. Placing drug cabinets high on the wall and locked, or securely fastened.

2. Keeping carbon tetrachloride, contained in dry-cleaning fluids and polishes, out of the way of children.

3. Keeping aspirin out of the reach of the young.

4. Checking the labels on children's toys to be sure that the paint used for the often bright and cheery colors is not deadly.

5. Determining whether or not unused medicine should be saved. To avoid hazards, unused medicine should be thrown away.

Accidents occur because of the human factor. Related to this at the elementary school age are essentially four elements:

1. Lack of knowledge and experience regarding the laws of cause and effect—the underlying reasons behind accidents and accident topics, i.e., fire, electricity, and water safety

2. Lack of skill in such activities as swimming, using playground apparatus, shop equipment, and crossing busy highways

3. Improper attitudes and personal traits—a "daredevil" or foolhardy manner that makes it easy to "take a chance"

4. Inadequate emotional health, coupled with unrestrained emotions and yielding an "accident-prone" state.

The last factor is especially interesting. A close study of accident causes shows too often that injuries are not as accidental as they first appear. A small number of people have a higher percentage of accidents. Even when they move to new locations they keep on getting hurt. These individuals are termed "accident-prone." They have an accident habit or pattern which usually develops early in childhood. Accidents have become their way of solving problems and frustrations. Thus the careless child who has frequent injuries and many minor accidents becomes the concern of medicine, psychology, and safety education. More specifically, this child has more emotional outbursts, lacks self-control to a greater degree, is apt to be more impulsive, and acts more hastily than other children.

What is suggested here should be quite clear; that is, avoiding accidents is not a simple matter. Overcautious teachers, for example, may fill a child's world with "don't"—"don't swim alone," "don't run down the stairs," implying that if he sits in the corner he will be safe. In reality his safety requires skill, judgment, and common sense to meet daily problems with successes. The relationship between feelings, emotions, and actions is fundamental. Thus accident prevention involves the promotion of good mental health, as well as day-by-day opportunities for children to practice safe behavior.

The school safety effort also calls for the provision of a safe school environment, one that is supervised and surveyed periodically. Across the land there are 800,000 accidental injuries to school pupils while under school jurisdiction. There should also be an accurate accident-reporting system. First aid, medical procedures, and fire drills must be set up on "standing orders." Community personnel must cooperate with the schools. And finally, the classroom instruction program must be carefully structured so that pupils completing a unit of work on safety will be quite aware of hazardous situations in the school and community and how to adjust to them satisfactorily.

At the primary and intermediate levels the accentuation is as follows:

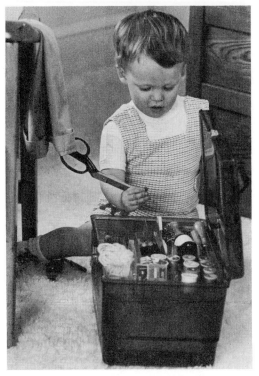

Figure 8–11 Children will talk about very curious toddlers.

Primary Level
1. Safety in the home
2. Safety to and from school
3. Classroom safety
4. Playground safety
5. School building safety

Intermediate Level
1. Safety patrols
2. Bicycle safety
3. Traffic safety
4. Fire prevention and drills
5. Home and farm safety
6. First aid procedures
7. Harmful substances

By the sixth grade more attention is directed toward firearms safety and other significant aspects of safety within the community. Certainly, in a town or city where there are a number of lakes and streams, some specific instruction is called for in the area of water safety. A growing number of the newer elementary schools have excellent swimming pools. In such cases instruction pertaining to personal safety is taught directly to pupils of all ages. This is done through the development of skills in swimming

and the handling of boats and canoes. These experiences in physical skills are followed by classroom discussions. This kind of "skill-knowledge" experience is extremely effective. Carryover value, in terms of habits and attitudes, is long lasting. Excitement-loving fifth and sixth grade boys and girls are sometimes repelled by the idea that being safe means avoiding all risks, but they may be intrigued with the idea that it takes smartness to recognize and appraise risks, and good judgment and skill to overcome them. Almost anything may be accomplished either in a hazardous or a comparatively safe manner. In class discussions teachers can help their pupils to realize that what counts in accident prevention is the ability to anticipate risks and the willingness to prepare to meet them with clear thinking and skill.

Teaching first aid to boys and girls permits the teacher to strengthen attitudes concerning how a person should react to emergency situations. Injury and sickness should be dealt with calmly and with an air of confidence. Fortunately, pupil interest is high. They give instant attention to accidents by asking, "Did he have to go to the hospital?" "Did he go in an ambulance?" "Will he be O.K.?" The teacher herself should have some training in first aid and be familiar with first aid supplies and the emergency practices in her school. She should also be able to capitalize on the curiosity aroused by individual first aid occurrences in the classroom. Taking advantage of interest by holding a group discussion on a topic growing out of an emergency situation is good teaching. As an example, an appropriate time to consider the control of bleeding and the precautions which should be taken to prevent it is when a pupil cuts his finger and requires immediate first aid. Likewise, when a child gets a blister or burns himself there is an opportunity to make safety education a vital subject in the health curriculum. A helpful booklet, *Teaching Safety in the Elementary School*, by Peter Yost, is available for the classroom teacher. It may be obtained from the Department of Classroom Teachers, N.E.A., Washington, D.C. 20036. Another excellent classroom teaching aid is the programmed instruction manual, *First Aid*, developed for sixth grade use by Behavioral Research Laboratories and distributed as a public service by Johnson & Johnson.

Considerable instructional assistance is available to any teacher who requests it from the National Safety Council. The materials are informative and are carefully designed to create and maintain student interest in personal health and safety. The 60-page booklet, *Improving Elementary School Safety—Here's How They Did It*, is a compilation of safety success stories, poems, songs, etc. from elementary teachers throughout the country. The Council periodically distributes leaflets illustrating unique experiences in elementary safety education. Teachers who want to meet real needs:

1. Make an analysis of the temporary and permanent hazards in the student's environment.

2. Make an analysis of the hazards connected with the pupil's activities.

3. Study the records collected through the usual student accident reporting system.

4. Study the hazards associated with the various seasons and with such special days as Fourth of July, Halloween, and Christmas.

5. Carefully consider individual student abilities, limitations, and difficulties.

Thus proper safety programs provide for many experiences in the classroom involving textbooks, audio-visual aids, and pupil-made materials. They also involve experience with school equipment, school buses, emergency drill, physical education activities, and such other major motivation items as junior safety councils, safety patrols, safety committees, monitors, and bicycle clubs.

It should also be pointed out that *Safety Magazine* is a periodical of high caliber which is worth reading each month for new ways and means of making this topic more effective with children.

No study of safety would be complete without referring to bicycle safety. The need for bicycle safety education is emphasized by the fact that three out of four youngsters between the ages of six and 15 ride a bicycle. There are more than 75 million bicycles on American streets and highways. Every 19 minutes, day and night, a cyclist is injured; every 21 hours a cyclist is killed by an automobile. It is recommended that all communities establish a sound procedure for testing, registering, and licensing bicycles. Four recommended practices, which the schoolteacher should know about, are as follows:

1. Test all bicycle owners for knowledge of traffic rules and regulations and skill in riding.

2. Inspect all bicycles for mechanical operation.

3. Register and license all bicycles.

4. Teach bicycle safety in the elementary school health program.

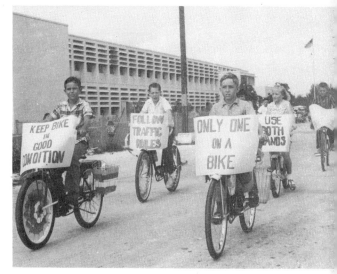

Figure 8–12 Bicycle safety project outside a Florida school. (Courtesy Dade County Public Schools.)

Numerous communities, working through the schools, have developed quite satisfactory bicycle safety programs. In Hamden, Connecticut, for example, a standard bicycle safety test record is kept on boys and girls. Once the examination is passed a wallet-size card is issued. Teachers interested in working out similar programs will discover the materials from the Bicycle Institute of America, Inc., quite exciting to use. The game book, *Bike Fun*, the *Bike Quiz Guide*, and the several colorful posters should be seen to be appreciated.

The suggested activities which follow on safety and first aid, instead of being grouped together, have been set up in categories. This is because safety embraces so many phases of the school and community environment. The categories are home and community safety, bicycle safety, school safety, playground and gymnasium safety, and first aid. Of course, some items overlap and tend to apply to more than one category. Bicycle safety, for instance, could easily have been incorporated under the home and community area or under school safety. However, because bicycle safety is such a major problem, the activities and experiences are treated separately.

Fire safety might well be treated as a separate topic. It is included here as an item under home and community and

school safety. With over a million fires a year, 11,000 fatalities (one third of them children), it becomes necessary to prepare lessons in fire prevention, many of which can be integrated with classes in history, science, and social studies. Significant fire safety materials for classroom use may be obtained for a small cost from the American Insurance Association in New York and the National Fire Protection Association in Boston. The latter organization has a great variety of materials prepared for school use; the *Sparky* fire prevention program is complete with a coloring book, posters, quizzes, and booklets. Helpful materials are also available from the American National Red Cross.

Suggested Activities

Home and Community Safety — Primary Level

1. Fires can be dangerous. Prepare an ordinary fire on the playground. Show that any child may put it out by pouring sand or water on it. Stress that children should not build fires by themselves.

2. In the winter, appoint several pupils to put sand or ashes on icy steps or pavement. Show young pupils how this reduces the danger of slipping. Show also how calcium chloride melts and helps break up ice.

3. Make an exhibit of familiar items

BICYCLE SAFETY TEST RECORD

	Initial of Inspector
Name of Pupil	
Written Test	
Mechanical Condition	
Test #1–Balance	
Test #2–Obstacle Course	
Test #3–Precision	
Test #4–Braking	
Test #5–Maneuvering	
Test #6–Hand Signals	
Certificate	

HAMDEN PUBLIC SCHOOLS
BICYCLE OPERATOR'S CERTIFICATE

This is to certify that

PUPIL'S NAME	SCHOOL

has passed an examination on Rules of the Road for bicycle riders and has passed the Bicycle Riding Test.

Matthew Barberi

SUPERVISOR OF PHYSICAL AND HEALTH EDUCATION	PRINCIPAL

which have rough surfaces to reduce the danger of slipping. This exhibit might include sport shoes, automobile tires, tires with snow treads, bicycle tires, rubber gloves, rubber backed throw rugs or mats.

4. Have pupils make suggestions relative to the causes of street accidents: not looking in either direction, running after a ball, dashing from behind parked cars, crossing the street diagonally or in the middle of the block (third grade).

5. Draw an imaginary street with intersections on the classroom floor. Use the children as buses and automobiles, a traffic officer, and people. Teach how to cross the street safely and obey signals (kindergarten or first grade).

6. Build with blocks. Make streets and sidewalks; place people, cars, and buses.

7. Use the sand table to build a community complete with streets, playgrounds, and houses. Put in traffic lights and stop signs. Use small toys for community equipment such as bulldozers, derricks, trucks, police cars, fire engines. Build an airport on the outskirts of the town. Use twigs and sticks as trees and telephone poles.

8. Make a stop and go sign for class use. Place a small inexpensive flashlight behind each piece of colored paper. Have the class practice operating and responding to the light changes.

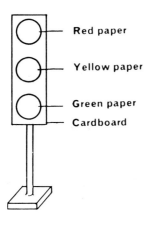

9. Visit such nearby places as the fire station, public playgrounds, railway stations, parks. Combine community health with safety education.

10. Play a game such as "grab bag game." Produce a big bag filled with various items. Have students draw from the bag pictures of pins, scissors, matches, nails, and sharp instruments, and tell how each should be taken care of.

11. Practice calling the fire department by telephone.

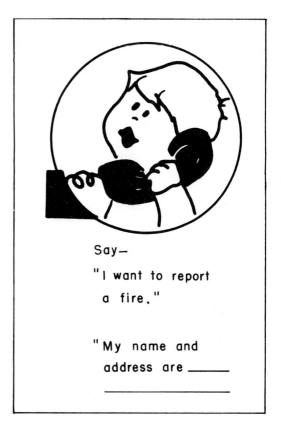

Say—

"I want to report a fire."

"My name and address are _____

_____

12. Build a model of a house that is open on one side, or borrow a large doll house for class demonstration of the relationship of space to accidents (third grade). Falls and poisonings may be traced to the unwise use of space. With the model show:

Small objects left on stairs
An open window on second floor
An open basement door
Medicines left where toddlers can "try" them

Electric toaster partly plugged into outlet

Ladder against the house

Milk bottles sitting on window sill

Bubbling coffee pot on edge of stove (with model of small baby standing under it)

13. Discuss "Our Friend the Fireman." Read or tell stories about brave firemen. Have children check off a list of fire hazards in their homes.

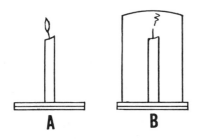

14. Demonstrate that a candle will not burn after it has used all the air under the glass jar which is put over it. Point out that if clothes catch fire, the fire can be smothered by wrapping the person in a rug (third grade).

15. Prepare an enlarged chart for a fire drill, marking exits in red. Talk over the importance of the fire drill and then conduct one.

16. Organize a fire brigade with the following duties:

    a. Inspect the school premises. Gather up papers and other waste materials and put them into metal containers. Watch for anything that might cause fires and report the condition to the teacher.

    b. Confiscate matches brought to school by boys and girls. Emphasize the need for thinking of others.

17. Have the class list ways in which falls may be prevented. Here are some examples:

Keep toys where they belong

Keep rugs straight

Ask grownups to reach things on high shelves

Keep shoelaces tied

Do not play on window sills and porch railings

18. Visit a drug store. Have the pharmacist point out poison labels and caution children regarding tasting substances they know nothing about (third grade). Return to the classroom, hang up a poison sign and talk about how children have put the following into their mouths:

Aspirin

Tranquilizers

Sleeping pills

Iron pills

Furniture polish

Cleaners and lye

Insect or rat poisons

Weed killers

Kerosene

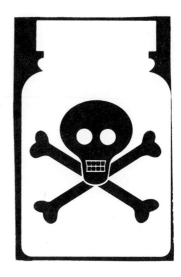

Home and Community Safety—Intermediate Level

1. Make a class survey of the community agencies for recreation. Discuss the facilities available and some of the hazards involved in their use.

2. Study the beaches and swimming pools with an eye to sanitation, supervision, safety devices, and the presence of lifeguards, and inform children about these conditions. The suggestions prepared by the American Red Cross may be quite helpful.

3. Build a model of a safe well, show-

ing that it should be dug properly, lined, and covered to protect the water from pollution; a model of the local inspection and purification plant might also be made by a committee of about three who would arrange to visit the plant manager and make sketches.

4. Encourage wide discussion on safety in the use of fire. Point out that over 2000 children die each year in home fires. Discuss lighted cigarettes, bonfires, electrical appliances, candles, gasoline and kerosene, rubbish, defective chimneys, stoves, fireplaces, and furnaces. Display the poster, *Don't Give Fire a Place to Start.* It may be obtained from National Fire Prevention Association.

5. Have a student demonstrate how to roll over and over on the floor in case the clothing is on fire. Have another pupil demonstrate how to wrap someone in a rug, blanket, or coat. "Never run. Inform an older person at once or turn in the alarm and wait for the firemen at the alarm box."

6. Demonstrate through group action such fire fighting methods as the bucket brigade and the volunteer system. Follow this with a description of the way the big city system is operated.

7. Invite the local fire chief or director of public safety to visit the class.

8. Have a pupil roller-skate into the class, preferably at a most inopportune time. Discuss roller-skating safety.

9. Have a pupil bring his pet dog or cat to a class. Talk about safe practices in handling animals and about avoiding strange dogs. Discuss rabies and, if appropriate (in the southern states), talk over animal hookworm.

10. Look into lead-based paints—especially with inner city children. Post a news clipping such as the one below to start discussion.

11. Plan a clean-up campaign in each home. Let the class hear some of the plans.

12. Check the daily paper for one week for accidents of all kinds. Note types of accidents and age classification.

13. Either organize a school safety council or consider ways of improving the one in existence (sixth grade).

14. Secure a list of city ordinances which pertain to public safety. Study these to find what they are all about.

15. An interesting activity, particularly for fourth graders, is to list and talk about dangerous products in our everyday life, which bring about 30,000 deaths and 20 million injuries every year. As studied by the National Commission on Product Safety in 1969 and more recently by the Senate Commerce Com-

FDA bans lead-based paints; urge anti-poisoning fund boost

The Food and Drug Administration last month published final orders banning lead from all household paints, while Congressional leaders urged an increase in federal funds to detect and treat lead poisoning and paint from ar

poisoning in the future problem of lead in Interior na level

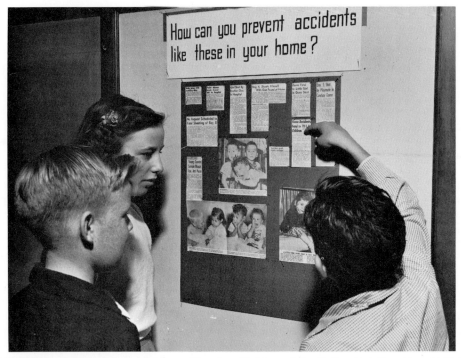

Figure 8–13 Hazards are everywhere. (Courtesy Safety and Youth Services Branch, Los Angeles Schools, California.)

mittee, among "unreasonably hazardous" products were: glass doors, color television sets, fireworks, gas-fired floor furnaces, glass bottles, high-rise bicycle handlebars, hot-water vaporizers, household chemicals, stepladders, power tools, football headgear, rotary lawn mowers, toys, wringer washing machines, electric blankets, electric driers, hot plates, bathtubs, extension cords, lead paints, propane gas, eyeglasses, swimming pools, boats, and aerosol containers. Look at each.

16. Discuss "the grownups." Do they always set a good example?

Display in front of the class the poster on page 207.

Tell the class that this is a reproduction of a jay-walking ticket actually distributed in Lakewood, Ohio. Discuss its implications (fifth or sixth grades).

17. Obtain and put up 11″ × 28″ colored posters from American Association of Poison Control Centers, c/o Academy of Medicine of Cleveland, 10525 Carnegie Avenue, Cleveland, Ohio 44106:

Little People Don't Read Labels
Avoid Accidental Poisoning: Keep All Medicines Here
Danger—Lead Poisoning Can Cause Death! (English or Spanish)

18. Discover the hazards of pesticides. They are potentially dangerous both in diluted and concentrated form. Accidental swallowing by children has been responsible for most deaths from pesticides.

Bicycle Safety—Primary Level

1. Display a large poster of a bicycle with lines going to all significant parts. Excellent posters may be obtained free

---

READ THE LABEL!
FOLLOW DIRECTIONS!

beam hits it and how it serves as a warning signal to protect *you* from unforeseen dangers. Show how the *basket* or *carrier* keeps the hands free for the proper control of the wheel. The Bicycle Institute of America will furnish an excellent four-color poster which wisely illustrates these bicycle aids.

3. Practice giving hand signals. Have several class members illustrate these by riding a bicycle on the playground for all to observe:

    a. Left arm *pointed up* for turning to the right.

    b. Left arm *straight out* for turning to the left.

    c. Left arm *pointed down* for slowing or stopping.

Posters in green and orange on bicycle hand signals may be obtained free from Bicycle Institute of America.

4. Bring a bicycle into class. Stand it on a table where all pupils can see it clearly. Discuss "How to care for your bicycle." Include the saddle, wheels, brake, handle grips, reflector, chain, pedals, warning devices, level of handle bars, fork bearings, light, spokes, tire pressure, and tire valves (third grade).

5. Have class members demonstrate the method of getting on a bicycle, the means of guiding it, applying the brake and coming to a stop, and parking the bicycle (first or second grade). Discuss using the horn or bell. Do not use the horn or bell as a brake.

6. Encourage pupils to send for safety materials from state motor vehicle departments and other sources. Materials

from the Bicycle Institute of America, Inc.

2. Talk about bicycle safety aids. Discuss the *bell or horn* as an important signaling device which should be used to warn of approach. Discuss the *headlight,* so essential for safe bicycling at night. Stress, however, that night riding should be held to a minimum. Illustrate how the *reflector* brightens when a headlight

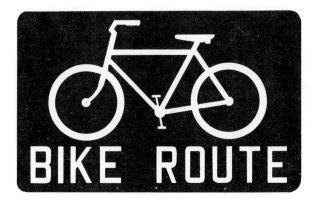

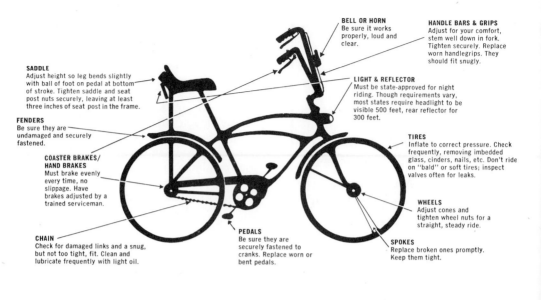

SADDLE
Adjust height so leg bends slightly
with ball of foot on pedal at bottom
of stroke. Tighten saddle and seat
post nuts securely, leaving at least
three inches of seat post in the frame.

FENDERS
Be sure they are
undamaged and securely
fastened.

**COASTER BRAKES/
HAND BRAKES**
Must brake evenly
every time, no
slippage. Have
brakes adjusted by a
trained serviceman.

CHAIN
Check for damaged links and a snug,
but not too tight, fit. Clean and
lubricate frequently with light oil.

PEDALS
Be sure they are
securely fastened to
cranks. Replace worn or
bent pedals.

BELL OR HORN
Be sure it works
properly, loud and
clear.

HANDLE BARS & GRIPS
Adjust for your comfort,
stem well down in fork.
Tighten securely. Replace
worn handlegrips. They
should fit snugly.

LIGHT & REFLECTOR
Must be state-approved for night
riding. Though requirements vary,
most states require headlight to be
visible 500 feet, rear reflector for
300 feet.

TIRES
Inflate to correct pressure. Check
frequently, removing imbedded
glass, cinders, nails, etc. Don't ride
on "bald" or soft tires; inspect
valves often for leaks.

WHEELS
Adjust cones and
tighten wheel nuts for a
straight, steady ride.

SPOKES
Replace broken ones promptly.
Keep them tight.

designed to assist those working with bicycle safety are available from:

a. American Automobile Association
   Traffic Engineering and Safety Department
   1712 G Street, N.W.
   Washington, D.C. 20006
b. Bicycle Institute of America
   122 E. 42nd Street
   New York, New York 10017
c. Insurance Institute for Highway Safety
   1725 DeSales Street, N.W.
   Washington, D.C. 20036
d. National Safety Council

425 N. Michigan Avenue
Chicago, Illinois 60611

7. Have the class draw and color road markers. Check on local variations by contacting the traffic police.

8. Talk over how to ride sidewalk vehicles:

a. Ride alone on a tricycle, not double.
b. Be especially careful when there are pedestrians on the sidewalk.
c. Watch cars backing out of garage or driveway.
d. Stay on sidewalks or in own yard—streets are made for fast-moving vehicles (kindergarten or first grade).

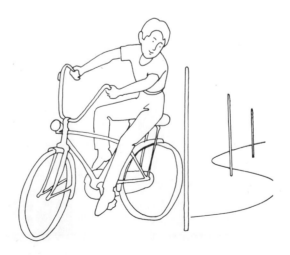

9. Play an obstacle game such as Bicycle Slalom. Set six poles in the ground about 10 feet apart. The participant races from the starting line about 20 yards to the first pole. He goes to the right or left of the poles to the finish line. Try a Potato Race or Tug-Of-War on bicycles. See *Bike Fun*, distributed free by Bicycle Institute of America.

Bicycle Safety—Intermediate Level

1. Administer a bicycle test at the start of this topic to see how much the class actually knows about their bicycles and how to use them. The *Bicycle Safety Quiz*, distributed (free) by Aetna Life Affiliated Companies, is a good one.

2. Post a readily visible list of bicycle safety rules on bulletin board. Typewritten rules on white paper pasted to a black background are easily noticed. Call attention to these rules and have the class check themselves to see how many they sometimes violate. Here is a sample list of rules:

    a. Observe all traffic regulations—red and green lights, one-way streets, stop signs.

    b. Never hitch on other vehicles, "stunt," or race in traffic.

    c. Have satisfactory signaling device to warn of approach.

    d. Ride at a safe speed.

    e. For night riding have a white light on front and a danger signal reflector on rear.

    f. Wear white or light-colored clothes at night.

    g. Give pedestrians the right of way.

    h. Avoid sidewalks; otherwise use extra care.

    i. Watch for car pulling out into traffic.

    j. Look out for sudden opening of automobile doors.

    k. Keep to the right, and ride in a single file.

    l. Keep a safe distance behind all vehicles.

    m. Do not carry other riders.

    n. Do not carry packages that obstruct vision or prevent proper control of the cycle.

    o. Slow down at street intersections; look to the right and left before crossing.

    p. Check the brakes for good working condition. Keep the bicycle in perfect running order.

    q. Ride in a straight line. Do not weave in or out of traffic or swerve from side to side.

    r. Always use proper hand signals for turning and stopping.

    s. Park the bicycle in a safe place.

3. Invite a safety specialist or member of the police department to talk on bicycle safety, including mechanical condition of the bicycle.

4. Organize a bike trip to a nearby park for lunch. Appoint a leader. Those who cannot go on bicycles may walk.

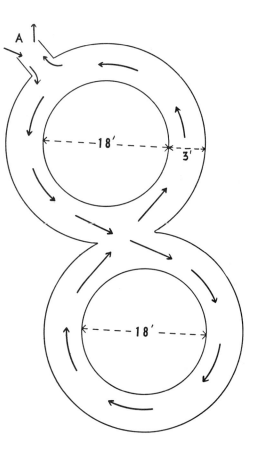

5. Prepare a bicycle skill test to be given on the school playground or play yard. Several of the pupils in the class

will be especially eager to help in such a project. The following test, for example, is not hard to set up.

    a. Begin at point A.

    b. Ride slowly, being careful not to touch border lines.

School Safety — Primary Level

1. Help the class analyze the essentials of good fire drill. Teach the importance of a cool and immediate response, how to send in the alarm in the community (in the absence of an adult), and where to find the fire hose and extinguisher in the school. Tour the school, corridor by corridor, to see these locations.

2. Talk about the safest route home from school. Early in the school term, practice crossing the street.

3. Play the little game, "Who Are You?" Line the class up in the front of the room. Appoint one pupil to ask the question of anyone he chooses, "Who are you?" The pupil selected gives his name, address, name of his school, and parents. If he does this satisfactorily, he becomes "it" next.

4. Use the school bus to practice safe behavior on a bus. Have the school bus driver speak to the pupils, especially in connection with a field trip.

5. Discuss what to do if a stranger offers a ride. Know that one should not accept rides from strangers.

6. Organize the class on a daily basis to put away their toys and other materials when they have finished using them.

7. Make an attractive cut-out to use with a school safety jingle. The one below, for example, could be used with third graders:

    a. Have the pupils step on a piece of colored paper. With a pencil trace the outline of the shoes.

    b. Cut out the footprints and in the space available write a safety jingle. See top of page for example.

School Safety — Intermediate Level

1. Discuss school fire hazards. Make a survey of the school building.

2. Prior to an extended vacation period (Thanksgiving, Christmas), make

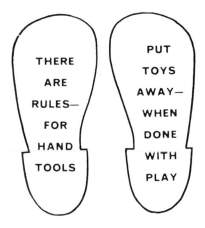

charts of safe practices to be followed during vacation activities. For example, what are the hazards to be aware of while on Christmas vacation, both indoor and outdoor?

3. Engage in safety poster construction. Each row or small group of pupils should be made responsible for a particular phase of safety; completed posters could be exhibited in the school corridor or multi-purpose room.

4. Participate in a school safety patrol. Train leaders so that everyone will eventually have a chance to be a patrolman; local traffic officials are usually available to assist the school safety patrol in setting up acceptable standards. This may well be a total elementary school project with classroom representation. Patrol standards and particulars are available from National Safety Council.

5. Describe an accident that may have happened in the school. Write down all the facts and decide what might have been done to prevent it. Compare pupil findings.

6. Safety is not an isolated topic. The help of a mother or a group of mothers may be enlisted in a discussion of school, home, and community safety. The children may enjoy preparing a play or reading a report on their safety activities before a group of interested adults.

7. Try "on the spot" safety messages over the school intercom system. A special event of the school day is connected to the safety message and relayed to the students.

Playground-Gymnasium Safety — Primary Level

1. Talk over the many sources of danger from playground accidents. Call attention briefly to items such as the following:

   a. *General:* Broken glass, protruding nails, tin cans left on ground. Unnecessarily rough play, tripping, pushing, climbing fences, shelters, trees. Congestion of activities. Bicycle riding across the playground, especially during games. Children with contagious skin diseases mingling with others. Activities not adapted to grounds. Dogs on grounds. Pools of water remaining after rain. Need for first aid kit.

   b. *Swings:* Jumping from moving swings, running or playing between or around swings. Climbing on frame while swings are in use. Holding baby brother or sister while swinging. Improper use of swings. Other activities too near swings. Swinging too high causing chains to slap and yank. Climbing across top of frame.

   c. *Sandboxes:* Glass, cans, and broken or unbroken bottles in boxes. Throwing sand or blocks; concealing hard or sharp objects in the sand. The use of a sandbox lid or cover when box is not in use. Looking for nails working loose and splinters.

   d. *Drinking fountain:* Pushing or crowding. Molesting the drinker. Unsanitary conditions of the bubbler.

2. Set up a number of situations to study. Refer to them as cases. Example:

CASE #1

Your town has just had a very heavy snowfall and schools are closed. You decide to go sledding with your friends. At the bottom of the steepest hill in your neighborhood is a busy thoroughfare. The police have not blocked off this street for sledding. *What should you do?*

---

3. Appoint a weekly clean-up squad for the play area.

4. In winter, when there is snow and ice, stress safe places to skate and slide. Point up the dangers of interfering with others. Encourage the use of targets in snowballing. Purposely set up targets and let everyone throw all the snowballs they want.

5. Plan an outing and, after the fun and food details have been considered, talk over the safety precautions:

   Provide safe transportation
   Use school bus if possible
   Have the school nurse go on the trip
   Check the availability of a telephone
   Take a first aid kit along
   Consider safe cooking, water supply, provisions for shade and rest
   Shelter from rain
   Protection from dangers of traffic

6. Study the natural surroundings at a picnic or outing area. Give information on such matters as poison ivy, poison oak, snakes, insects, and overexposure to the sun.

7. Select from several volunteers a group of children to help mark off the danger area around swings and to warn other children about entering it while swings are being used. Consider, also, other safe practices and equipment safety rules.

8. Demonstrate the importance of proper footwear on a gymnasium floor. Stress that sneakers are cleaner than shoes, that they give better traction while shoes slide, that it is difficult to be agile and quick when wearing shoes, and that our athletic skill is improved when we wear good sneakers.

Playground-Gymnasium Safety — Intermediate Level

1. Appoint a small committee to inspect the playground or gymnasium area, its equipment, and game boundary lines. Have these people report back to the class. Point out that faulty and hazardous conditions should be remedied immediately, or the play area should be closed from further use.

2. Have boys and girls discover how clear rules and definite boundary lines help make a game safe.

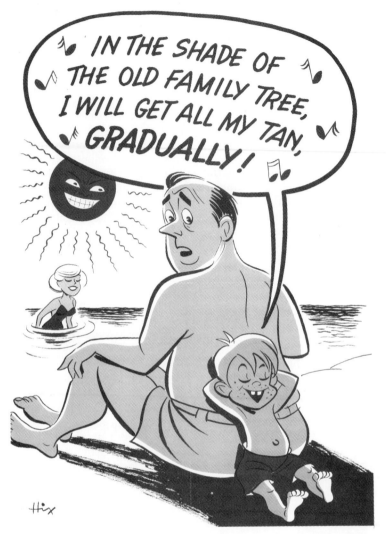

Figure 8–14 Posters promote both laughs and questions. (Courtesy Employers Mutuals of Wausau.)

3. Indicate the relationship between properly developed game skills and safe performance. This may be illustrated by having two boys throw a ball accurately in dodgeball or handle themselves on a dodging run in a relay-type activity.

4. Have a painting project. Gaily colored swings and slides help reduce playground injuries. In addition, the attractive colors help entice youngsters to the playground and away from the street.

    a. Slides—paint them green to counteract excessive sunlight. Paint the steps to the top of the slide yellow to draw the children's attention.

    b. See-saws—paint green, with edges painted yellow to give greater visibility and reduce chances of children running into them.

    c. Swings and swing rings—paint seats and swings yellow. Green is best for upright and overhead bars.

    d. Sandboxes—paint green.

    e. Jungle gyms—paint a cool restful blue.

f. Trash cans—paint gray with a white star. This emphasizes neatness and encourages youngsters to help keep the playground or gymnasium area tidy.

5. Have pupils make a list of the many sources of danger on playgrounds and in gymnasiums, such as:

a. *Baseball:* Playing too near the street and chasing balls into the street. Spectators too near baseline during a game. Batting fly balls in too small an area. Throwing the bat after hitting the ball. Playing catch too near swings, sandboxes, and other activities. Older boys playing on an area adapted only for younger children.

b. *Horseshoes:* Running in front of the pitcher. Careless pitching and throwing too near other activities. Pitching distance too great for control. Locating stakes where children are likely to pass between.

c. *Gym Floor:* Unnecessary running and pushing. Interfering with others who are on equipment. Playing unsafe games. Wearing shoes without rubber soles in gym. Wearing poor quality sneakers, especially for heavy children. Safe playing facilities: Do doors open outward? Are end walls padded? Is the heat of the water in the shower room automatically controlled? Are the radiators screened or set back into the wall? Does the gym floor have a smooth, non-slip surface?

6. Show the relationship between good sportsmanship and safe play activities.

7. Demonstrate with pupils the safety rules for the most popular games. Example: Soft-ball: (a) The batter who throws the bat is automatically out, (b) catching behind the bat without a mask is prohibited, (c) sliding into a base is not permitted, (d) always signal that you are about to catch a fly ball so that someone else will know that you are after it and avoid a collision.

First Aid—Primary Level

1. Discuss the ways in which small children may get burned. Example:

a. Surface burns may be caused by falling on hot radiators, touching hot stoves or electric irons or toasters.

b. Burns may be caused by hot liquids falling off the stove, by bumping into a person with a hot substance, and by careless playing with matches.

Point out what to do when a burn occurs.

2. Show pictures or exhibit real cans of varnish, paint, kerosene, and gasoline. Have pupils give reasons for not touching or tasting these liquids.

3. Dramatize proper procedure to follow in case of an accident in the school, the house, at the beach, or on the playground. Keep calm. Call an adult. Be of help where you can.

4. Find out about accidents and emergencies that should be reported to adults.

First Aid—Intermediate Level

1. Plan and equip a first aid cabinet for the school. Consider also the items one might need on a day-long hike or trip into the country. Local needs should be considered.

2. Read about poisonous plants. Study how to prevent poison ivy, and stress what to do if one has been exposed to it. Show plastic replica of poison ivy, oak, and sumac available from Eli Lilly Company.

3. Discuss the ways of acquiring a sun tan. Refer to the dangers.

4. Demonstrate care of ordinary cuts and bruises.

5. Practice the control of bleeding (fifth or sixth grade).

6. Practice giving artificial respiration. Blankets or heavy paper may be placed on the floor, children divided into pairs to work on each other. See the American Red Cross Water Safety or First Aid Manual for the approved manner in giving the Holger-Neilson (arm lift—back pressure) method of artificial respiration. Refer also to mouth-to-mouth breathing. (ARC Junior Life Saving material.) Complimentary copies of *The Breath of Life,* with clear drawings of

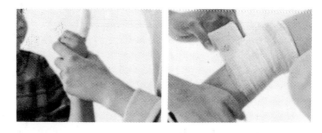

how to give mouth-to-mouth breathing, may be obtained from Aetna Life Insurance Co. Johnson and Johnson, Metropolitan Life Insurance Company, and American Insurance Association, all make first aid guides available at no cost. The Johnson and Johnson film, *First Aid Now,* is also appropriate (no charge).

6. Have the class print markers for poison containers that should be left alone. These may be done on adhesive tape. Have the pupils take the markers home and ask their parents to put them on medicine bottles and boxes.

7. Make a list of first aid practices that might be employed in the winter sports scene. Consider accidents while coasting, skiing, and skating. Do the same thing for summer safety. Discuss diving into unknown waters, picking strange fruit, treating sunburn, and dangers involved in using an axe or knife.

8. Practice putting bandages on fingers and knees.

8. MENTAL HEALTH

Behavioral Objectives (Primary Level)

Explains what it means to be accepted by classmates and school.

Demonstrates some ability to adjust in part to the demands of daily living, and establish satisfactory relationships with others.

Identifies new interests and new friends.

Shares work and play materials with others and accepts some responsibility for actions.

Overcomes difficulties and adjusts to minor disappointments.

Chooses to help others, and gains personal satisfaction.

Behavioral Objectives (Intermediate Level)

Distinguishes between responsible and irresponsible actions as a member of the school and member of a family.

Employs ways of showing specific regard and respect for the welfare of others and for oneself. Serves sometimes as a leader and sometimes as a follower in school situations.

Enjoys working with others in play and work activities, and realizes that routine changes and unexpected failures and successes are to be taken in stride.

Explains how mental health and personal feelings have a bearing on the way the whole body works.

Describes the fine relationship between mental health, recreation, and rest.

Sets personal goals and shows how to attain them while maintaining proper mental health.

Comments

Learning to live together harmoniously is still the number one problem for the people of the world to solve. Moreover, the hospitals and physicians' offices of the country are crowded with thousands of people (vast numbers of whom are children) who are ill enough to seek the assistance of a physician, but whose illnesses are emotionally conditioned and frequently do not involve organic disease. This area of medicine is concerned with somatic symptoms (pain, rapid heart, loss of appetite, undue fatigue) and psychological or emotionally induced reactions. Every other person today who seeks the help of a physician has emotionally induced illness. Such individuals may be classed in one way or another as emotionally immature; they are not able to face life as it really is, and their illness serves as a measure of their vulnerability to these stresses. Unfortunately, the steadily rising tempo of American life brings on growing tensions, frustrations, and complexities.

Mental health is more than the absence of mental illness. It is a style of life characterized by a capacity to adapt—a growth of the ability to cope with a wider range of changes in a complicated culture. Moreover, individual evidences of failure to adapt not only can be interrupted and reversed, but they can be *prevented.* This is why human dignity must be nurtured right in the local community, especially if children are to be guided toward sound mental health. In the larger areas teachers can get help from the Community Mental Health Centers established by Congress to intercept emerging crises in the home community.

There are few endeavors in the school curriculum of more importance than the one concerned with the development of mental health. This is admirably set forth in *Mental Health in the Schools.*[16]

When a realistic perception of self is added to a realistic perception of the world, the possibility of effective and productive interaction is reasonably assured. The mentally healthy person's relationships with people and the world produce certain constructive consequences. Two consequences are especially significant to the school. First, the mentally healthy person perceives reality with minimal distortion and is able to communicate these perceptions effectively. Second, the possession of self-esteem contributes to intellectual functioning.

Back of the teenage difficulties and the compulsive search for happiness are unresolved problems that have to do with living with oneself and others during the formative elementary school years—when the classroom teacher's influence in the child's community is most effective. In the early grades there are opportunities to encourage children to come out of isolation so that they can find themselves. When Ivan Illich talks about "de-schooling," he is stressing the need to get away from institutions and toward individuals. Silberman in *Crisis in the Classroom* calls for the same thing and, each in his own way, Piaget, Erickson, Bruner, and even John Dewey have made the same point.[17]

Although sound mental health is related to the family background, the elementary school is in an excellent position to influence boys and girls. The chief reason for this is that personalities are defined early, and children frequent the elementary grades during the most formative years. Early habits of response to teachers and classmates, to simple requests, to ideas, and the like are established during these elementary school years. The needs of children and the interrelationship of these needs are impressive at this time. Mental health activities must be taught in the light of these needs; children have real feelings even if they are not aware of them at the time. Maslow suggests six groups of needs to keep in mind when teaching. These are: (a) physical needs, (b) safety needs, (c) love needs, including the need for affection, belonging, and mutuality, (d) esteem needs, including the needs for mastery, achievement, recognition, approval, and self-respect, (e) the need to solve problems and have sources of information, and (f) the need for self-realization, including the need to develop a sense of personal identity, to accomplish the tasks for which one is best fitted, and to function at a level in keeping with one's capacities.[18]

Setting up a health curriculum that includes instruction in mental health is both challenging and formidable. It simply is not easy to teach personality adjustment and wholesome participation in the classroom, although this is where the child spends most of his time outside of

---

[16]Joint Committee Report. *Mental Health in the Schools*, 32 pages, 1966. Available from Chief State School Officers (NEA), 1201 16th St., N.W., Washington, D.C. 20036.

[17]For greater detail see "Mental Health at an Early Age" by Carl E. Willgoose, *Instructor*, *81*:58–59, October 1971.

[18]Maslow, A. H. "Theory of Human Motivation," *Psychological Review, 50*:370–376, 1953.

the home. This is the place where he is often deeply affected by his daily experience. Instruction in mental health, therefore, must permeate the *total* program. In a sense, it is not a subject at all, but a way of teaching. Curriculum cannot be divorced from method.

Since the human personality cannot be compartmentalized, every subject-matter area has experiences and activities, often too subtle to measure, which consciously and unconsciously promote mental health. Every essential skill and learning, when coupled with worthwhile feelings and attitudes, tends to build a wholesome personality. Practically all classroom and school environment activities serve as social science experiences. In the laboratory of the classroom, gymnasium, lunchroom, workshop, and playground are to be found opportunities for attaining emotional maturity. Mental health is fostered through learning the rules of sportsmanship and learning to play together in physical education. It is enhanced when pressures to succeed are relaxed a bit in arithmetic and reading. It is encouraged when scientific appreciations are deeply felt, for personal adjustment in the modern world is more than slightly related to our understanding of scientific advances. Music and art, when taught as recreational or diverting activities to be enjoyed, are rich items in the promotion of mental health. In addition, it seems true that the *way* we teach has much to do with relieving "pressures" and permitting the pupil to work up to his potential.

Instruction in mental health requires that the teacher know the pupils, not as entities in the classroom but as living personalities. The instruction, to be effective, must involve each pupil in a number of activities designed to bring out his personality. This is an ongoing process which is further enhanced by the teacher's own mental health. By example and precept she helps children make optimum adjustments in school; and most of all she makes them *feel wanted.* Youth is a time for reaching for human touch points; a time for searching. It is not always a joyous time, for sometimes one reaches and there is no one to touch. As one older pupil said, when looking back on his elementary school years: "I felt alone . . . I felt different . . . I was popular on the outside but shy and insecure on the inside . . . I needed friends . . . I needed to be accepted . . . I needed to feel valuable and important somewhere . . . I needed to be close to someone. . . ." At any age life is bound to be full of disappointments. Even so, wrote the Irish playright Sean O'Casey, ". . . each of us one time or another, can ride a white horse, can have rings on his fingers and bells on his toes, and if we keep our senses open to the scents, sounds, and sights all around us, we shall have music wherever we go." How to help young people discover the "scents, sounds and sights" is the inspiring task here.

Primary grade children love movement. They love to play. In fact, they play because they must. Their running, jumping, and dodging have potential val-

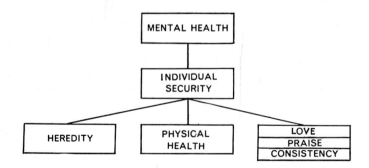

ues beyond the purely physical ones. Play contributes immeasurably to personality growth. Play and game situations in the classroom, therefore, have a vital part in building mental-emotional health.

Primary grade instruction and learning activities foster and deal primarily with:

A feeling of belonging
Inspiring self-confidence
Assuming responsibility
A feeling of importance
Making decisions
Realizing limitations
Learning to profit by mistakes
Consideration for others
Making others happy
Affection
Respecting the rights of others
Etiquette
Facing up to fears
Keeping healthy
Pride in family
Getting along with others
New experiences

Exploring these kinds of mental health activities should provide a degree of built-in motivating power that will foster some creative ways of learning. Research has indicated for years that almost any kind of human functioning can be improved by increasing motivation. In this instance creative growth is the issue. Torrance and Myers make it clear that one of the most important conditions for creative growth is that pupils feel that *their* teacher is on *their* side.[19] Following along from this point Sylwester and Matthews would have the children ask many questions—especially these four:[20]
1. What am I like?
2. How am I changing?
3. What will I be like?
4. How will I affect others and how will they affect me?
Peeking at one's feelings at the primary level may even be more important than

waiting until later on. In the Brookline, Massachusetts schools, for example, the emphasis on mental health and personality development has been shifted from the junior high level to the elementary. Here, the Dimensions of Personality series is used.[21] In the third grade text, *What About Me,* the discussion topics are: 1) I Belong Here, 2) I'm Somebody Special, 3) My Feelings Are Me, 4) Who's Afraid, 5) I Feel Mean, 6) I Like Me, and 7) Becoming Me. In the intermediate grades this particular series is loaded with ideas for understanding mental health. For one thing, it helps the teacher be more *personal* in teaching. It gets at emotions, awareness and self-image in an interesting fashion. Paperback books for the students include: *Here I Am* (Grade Four), *I'm Not Alone* (Grade Five), and *Becoming Myself* (Grade Six).

Additional intermediate grade instruction and learning activities which promote mental health deal primarily with:

Leadership and ability to follow
Assuming responsibility
Knowledge of how to act
Desirable personality traits
Worthwhile interests
Extending areas of interest
A chance to create something
Accepting oneself
Emotional controls
Interest in others
Making friends
Working together

A number of sources of substantive information and teaching ideas are available relative to the topic of mental health which are readily available to teachers. The Child Study Association of America, the American Medical Association, and the American School Health Association have printed materials. There are many excellent films such as "Mr. Finley's Feelings" (Metropolitan Life Insurance Co.) and filmstrips for elementary school use. The colorful film-

[19]Torrance, E. Paul and R. E. Myers, *Creative Learning and Teaching,* New York: Dodd, Mead & Company, 1971, p. 110

[20]Sylwester, Robert and Esther Matthews, "Four Big Questions Children Need To Ask," *Instructor,* 81:46–50, February 1972.

[21]Published by Pflaum/Standard, 38 West Fifth Street, Dayton, Ohio 45402.

strips on mental health topics of prejudice, envy, and criticism are part of a seven-part series designed by Image Publishing Corporation (Box 14, North Station, White Plains, N.Y. 10603) to develop deeper insights regarding mental attitudes.

In order to pinpoint more specifically what has already been stated rather generally, the following *teacher activities* are set forth as follows:

1. Create a desirable classroom atmosphere by making the room as cheerful, attractive, and healthful as possible.

2. Observe the relationship between each child and his companions. Where a pupil avoids another, or fails to make friends, attempt to discover the cause.

3. Arrange group activities so that children showing the greatest difficulty in making friends may have a chance to participate.

4. Encourage the confident child to make friends of the timid.

5. Promote good fellowship through the art of listening and of cooperating in carrying out group ideas.

6. Develop opportunities for leadership. Group children so that all have a fair opportunity for recognition. Change groups so that leadership is not restricted to just one of two children whose leadership qualities are already developed.

7. Plan for children to share to a maximum degree in planning classroom activities. Try to give each child the feeling that he has something to contribute.

8. Provide opportunities for original effort. Avoid doing things for children which they can do themselves.

9. Give credit to pupil ideas and suggestions.

10. Challenge the pupil's creative imagination by having available a number of simple craft materials such as wood, fiber, plaster, and metal. Provide a time and place to work with these materials in an atmosphere conducive to creative work.

11. Encourage wholesome curiosity. Aid children who wish to explore and ask questions.

12. Use tests to help judge each pupil's intellectual capacity so that neither too much nor too little is expected of him.

13. Create a classroom atmosphere of fairness. One should see that rules and regulations are reasonable. Have only a few rules, but see that all observe them. This is also true in games played in the gymnasium or on the playground.

14. Keep the classroom atmosphere calm and serene, businesslike but unhurried.

Suggested Activities

Primary Level

1. Hang a printed sign or large poster in front of the class for a few hours prior to discussing its meaning:

> A GOOD LAUGH
> IS SUNSHINE
> IN THE HOUSE
> —William Makepeace Thackeray

2. Explain something that is painful to the teacher. Have the class suggest means of solving it.

3. Talk about self-awareness: What am I like? (3rd grade)

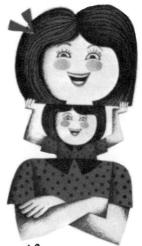

self-awareness

4. Make a list of the qualities admired in other people.

5. Use every opportunity to practice using terms such as "please," and "thank you" (kindergarten or first grade).

6. Share toys and materials.

7. Send cards, pictures, or class letters to classmates who are ill.

8. Read and discuss stories which show thoughtfulness of others.

9. When a new pupil joins the class, plan several ways to make him feel at home.

10. Bring pets to class and talk about how one treats his pets.

11. Work as a group on several projects. Point out to the class what each individual has done so that everyone will appreciate the contributions of others.

12. Encourage serving on committees and taking turns as leader.

13. Encourage children, especially at the start of the school year, to talk about themselves, what they like most at home, and what they think they will like around school.

14. Cooperate in keeping the room attractive.

15. Plan picnics and school parties. Talk about and demonstrate good manners and decide how everyone should act on the bus, on the street, in the stores, and on visits.

16. Do something about others less fortunate. Secure large scrapbooks from the ten-cent store and let the class cut colorful pictures from magazines and paste them in the books for sick children in the hospital.

17. Talk over taking turns on playground equipment.

18. Permit pupils to talk about their families. Encourage them to tell what they do to keep their home a happy place.

19. Try role-playing. Describe the rules, select volunteers. After acting out the sociodrama ask other class members if the enactment was realistic.[22]

20. Keep a collection at school of something that each child cherishes.

21. Collect and post pictures of people showing kindness, and of happy children and families.

22. Draw cartoons of various facial expressions in order to show feelings.

[22] See steps set forth by Lynn Teper, "Role Playing as a Tool in Mental Health Education," *School Health Review*, 2:31–32, February 1971.

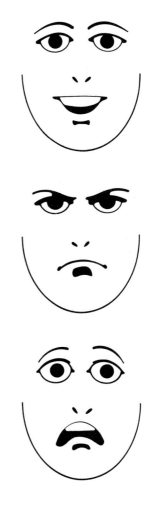

Intermediate Level

1. Write, tell, read, and discuss stories about emotions. Particular instances of interest may be dramatized.

2. Discuss spontaneous situations that arise to develop understanding of emotions of other children. Use interesting stories involving emotional problems to stimulate discussions on the importance of controlling our emotions.

3. Participate in creative activities, such as finger painting, drawing, painting, clay modeling and rhythmics, as acceptable means of expressing emotions. "Talk it out" with sympathetic listeners.

4. Arrange for parent and child to each explain his feelings toward the other on a tape recorder and listen to each other's tapes (5th-6th grades).

5. Send a sunshine package to some-

one who is ill. This may contain cards, pictures, and various objects presented by the class.

6. Share hobbies. Have pupils tell about and demonstrate their special hobby before the class (sixth grade).

7. Make up some everyday problems, and give correct and incorrect ways of solving them. Also use "open-end stories" regarding a problem, using class names.

8. Choose a class hospitality committee and set up a procedure for operation.

9. Have each class member pick out his worst habit or worst fault and tell how he hopes to overcome it.

10. Set up a question box and encourage questions concerning worries and fears of class members. "What's on Your Mind?" box precipitates some excellent discussion.

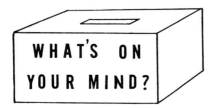

11. Hear reports on famous handicapped persons such as Keller, Edison, and Baruch, who have succeeded in spite of their handicaps.

12. Have several boys and girls tell how someone helped them to feel better or to gain self-confidence (sixth grade).

13. Collect newspaper clippings depicting cases of mental problems. Note, also, the numerous articles which appear in the paper and have to do with personal unhappiness. In the course of a week, check to see if news items of an unhappy nature are more or less prevalent than those of a happy nature (sixth grade).

14. Have each pupil make a list of several things he likes about (a) girls and (b) boys. Make a similar list of dislikes. Do the likes outbalance the dislikes?

15. Look up the meaning of the word "please." Say the word "please" in the following manner: when angry, when happy, when pleased, when worried, when anxious.[23]

16. Emphasize good sportsmanship and fair play. This may be done through a project on accident prevention on the playground.

17. List the characteristics of people who are able to get along well with others. Discuss famous people, their lives, achievements, and characteristics. Show the effect of a good personality as a positive force in living together harmoniously.

18. Find out why fatigue or illness can make us "fussy" or irritable.

19. Through careful "soul-searching" discover that everyone is good at something.

20. As a class, "adopt" a younger child who needs help. This should help encourage an awareness of, and sensitivity to, the feelings and difficulties of others less fortunate.

21. Put a notice on the front blackboard. Ask a 5th or 6th grade group what it might have to do with mental well-being. (See top of p. 221.)

22. In a fifth-grade Cincinnati school classroom, the topic of mental maturation was discussed, with students in the leadership role. The leader had a 3' × 4' chart entitled "How Mature Am I?" It carried the following list:

1. When someone pokes fun at me.
2. When someone disagrees with me.
3. When I want attention.
4. When I am confused.
5. When I don't get what I want.

At the right was a column for each day of the week, in which ratings could be entered.

23. On a piece of paper put down some personal items. It will be kept secret by being put in a large envelope with the others in the class. Two or

---

[23]See also Genelle K. Mantz, "Can Mental Health Be Taught?" *Journal of School Health,* 42:398–399, September 1972.

HELP I'M BEING HELD
PRISONER BEHIND
THE BLACKBOARD

three months later it can be returned. The changes will be interesting—if not amusing (4th or 5th grade).

	Now	Later in Time
My name	_____	_____
My weight	_____	_____
Best friend	_____	_____
Newest friend	_____	_____
Favorite song	_____	_____
Favorite food	_____	_____
Favorite game	_____	_____
What I worry about most	_____	_____
Other items	_____	_____

9. SEX AND FAMILY LIVING EDUCATION

Behavioral Objectives (Primary Level)

Describes a happy home and explains how one acts in it.

Shares work as well as recreation in the home.

Explains how animals protect and feed their babies.

Identifies with other living things— life with life, both plant and animal.

Investigates how living things come from other living things—plant life, baby animals, mothers and babies.

Chooses a variety of activities that bring about good times in the home and family living.

Behavioral Objectives (Intermediate Level)

Evaluates the specific role of each family member in maintaining a happy home.

Interprets the cooperative and unique contributions of both sexes to society.

Relates how life begins and how physical growth advances.

Describes the relationship of boy and girl behavior to social living and to family-community life in general.

Analyzes the different interests and activity choices of boys and girls.

Describes the function of menstruation and conception, and how life begins from a single cell.

Employs several means to demonstrate that social and emotional growth is an essential part of the process of maturation.

Comments

It has been wisely stated that sex is not something we do—it is something we are. Therefore, sex will never be thoroughly understood until it is related to the total adjustment of the individual in his family and his society. Ultimately, everyone must define his sexual role and establish a value system. The combined efforts of the home, church, and school are required in order to bring about a full understanding and acceptance of human sexuality at all age levels.

Interest in sex occurs at all ages. Whether sex education is formal or informal, a part of the home life or a part of the "gang talk" on the street corner, it is of vital concern to all growing boys and girls. Knowledges and appreciations in this area are every bit as important in terms of future behavior as they are in other health areas. More and more research indicates that the school is in an excellent position to carry out a sound sex education program. Here children gain values from peer-group discussions under competent leadership which is difficult for parents to duplicate.

Since attitudes are formed at an early age, it is important to start sex education at a time prior to the building up of personal inhibitions — inhibitions which tend to limit frank discussion. Foster has shown in a study of age and grade level inhibitions that children at the fifth grade level or below normally do not possess reticence toward matters of sex. He states that, "only if sex education is delayed . . . will the feeling of improperness influence his thinking since the child will have incorporated all of the fears and incorrect thoughts of his peers and perhaps his family. . . . It is better to be a year early in our provision of sex education during pre-adolescence than to be a day too late in adolescence."[24]

There is an immediate need for an educational program to offset the half-truths and general misinformation that children are constantly exposed to through the commercial exploitation of sex and erotica by modern mass media. Children have grown up to become adults who believe that sex is simply a plaything, or at best a biological phenomenon — a reproductive item. They have not understood it as an integral part of total personality. Quite the contrary, they see it as genital-centered — the exact opposite of what should be the goal.

It is difficult to develop responsible sexual morality in personal and family situations when the "anything goes" philosophy of life permeates the minds of primary graders and adults alike. As the old taboos die and the permissive society takes shape, only a calculated sex and family living education can hope to be an effective counteracting agent. This is not easy. It is a difficult undertaking in an era of endless seductions, obscene language, increasing nudity, suggestive posters and films, homosexual frankness, and an almost constant celebration of the erotic life.

Confusing genital-centered sex with true sexuality is recognized by the major faiths and parent groups as an unfortunate contemporary fact. Its relationship to sexual experimentation, venereal disease, promiscuity, pregnant teenagers, and unwed mothers is clear. The statistics are frequently overwhelming. (Review the evidence in Chapter 1.) Moreover, the numerous expressions of sex are as important to the health of the marital relationship and to the solid foundation of the family in twentieth century society as are its procreative aspects.

The Role of the School

It is the function of the school to cooperate with community leaders in the early exploration and planning of a curriculum in sex and family living education, from the kindergarten through high school. Failure to do so has almost always resulted in misunderstandings and less than adequate programs. Local groups of citizens should realize that they do indeed have a say in what the school does. Also, they have a responsibility to back the school in its efforts.

From the start it should be made clear that the objective is to eliminate anxieties and misunderstandings pertaining to

---

[24]Foster, Greg R. "Sex Information vs. Sex Education: Implications for School Health," *Journal of School Health,* 37:248–250, May 1967.

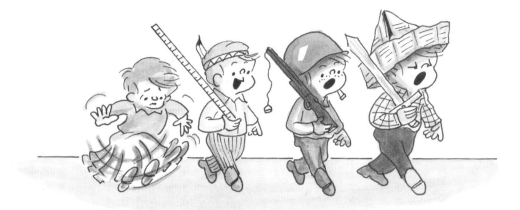

Figure 8–15 "Hut, Toop, Threep, Forp, Fiivp, Sex, Sevm, Hate, Niieen, Tem! Hut, Toop, Threep . . ." (Courtesy, *Instructor* magazine and Ford Button.)

sex through the development of an adequate knowledge of the physical, mental, social, emotional, and spiritual processes involved.

Sex education is to be distinguished from sex information. It implies that man's sexuality is integrated into his total life development as a health entity and a source of creative energy.

Historically, the learned organizations and their prophets have been urging the schools to get started. In 1941 the American Association of School Administrators recommended that sex education be included in the school curriculum. It was recommended again in 1960 at the White House Conference on Children, and by the middle 1960's a number of state and national groups called for action. Several states have developed excellent policy statements regarding sex and family living education. One of the finest, put forth in a 24-page booklet and complete with 26 admirable objectives, is the one from Illinois.[25] Another policy statement, short and clear, was prepared by the New Jersey State Board of Education and given wide distribution throughout the state and beyond. The full statement follows:

---

[25] Illinois Sex Education Advisory Board. *Policy Statement on Family Life and Sex Education,* Springfield, Illinois: Office of the Superintendent of Public Instruction, 1967.

A POLICY STATEMENT ON SEX EDUCATION

(ADOPTED BY THE STATE BOARD OF EDUCATION ON JANUARY 4, 1967)

Sex education is a responsibility which should be shared by the home, church, and school. The State Board of Education and the State Department of Education support the philosophy that each community and educational institute must determine its role in this area. Therefore, the State Board of Education recommends that each Local Board of Education make provisions in its curriculum for sex education programs.

Sex is a major aspect of personality. It is intimately related to emotional and social development and adjustment. Being boy or girl, man or woman, conditions one's sense of identity, ways of thinking and behaving, social and occupational activities, choice of associates, and mode of dress. Sex cannot be understood simply by focusing on physiological processes or classifying modes of sexual behavior. Human sexuality—the assumption of the individual's sex role—can best be understood by relating it to the total adjustment of the individual in his family and society.

The primary purpose of sex education is to promote more wholesome family and interpersonal relationships and, therefore, more complete lives. It is not a subject that lends itself readily to "lecturing" or "telling." An approach which encourages open discussion and solicits the concerns of the individual is needed to help young people develop appropriate attitudes and understandings regarding their sex roles. This approach is possible if parents, clergy, teachers, health personnel, and others responsible for the education of children are informed and secure in their own feelings about sex.

Sex education is a continuing process throughout life and therefore must be planned for during the entire school experience of the child. Schools are important agencies in the development of healthy habits of living and moral values. Therefore, the Department of Education recommends that appropriate programs in sex education be developed by educational institutions cognizant of what is desirable, what is possible, and what is wise.

An early start in the sex and family living area builds a firm foundation of understandings and attitudes before complex and emotional problems confront boys and girls in their teens. Thus, Glen Cove, New York kindergarten children discuss the coming of a new baby into the family group. Moreover, the baby was not "got" at the hospital, but grew inside the mother until the doctor helped bring it out.

In numerous elementary schools programs have been carefully planned to meet local needs. These needs are much the same everywhere. Whether it is Washington, Illinois, or Oregon, the teacher is the key to a good program. No teacher should be forced to teach in an area in which she feels uncomfortable. Fortunately, many elementary school teachers are usually "at home" discussing the world of persons and families, both formally and informally in their classrooms.

The following selected references are especially useful in building a rationale for teaching sex and family living education early in the grades, and for appreciating the need for a sequence of experiences which will contribute to the development of appropriate concepts of sexuality in the later years:

Benell, Florence B. "Eliminating Barriers to Sex Education in the Schools." *Journal of School Health*, 38:68–71, February 1968.

Bracher, Marjory. "The Martinson Report: Implications for Sex Education." *Journal of School Health*, 37:491–498, December 1967.

Breiner, S. J. "Psychological Principles of a Sex Education Program for Grades K Through 12." *Journal of School Health*, 42:227–230, April 1972.

Broderick, Carlfred B. "Sexual Behavior Among Pre-Adolescents." *Journal of Social Issues*, 22:6–21, April 1966.

Brower, Linda and Southworth, Warren H. "A Guideline for Discussion of Sexual Behavior." *Journal of School Health, 39*:715–720, December 1969.

Calderone, Mary A. "Planning for Sex Education: a Community-wide Responsibility." *NEA Journal*, January 1967.

Guidance Associates. *Sex Education U.S.A.: A Community Approach*. New York: Harcourt, Brace & World, 1968.

Hawkins, Barbara. "The Family Life Education Program in the Chicago Public Schools." *School Health Review*, 2:33–35, April 1971.

Kirkendall, Lester A., and Cox, Helen M. "Starting a Sex Education Program." *Children*, August 1967, p. 136.

Lennon, Mary Louise. "Selection of Family Life Education Materials Used in the Chicago Public Schools." *Journal of School Health*, 42:233–237, April 1972.

Levin, Barbara B. et al. "A Peek at Sex Education in a Midwestern Community." *Journal of School Health*, 42:462–465, October 1972.

Levine, Milton I. "Sex Education in the Public Elementary and High School Curriculum." *Journal of School Health*, 37:30–38, January 1967.

Simon, William, and Gagnon, John H. "The Pedagogy of Sex." *Saturday Review*, November 18, 1967, p. 79.

Teachers Publishing Corporation. "Sex Education: How It Is Being Taught in Elementary Classrooms." *Grade Teacher*, May-June 1967.

Uslander, Arlene S. "Study of People in Skokie." *Instructor, 80*:78–80, November 1970.

There is a reasonably good amount of experience to draw upon when it comes to structuring a program. The list of communities with effective elementary programs is rather extensive. Well prepared curriculum guides such as the following may be obtained at moderate cost:

Sex Education—a Working Design for Curriculum Development and Implementation, Grades K–12. The Education Council, 131 Mineola Blvd., Mineola, N.Y., 11501.

Curriculum Guide for Family Life and Sex Education, Great Neck Public Schools, Great Neck, N.Y.

Guide to Health and Family Life Education, Grades K–12, San Francisco Unified District, San Francisco, California.

Guidelines for Family Life and Sex Education, Grades K–12, Curriculum Bulletin No. 32, State of Minnesota, Dept. of Education, St. Paul, Minnesota.

Personal and Family Living for the Elementary School, Curriculum Resource Bulletin, Public Schools District of Columbia, Administration Annex No. 7, North Street, N.W., Washington, D.C. 20007.

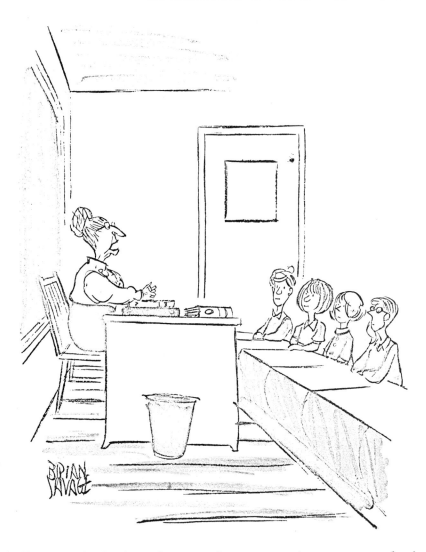

*"The Board of Education requires me to give you some basic
information on sex, reproduction and other disgusting filth."*
(Reproduced by special permission of PLAYBOY Magazine; copyright © by HMH Publishing Co., Inc.)

Interest surveys tend to help teachers structure the curriculum. In the *Teach Us What We Want To Know* study (Connecticut State Department of Education, Hartford, Connecticut) there was tremendous interest among second and third graders relative to babies — "Where do they come from?" "How do they get out of the mother's stomach?" "Why can't babies talk and walk?" "Why do they cry?" By the fifth grade the children ask, "Why do only girls have babies?" "Does smoking have anything to do with babies being formed wrong?" and "What makes it a girl or a boy?" In the Skokie, Illinois study, first and second grade children asked:[26]

------

[26]Uslander, Arlene S. "Study of People in Skokie," *Instructor, 80*:78–80, November 1970.

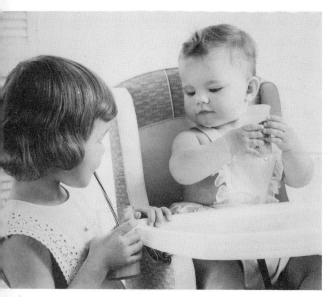

Figure 8–16 Primary grade children like pictures of babies—to view and talk about. (Courtesy Gerber Baby Foods.)

Does it hurt the mother to have a baby?

How does the mother know when the baby is ready to be born?

How does a father help to make a baby?

Significantly, these questions are asked at an age when straightforward answers are effective and accepted as matter-of-fact.

Intermediate graders can ask keen questions calling for detailed answers. Levine discovered that sixth grade students want to know about miscarriage and artificial insemination. They ask: "Why do some girls develop before others?"; "Is something wrong with me? I like sports better than going with girls."; "Sometimes in the movies or on television, a woman tells her husband, 'We're going to have a baby!', why didn't he know about it?"

After studying a great number of curriculum guides and working with adolescents concerning sex education, Deryek Calderwood concluded that the most common complaint was that their education came too late. Student interest in sexuality is so high at an early age that much sex education comes "after the

fact" for young people, rather than preparing them for their psychosexual development and socio-sexual experiences. In short, young people's readiness for effective sex education far exceeds most adults' cautious willingness to provide it. Yet, when it is done well there are deep felt appreciations. A fifth grade boy in the Chicago program says, "Family life has been the most interesting study I ever had in school. I never realized how wonderful our bodies were." This boy's program received a high rating in a Northwestern University study that covered 54 elementary schools.[27] Some 12,230 children received instruction. Only 43 were withdrawn at the request of parents; 378 classroom teachers were involved. Evaluation by parents was 91 per cent favorable; evaluation by principals was 98 per cent favorable; and there was a solid 100 per cent favorable report by the teachers.

The Program

The finest education relative to sexuality and family living probably takes place in the home itself under the guidance of informed and sympathetic parents. Unfortunately, not all homes function in a way to promote optimum family living. In fact, some of them promote anything but optimal family living. However, prior to initiating a school program all parents should be oriented relative to what the school proposes. The clergy and other leaders in the community should give their support as well. A local elementary school Parent-Teacher Association can be very helpful in the process. It also provides classroom teachers with a little help through an in-service training program. Carefully selected and well-prepared teachers increase support and cooperation of the public in this program.

The question of what to teach and how to teach it is the next consideration. Everyday classroom experiences are suit-

[27] Hawkins, Barbara. "The Family Life Education Program in the Chicago Schools," *School Health Review*, 2:33–35, April 1971.

able for integrating information about the beginning of life and the care of the young. At an early age children are curious about life in all of its many manifestations—how it originates, how it grows, and how it perpetuates itself. Children's questions are generally not difficult to answer, but they do require that the teacher have the ability to answer them honestly, unemotionally, and accurately. Instruction must be conducted with dignity and discretion. Sex is a life function that is normal, clean, respectable, and admirable. Here are some guiding principles to follow.[28]

Sex education in schools should be integrated with the total health education program at all grade levels. It should not be singled out for separate or undue emphasis.

Example on the part of parents and teachers is far more effective than precept.

Sex education should be couched in terms easily understood by the child and should make use of examples within his experience.

Sex information should not be forced upon the uninterested child but should be adapted to his maturity level at each stage of growth.

Sex should be presented in a dignified vocabulary.

Sex should be taught positively by showing its nobility in terms of creative drive and family happiness rather than negatively through the enumeration of horrible examples of immorality.

Sex anatomy and physiology (upper grades) should be treated as just another body system; due allowance must be made for modesty.

The many relations of sex to all phases of normal, private and public life must be discussed in an objective manner.

Although the emphasis differs, there is a fair amount of agreement as to primary and intermediate grade content in sex

and family living education. This is particularly true when one compares the courses of study that have been periodically revised in the several communities where established programs have been in operation for some time.

Some idea of the scope of the program, kindergarten through sixth grade, can be appreciated by looking over the Sex and Family Living Education outline, set up by concepts and arranged by the author for the Massachusetts guide.

Kindergarten

I am a member of a family.
Families do many things together.
Boys and girls are important in families.
Mothers and fathers are important too.
Children and parents working and playing together help to make home a happy place in which to live.
Family members show love for each other.
I am a member of a school family.
Every person needs to feel wanted at home and at school.
Our bodies are wonderful and there is nothing shameful about any part of the body.
There are proper names for the body parts concerned with elimination.
Everyone has a right to privacy at some times.
Each person should respect the privacy of others.
Show caution when dealing with strangers.

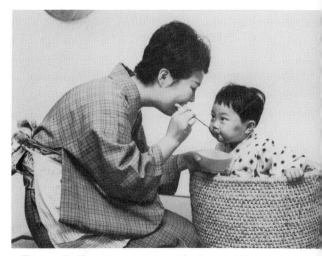

Figure 8–17 Understanding families, children, and love are needs the world over. (Courtesy Gerber Products Company.)

[28]Adapted from the Joint Committee, National Education Association and American Medical Association. *Health Education*, revised 1967. National Education Association, 1201 Sixteenth St., N.W., Washington, D.C. 20036.

Grade One

Animals are members of animal families.
All life comes from life.
All living things grow and reproduce.
Plants grow from seeds.
Some animals hatch from eggs and others develop inside the body of the mother until birth.
Cats have kittens; humans have babies.
In the beginning every child has a mother and father.
Babies come from mothers.
Both animal and human parents try to keep their young safe, fed, happy and healthy.
Girls and boys are alike in some ways and different in some ways.

Grade Two

Different animals need different amounts of time to get ready to be born.
Mice, cats, dogs and cows are born live through a special opening in the mother's body.
Both human and animal parents take care of their children until they are able to take care of themselves.
Animal and human babies need good food in order to grow properly.
Growing older means more responsibility at home.
Helping at home and in the community helps us learn more about ourselves, other people, and the world we live in.

Grade Three

Every living thing grows and reproduces.
An egg cell develops in the mother to become a baby.
The baby is born through a special opening in the mother's body.
Human beings grow in many ways — physically, mentally and socially.
We inherit many of our physical and mental characteristics from our parents.
Living things are alike in many ways — requiring air, light, food, rest, water, etc.
Each parent contributes something to its offspring.
Children are both alike and different from their parents.
Growing older means more than just getting bigger.

Grade Four

Family patterns differ throughout the United States.
Families may have problems, but they can work together to solve them (broken homes, death, physical and mental handicaps, unemployment, etc.)
How life begins is a wondrous miracle.
The mother's egg (ovum) is fertilized by the sperm of the father.
The fertilized ovum divides into many cells which have a special function to perform.
Both parents contribute their own particular characteristics to their offspring.
All living things develop from a single cell.
When the baby has been in the mother nine months it is ready to be born.
As the baby grows certain glands control its growth and development.

Grade Five

Glands which produce hormones help control body growth and development.
Sex glands at puberty bring about certain physical and emotional changes.
There is a time when girls may be taller than boys, but later on the boys usually catch up to the girls in height.
Menstruation occurs as a natural part of a girl's growing up.
Menstruation indicates that a girl is becoming a woman who will be able to conceive and have children.
Seminal (nocturnal) emissions occur as a natural part of a boy's growing up.
Though nature readies the body for reproduction at puberty, several years more are needed to prepare for marriage and the responsibility of parenthood.
Menstruation does not occur when the ovum has been fertilized by the male sperm.
As the fetus grows inside the mother, the placenta and umbilical cord bring it food and oxygen from the mother, and carry away the waste products to the mother for elimination.
The baby's blood and circulatory system is separate from the mother's.
Through the process of osmosis oxygen and food are exchanged between mother and baby.
Before being born the baby is well protected by the amniotic sac and fluid in the abdomen of the mother.
The uniqueness of boys and girls is expressed in one's sexuality, not only through the reproductive process but within the framework of the family.

Grade Six

Femaleness and maleness refer to biological characteristics unique for each person.
No person is totally male or totally female; there are characteristics of the opposite sex in both males and females.

Understanding the role of men and women in our society is part of becoming a mature person.

Mature boys and girls learn to control their feelings and emotions.

There are proper and improper ways of expressing emotions.

The endocrine glands secrete hormones that prepare the body for many kinds of actions during periods of emotional stress.

Both boys and girls have natural emotional feelings of affection toward the opposite sex. There are acceptable ways to express these feelings.

Because one has a responsibility for personal relationships, sexual feelings are controlled.

Recreational activities contribute to the development of wholesome boy-girl relationships. They also help family morale.

It is important to learn to make some decisions early in life and accept the consequences.

A further example from an on-going program in Glen Cove, New York appears below:

GLEN COVE PUBLIC SCHOOLS, N.Y.

HEALTH GUIDANCE IN SEX EDUCATION— AIMS AT EACH LEVEL

Kindergarten

1. Know sex differences between girls and boys.
2. Give direction toward male or female role in adult life.
3. Learn correct names for body parts and terms concerned with elimination.
4. Understand that human baby develops inside body of mother.
5. Understand baby gets milk from mother's breast by nursing.
6. Appreciate that there are good body feelings.
7. Learn to recognize signs of love and devotion within family.
8. Develop idea of continuity of living things— incubate eggs.

First Year

1. Understand egg cell is basic to new life.
2. Learn that some animals hatch from eggs and others develop inside body of mother until birth.
3. Appreciate wonder of human body.

4. Develop sense of responsibility for own body.
5. Appreciate efforts of mother and father for family members.
6. Recognize influence of emotions on body health.

Second Year

1. Learn that different animals need different amounts of time to get ready to be born.
2. Understand that the egg cell does not develop into a baby by itself—role of father.
3. Learn that some animals are born live through a special opening in the mother's body.
4. Recognize that growing up brings responsibility.
5. Appreciate importance of mutual love and consideration in family.
6. Understand composition of family does not necessarily determine happiness of family.

Third Year

1. Understand that each person's unique heredity is determined at moment of fertilization.
2. Observe influence of heredity in your family.
3. Know that growing up means more than just getting bigger.
4. Develop increasing sense of responsibility to self and family.
5. Understand relationship between a healthy body and mind.
6. Study life cycles of various animals, including humans.

Fourth Year

1. Learn that certain glands control body growth and development.
2. Recognize importance of protecting vital body parts from injury, i.e. during sports.
3. Appreciate miracle of reproduction and maternal care among various forms of animal life.
4. Appreciate superiority of brain of man over instinct reaction of animals.
5. Learn meaning of responsible behavior in peer and family groups.
6. Study circulatory and digestive systems and realize their functional potential is influenced by habits being developed.

Fifth Year

1. Learn role of sex glands at puberty and emotional changes they bring.

2. Understand menstruation occurs as a natural part of a girl's growing up.

3. Understand seminal emissions occur as a natural part of a boy's growing up.

4. Learn that although nature readies our bodies for reproduction at puberty, several years more are needed to prepare for marriage and responsibility of parenthood.

5. Discuss importance of wholesome life attitudes and values as manifested in responsible behavior.

6. Discuss acceptable and unacceptable ways of showing emotions.

One of the most thorough reports to appear in recent years was prepared by the Committee on Health Guidance in Sex Education of the American School Health Association.[29] An outstanding feature of this extensive publication is that specific concepts and attitudes are set forth for each grade level in a manner readily understood by the teacher.

AMERICAN SCHOOL HEALTH ASSOCIATION

Kindergarten and Grade One

A. **Concepts.** As a product of their experiences in the study of this unit, it would be hoped that some such concepts as these would be formulated by children in kindergarten and the first grade:

1. All living things reproduce. Life comes from life.
2. The creation of new life is one of nature's greatest miracles.
3. Every child has a mother and a father in the beginning.
4. Every person needs to have a feeling of belonging.
5. Each member of a family is an important member. Children and parents working and playing together help to make a home a happy place to live. There are many ways in which children can help to make their homes happy ones.

6. Each member of a family is interested in the well-being of every other member.

7. Using good manners lets other people know that we like and respect them. Thoughtful boys and girls are courteous to each other, to their mothers and fathers. their brothers and sisters, and to everyone else.

8. Every person desires privacy at some times. Each person has a right to privacy, and each should respect the privacy of others.

9. Each part of the body is an important part of the whole person, and there is nothing shameful about any part of the body.

10. We should be cautious in dealing with strangers. Although some strangers who offer rides or candy to children are trying to be kind, others are not. We should always refuse such offers and should tell our parents and teachers about them.

B. **Attitudes.** As an outcome of this unit, it is to be hoped that the student will form some such favorable attitudes as these toward himself, others, family living, and reproduction:

1. An appreciation for the role of each family member.
2. An appreciation for his own importance as a member of his family and a desire to contribute to his family's well-being.
3. A respect for the rights of others.
4. A sense of wonder in regard to reproduction.
5. A wholesome respect for all parts of the body and a desire to learn and to use correct terminology in referring to them.

Grades Two and Three

A. **Concepts.** As a product of their experiences in the study of this unit, it would be hoped that some such concepts as these would be formulated by children in the second and third grades:

1. All living things grow and reproduce.
2. Every child has a mother and a father in the beginning.
3. Parents or guardians take care of their children in many ways until

[29]"Growth Patterns and Sex Education: a Suggested Program K-12," *Journal of School Health*, May 1967. This total in-depth issue of 136 pages is available for a small cost from American School Health Association, 515 E. Main St., Kent, Ohio 44240.

children grow up and are able to take care of themselves.

4. Human babies and children live with their parents or guardians for many years because it takes a long time for them to grow up and to learn how to do for themselves all the things that parents do for them while they are young.

5. Human beings grow in many ways—physically, intellectually, emotionally, socially, spiritually.

6. All living things have basic needs which must be fulfilled for optimal growth.

7. We need many different kinds of food to help us grow.

8. The food we eat is changed and used by our bodies to help us grow.

9. Optimal growth depends in part upon how well we utilize the food we eat.

10. Babies need special foods for optimal growth.

11. Everything we do helps us to learn more about ourselves, other people and the world we live in.

12. We can do our best work and have the most fun when we are happy.

13. Being neat and clean helps to make us feel good about ourselves.

14. Boys and girls enjoy playing and working with other boys and girls who are neat and clean.

15. There are many ways that mothers and fathers and children can show that they love each other.

16. Using good manners is one way we can let members of our families, other grown-ups, and other boys and girls know that we like them.

17. Fathers do many kinds of work in the community, and all of them can help to make the community a better place in which to live.

18. Mothers help the community in many ways—by making the home a healthy and happy place to live, by working at jobs outside the home, or by participating in community activities which they enjoy.

B. **Attitudes.** As an outcome of this unit, it is to be hoped that the student will form favorable attitudes toward himself, others, family living, and reproduction.

1. An appreciation for the roles of each member of the family as an individual and as a contributing member of the family unit.

2. A desire for optimal nutrition.

3. A desire to develop or to continue personal practices which lead to cleanliness and good grooming.

4. An appreciation for clothing that is clean and functional, regardless of its "fashionableness."

5. A respect for other persons as individuals and a desire to show respect for others by treating them courteously.

6. A growing regard for masculine and feminine roles in our society.

7. An appreciation for the ways in which adult men and women contribute to the community and the desire to become future contributing adult members of the community.

8. A sense of wonder concerning the complex nature of the human personality and its development.

9. An appreciation for the effect that a pleasant manner has upon one's relationship with others.

Grade Four

A. **Concepts.** As a product of their experiences in the study of this unit, it would be hoped that some such concepts as these would be formulated by children in the fourth grade:

1. We are made of many cells which have important tasks to do in making it possible for us to live and grow.

2. Blood carries food to the cells and waste products away from the cells to places where they can be collected and excreted.

3. A person's heredity refers to those personal characteristics that have been passed down to him from his parents through genes and chromosomes.

4. Each person receives half of his inherited characteristics from his mother and the other half from his father.

5. Each person's inherited characteristics are determined at the moment of conception when his father's sperm fertilizes his mother's ovum.

6. A person's heredity influences the way he grows, what he will look like, and how tall he can grow to be.

7. What a person becomes is determined by his heredity, his environment and, to some extent, what he wants to be.
8. Each member of a family contributes to the well-being of the whole family and each of its other members.
9. The health of each family member affects the well-being of all family members.
10. There are many activities that all members of a family can participate in and enjoy together. Playing together and working together helps mothers and fathers and children know each other better and strengthens the family as a unit.
11. Having a hobby is one way a person can use his leisure time constructively. Hobbies add enjoyment to living. Sometimes the members of a family enjoy sharing the same hobby.
12. A friend is someone who likes you and whom you like. A person can have many different kinds of friends among people of all ages.
13. One of the best ways to make new friends is to be friendly to other people. Being friendly lets others know that we would like to have them as our friends.

B. **Attitudes.** As an outcome of this unit, it is to be hoped that the student will form favorable attitudes toward himself, others, family living, and reproduction:

1. An appreciation for one's family heritage, both hereditary and environmental.
2. An appreciation for the influences that heredity and environment have upon growth and development.
3. An appreciation for the ability one has to control the direction of his own development and a desire to exercise this control to the greatest extent possible.
4. A regard for the effect that the health of each family member has upon that of all other family members and upon the family as a unit.
5. A desire to have one's own health status and practices contribute to rather than detract from family well-being.
6. A willingness to understand and

adjust to the health problems of all members of the family.
7. An appreciation for the contribution that children this age can make to the leisure-time activities and fellowship of the family and a desire to help plan and participate in such activities with other members of the family.
8. An appreciation for the values and enjoyment that can be gained from constructive solitary activities.
9. A desire to select and pursue some activities that one can do on his own.
10. A respect for the desire others have to engage in solitary activities and a regard for their right to do so.
11. An appreciation for the different kinds of friendships one can develop with many different persons of various ages.
12. A desire to be a friend to others.

Grade Five

A. **Concepts.** As a product of their experiences in the study of this unit, it would be hoped that some such concepts as these would be formulated by children in the fifth grade:

1. Although the general pattern of growth and development is the same for everyone, each person follows this pattern at his own individual rate.
2. At some times in their lives, girls are taller than boys, but boys catch up later and usually become taller than girls.
3. A person's growth and development are determined by hereditary potential for growth and development and by the influence of the many kinds of experiences he has in his environment.
4. Hormones are responsible for the changes in appearance that occur as boys develop into men and girls develop into women.
5. Hormones influence not only a person's growth and physical development, but also the way he feels and behaves.
6. As boys and girls become men and women, their feelings and actions toward themselves and others change.

7. As people grow older they are able to assume more responsibility for their own care and for the well-being of others.
8. Although most habits are helpful to us, some of the habits people form can interfere with their well-being and ability to get along with others.
9. Seminal emissions are nature's way of releasing stored-up sperm.
10. Menstruation is a normal, healthful function which indicates that a girl is becoming a woman who will be able to conceive and have children.
11. The creation of a new life is one of the most wonderful acts of Nature.
12. Parenthood is a privilege and a responsibility.
13. Each new life begins with the union of a single sperm from the father and a single ovum from the mother.
14. The fertilized ovum divides into many cells which have different structures in order to assume different tasks. Cell division and differentiation begins at the time of conception and continues in order to form a fully developed human being.
15. As a baby lives and grows and develops inside the mother, the placenta and umbilical cord bring it food and oxygen from the mother and carry its waste products to the mother for elimination.
16. The blood of a developing baby is formed in its own body. Its circulatory system is separate from the mother's. Food and oxygen and waste products are exchanged between mother and baby through the process of osmosis.
17. The amniotic sac and fluid create an environment which protects the fetus until it is ready to be born.
18. The best way to assure that one's body will continue to function efficiently and well is to give it the normal care and attention it requires.
19. As a person grows and develops from a child into an adult, his changing body requires additional kinds of care in order to keep functioning at its best.
20. Although some children do not grow as rapidly as others, this is not an indication of any abnormality.

B. **Attitudes.** As an outcome of this unit, it is to be hoped that the student will form favorable attitudes toward himself, others, family living, and reproduction:

1. An appreciation for normal individual differences in rates of growth and development and an acceptance of one's own rate.
2. A desire to seek information pertaining to sex and sexuality from reliable sources as replacement for unscientific information and hearsay.
3. A persistent regard for medical services and health consultation from scientific sources.
4. An appreciation for the uniqueness of each individual and for the ways in which all individuals are similar.
5. An appreciation for the contributions that families make to the total development of each person.
6. A desire to contribute to wholesome family living by participating in family activities.
7. An appreciation for the constructive expression of one's sexuality through the reproductive processes and within the framework of the family unit.
8. A desire to respond to increased privilege by displaying a growing sense of responsibility for self and others.
9. A desire to form habits which will contribute to one's well-being and to eliminate or avoid developing habits that may be destructive to optimal growth and development.
10. An appreciation of one's sexuality as a healthful expression of his personality.
11. A wholesome acceptance of oneself as a sexual being and of those physiological processes (e.g., menstruation and seminal emissions) related to this aspect of one's being.
12. A regard for both the privileges and responsibilities attendant upon parenthood.
13. An increasing appreciation for the complexity of the human personality.
14. A persistent regard for the nature of the phenomena involved in the creation of a new life.
15. A respect for one's body as a tool for creative self-expression and the desire to give it the care it requires and deserves as such.

Grade Six

A. **Concepts.** As a product of their experiences in the study of this unit, it would be hoped that some such concepts as these would be formulated by children in the sixth grade:

1. Cells have different kinds of structures which enable each kind to perform its specialized function.
2. A person's emotions affect the way his body functions.
3. The hormones secreted by the endocrine glands regulate many physiological functions. They prepare the body for action during periods of emotional stress.
4. Emotions are natural human feelings existing in all persons. They are aroused in response to other people and to situations in one's environment.
5. Emotions need to be expressed in some way. There are constructive and destructive ways of expressing emotions.
6. Emotions can be expressed in the most constructive way when their expression is controlled by the use of one's ability to reason.
7. One of the tasks involved in becoming a mature person is that of learning to control the emotions in such a way that their expression helps, rather than hurts, both oneself and other people.
8. Maleness and femaleness refer to biological characteristics unique for each individual.
9. Although boys are mostly male and girls are mostly female, no person is all male or all female. There is some degree of femaleness in all boys and some degree of maleness in all girls.
10. Masculinity and femininity refer to patterns of behavior that are characteristic of males or of females in a particular culture. These patterns of behavior are not present at birth, but are learned through the experiences one has in his family, his school, and his community. As boys and girls grow up, they learn how to be masculine or feminine by observing and behaving like the men or women they know and admire.
11. The process of growing and developing from children into adults is very complex and involves many physical, emotional and social changes and adjustments.
12. The growth and development of a baby from one fertilized cell into a complex human being is one of nature's greatest and most miraculous achievements.
13. An appreciation of "maleness" and "femaleness" is an important aspect of becoming an adult.
14. There are such normal variations in physiological activity in each individual that it is important to recognize, understand and accept the many characteristics which may be common to both sexes.

B. **Attitudes.** As an outcome of this unit, it is to be hoped that the student will form favorable attitudes toward himself, others, family living, and reproduction:

1. An appreciation for the integrated nature of man.
2. An acceptance and appreciation of the emotional dimension of being and of the human quality that emotional expression gives to personality.
3. A desire to express one's emotions in constructive ways.
4. A willingness to explore a variety of alternatives in the attempt to learn how to channel one's emotions into constructive outlets.
5. A growing acceptance of and appreciation for the sexuality of oneself and others.
6. A desire to adopt the behaviors natural to and characteristic of one's assigned sex role in our culture.
7. A sensitivity to, acceptance of, and appreciation for behavioral characteristics which may be exhibited by members of both sexes, which are natural to both sexes, but which may be culturally expected of one sex rather than of the other.
8. An acceptance of and appreciation for the complex physical, emotional, and social changes that one undergoes in the process of growing and developing into an adult.

Here is an outline of five lessons for sixth graders from the San Diego Public Schools Teaching Monograph. Note how vital the topics are and how they develop:

How we grow, differences in the growth patterns of boys and girls, responsibilities of growing up, the importance of caution with strangers, how to choose the right friends, your appearance, glands that are responsible for growth and changes in our bodies, good attitudes, and the right names of the body's organs and functions. Questions and answers.

LESSON 2

Films on animal reproduction *(The Sunfish, The Snapping Turtle, Snakes Are Interesting)*. Questions and answers. This is a fine impersonal introduction to human reproduction; it helps boys and girls understand that in most animals a male cell and a female egg must join before a new life can begin.

LESSON 3

Read a short book or monograph on human reproduction.[30] Questions and answers.

LESSON 4

(Girls) Review the sex organs, discuss menstruation, discuss reason for body changes, sex relations, and self-control (a film may be used).[31]

LESSON 5

(Boys) Discuss glandular changes, growth of sex organs, formation of sperm, seminal emissions, masturbation, reasons for body changes, and use of self-control. Questions and answers.

LESSON 6

Show the film *Human Growth* to review and clarify previous lessons and to set the stage for further discussion of such things as strengthening right attitudes toward sex and growing up,

---

[30]One of the finest booklets written, with colored animated drawings, is distributed by the New York State Health Department, Albany, N.Y. Entitled *The Gift of Life*, it has the support of Catholic, Protestant, and Hebrew clergy.

[31]The excellent filmstrip, *Confidence Because—You Understand Menstruating*, may be obtained free for permanent use from Personal Products Corporation, Milltown, N.J.

correct terminology, cell division, twins, sex determination, heredity, boy-girl relationships, moral and spiritual values. Question and answer period.

Help for the new teacher concerned with teaching sexuality may be found in many places. Guidance Associates of Harcourt, Brace and World put out *Sex Education U.S.A.: A Community Approach*, a filmstrip-record-manual designed to present the sex education curriculum. Warren Schloat Productions, Inc. distributes several useful filmstrips for primary and intermediate level classes under the general title of *Human Birth, Growth and Development: Facts and Feelings*. These have had wide use, and the Teacher's Guide is especially helpful. The same may be said for the *Sex Education Resource Units, Grades K, 1, 2, 3, 4*, produced by the American Association for Health, Physical Education and Recreation. Revised in 1971, the American Medical Association booklet, *A Story About You*, is just wonderful for school use. The fifth or sixth grader as well as the teacher will profit from reading it.

Rather than list a number of books for the teacher to use, only four are mentioned here because they are superb in presenting programs, teaching ideas, and pupil activities. An understanding of these references will do much to insure a proper program of sex education:

Teachers Manual, *A Curriculum Guide on Sex Education for Elementary Grades 5-6*, Commonwealth of Massachusetts, Department of Public Health, Boston, Massachusetts, 1970.
Sex Education in the Schools, by H. Frederick Kilander, Macmillan Co., New York, 1970 (a study of objectives, content, methods, materials and evaluation).
Ideas and Learning Activities for Family Life and Sex Education, by Mark Perrin and Thomas E. Smith, William C. Brown Co., Dubuque, Iowa, 1972.
Family Life and Sex Education: Curriculum and Instruction, by Esther D. Schulz and Sally R. Williams, Harcourt, Brace and World, New York, 1969.

There exists in Cleveland, Ohio, the now famous Cleveland Health Museum. It is unique among educational agencies in the way it has informed the commu-

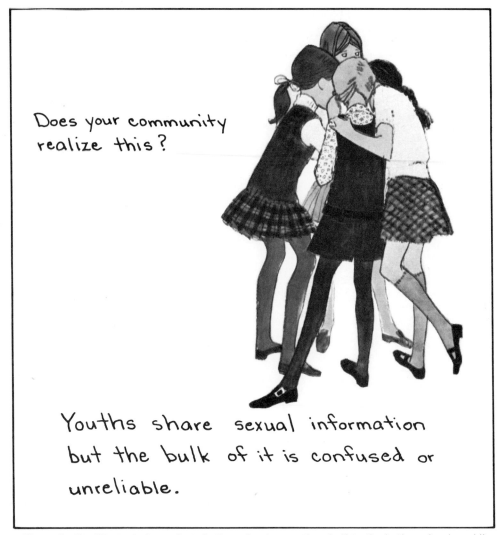

Does your community realize this?

Youths share sexual information but the bulk of it is confused or unreliable.

Figure 8–18 "Better to learn *facts* in the school room than half-truths in the school yard."

nity about personal and public health. *Sex and family living education is the mainstay of this institution.* The visitors at every age are motivated not by a love of esthetics as in an art museum or a curiosity about nature as in a natural history museum, but by a strong interest in their own physical and mental well-being. It is in this museum that sex has a unique setting, and it is in this area that the museum has made a lasting contribution over the years. Within 50 miles of Cleveland there are a large number of Ohio counties consisting of hundreds of

schools that make at least one museum trip a year for a lesson on human reproduction. Elementary schoolchildren study the pictures and incomparably fine models for an experience conducive to a high retention of facts in an atmosphere with a minimum of emotional trauma. So high does interest in these exhibits run, in fact, that one often finds a youngster explaining them to his parents on a Sunday afternoon following his class visit.

The famous birth series models are now available for purchase from the Cleveland Museum. These lightweight, durable polystyrene models present the growth and development of a baby sculptured in three dimensions for teaching purposes.[32] They are a superb teaching aid.

There will be times when it seems necessary to separate boys and girls, particularly in the fifth or sixth grade when a discussion of menstruation arises. As a general rule, sex instruction should be in mixed classes and the materials and methods of instruction adapted to the situation. When a topic is peculiar to a single sex, it might be more convenient to meet the sexes separately. Menstruation, for example, is so full of mystery and misconceptions that both preadolescent boys and girls should know something about it. There should be open classroom discussion regarding superstition, primitive beliefs regarding "uncleanliness" associated with menstruation, and the fear of blood. This topic is a normal part of growing children's lives. Mature attitudes begin early when the need for teaching first occurs. So we teach the life cycle and the menstrual cycle, that menstruation is normal, and we answer the question, "What is happening inside?"

Three very good films for fifth and sixth grade use are:

The Story of Menstruation. Kimberly-Clark Corporation, Neenah, Wis., color, sound, ten minutes. Delightful Disney animated film, showing causes and characteristics of menstruation. The same company distributes (free) the booklet, *Growing Up Young,* for parents and teachers of the retarded girl. Also, English and Spanish versions of *Very Personally Yours* teach basic menstrual health. This company distributes, at a modest cost, thought-provoking colored transparencies, *The Me I Want To Be,* and a teacher's guide for elementary school use. It is designed to stimulate open-ended discussion about physical and emotional growth. An extremely attractive booklet from Personal Products Company is *Growing Up and Liking It.*

Three girls keep in touch with each other by writing letters, chiefly about growing and menstruation. Braille booklets are also available. The same company has both an English and Spanish translation of the film *It's Wonderful Being a Girl (Es Maravilloso Ser Mujer).*

An especially useful booklet entitled *World of a Girl* is distributed (free) by the Scott Paper Company in Philadelphia. It is designed for fifth and sixth grade girls, to enable them to understand and respond wholesomely to the miraculous changes that begin their grownup life. A detailed teacher's guide is available for use with the booklet.

Another highly successful booklet for girls is *Accent on You,* distributed (free) by Tampax, Incorporated, 5 Dakota Drive, Lake Success, New York 11040.

Chapter 11, which deals with source materials, contains a number of films useful for primary and intermediate grade pupils. For the primary grades, *Baby Animals* (McGraw-Hill Text Films), *Farm Babies and Their Mothers* (Film Associates), and *Human and Animal Beginnings* (E. C. Brown Trust Foundation) are especially well done and effective with children. For older pupils the films *Growing Up* (Coronet Films), *Boy To Man* (Churchill Films) and *The Miracle of Reproduction* (Sid Davis Productions) are noteworthy.

Suggested Activities

Primary Level

1. Keep a pet cat with kittens or a dog with young puppies in the classroom for several days for general observation.

2. Discover how many children have a baby brother or sister. To class: What is your favorite way to help with the baby? What are some things your baby can do?

3. Visit the zoo, a health museum, or any place where baby animals may be observed and talked about.

4. Visit a local dairy farmer shortly after the birth of a calf. Children never fail to appreciate such a visit.

5. Keep a pair of canaries and observe the building of the nest and laying and hatching of eggs.

---

[32]Cleveland Health Museum, 8911 Euclid Avenue, Cleveland, Ohio 44106.

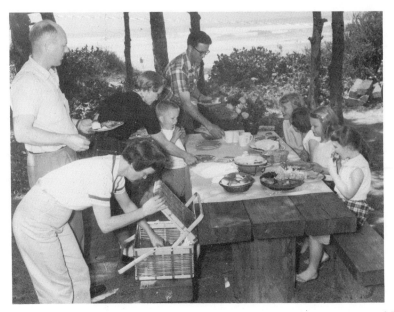

Figure 8–19 Family life—cookout at the seashore. (Courtesy American Institute of Baking.)

6. Raise guppies. These live-bearing fish are inexpensive and most interesting. The young may be seen inside the female late in pregnancy. Collect tadpoles or grow eggs in the spring.

7. Have pupils describe family vacations and ways of having a good time at home. (See Figure 8–19.)

8. Build a list of ways that children can help to make home more pleasant. Such a list should be posted with art work to illustrate this type of activity in action. A few examples of items that might appear on the list are:

Run errands willingly
Care for younger children
Come on the first call so Mother does not have to raise her voice or get angry
Help Mother with the cleaning
Hang up our clothes
Pick up our toys
Share good stories with the family

9. Talk about the effect of a happy home at mealtime, at bedtime. Set up a role-playing situation.

10. Read a pleasant story or poem to the class about family living and good times.

> We scrub the big potatoes
> That Mother wants to bake
> We pour the milk and water,
> We cut the bread and cake.
> When supper's almost ready,
> We rest a little while,
> And think of something funny
> That will make the family smile.

11. Draw body outlines of children on large pieces of paper. Do it again toward the end of the school year and note growth changes.

12. Compare families around the world.

13. Show a picture of a new baby coming home from the hospital. Ask: "Why do the grown-ups look so excited? Why are they happy? What do you like best about having a baby in a family?"

14. Read the story to class: *Laurie's New Brother* by Miriam Schlein. The joy of the new baby is depicted.

Intermediate Level

1. Raise tropical fish or collect caterpillars for the room terrarium. Watch the development of the cocoon.

2. Show pictures of tiny babies. Discuss special care needed for small babies. Listen to student experiences. Use the wall chart, *How A Baby Grows*, available (free) from Johnson & Johnson. It shows clearly body and hand language and social development.

3. Examine charts of high grade animals such as certain breeds of cows or dogs. Study the characteristics looked for in breeding these animals. Seek help from a 4-H club leader.

4. Examine the word "love." Ask: *What is Love?* What does Ashley Montague mean here?: "Love is the principal developer of one's capacity for being human, the chief stimulus for the development of social competence, and the only thing on earth that can produce that sense of belongingness and relatedness to the world of humanity which is the best achievement of the healthy human being,"[33] (sixth grade)

---

[33]Montague, Ashley, in *Age of Aquarius* by K. Jones, L. Shainberg, and C. Byer, New York: Goodyear, 1971.

5. Study the teacher guide struation and menstrual health, *Fiction to Fact*, published by Tamp Incorporated, New York. This is filled with excellent teaching suggestions, for boys and girls together and separately. See also the booklet, *Accent on You*, published by and distributed free by the same company.

6. Discuss (with fifth and sixth grade girls) the question of good menstrual health as a necessary part of a girl's growth into womanhood. Clear up misconceptions relative to cramps, water taboos, exercise restrictions, and the period itself. (Obtain illustrative materials from Personal Products Corp., Milltown, N. J.; Tampax Incorporated, and Kimberly-Clark Corp.)

7. Set up a question box to be used, especially during the unit on family relations. This encourages the pupils who do not feel free or comfortable enough to ask questions in class (sixth grade).

8. Develop an appreciation for the human body. Teach the intricacies and the beauty and the mechanism. Without stress, indicate the marvelous role of each sex.

9. Follow the NEA-AMA booklet, *A Story about You*, and hold a question-answer period.

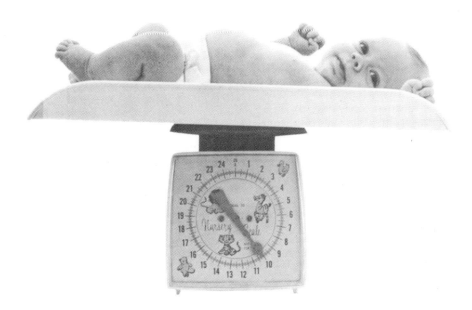

ts at the local
de a basis for a
relations. This
eloping desirable
good friend and
mber.

vacations. Have
ey like about their
m add to this what
they ~~ to earn a living in
the future.

12. Talk over the relationship of family health to family happiness. Show also how fear, prejudice, outbursts of anger, and other similar items keep a home in a state of unpleasantness. List socially acceptable ways to counteract these feelings.

13. Chart the combination of chromosomes (23 in the ovum and 23 in the sperm). Discuss hereditary influences and bearing on "how we look." Students should bring pictures to class to illustrate differences in height, weight, color, ears, eyes and other body structure items.

14. Plant a fast-growing green bean seed in fertile soil and water it in class. Put the other on the windowsill. Relate this experiment to nutrition and reproduction.

15. Show film *Growing Into Womanhood/Growing Into Manhood* (Guidance Associates)—a study of male and female reproductive systems relating to puberty. A slightly more advanced film is *Becoming A Woman/Becoming A Man* (Revised).

16. Have girls read the colorful booklet of letters, *Growing Up and Liking It* (obtained free from Personal Products Company, Milltown, N.J. 08850). Read and respond to what is said about menstrual cramps and try the exercises in Figure 8–20.

10. ENVIRONMENTAL HEALTH

Behavioral Objectives

(Primary Level)

Explains how one person's health practices can affect the health of other people.

Investigates how to keep the school, home and community environment reasonably clean.

Selects community services having a bearing on the welfare of himself and others in the class.

Relates how firemen and policemen protect children, adults and property.

Identifies ways in which milk is kept clean, fresh and safe to drink.

Describes briefly how all living things somehow relate to the happiness and health of children as well as adults.

Behavioral Objectives

(Intermediate Level)

Investigates the health services in the community with a view toward using them when necessary.

Explains the contributions made by people such as medical and dental personnel, barbers, sanitarians, street cleaners, opticians, public works engineers, conservationists and others.

Differentiates between public health personnel and other health-related people in the community.

Chooses hospital services as a significant community agency necessary in every part of the country.

Develops some responsibility for promoting health in the total environment through cooperative and independent activities.

Distinguishes between proper and improper food inspection, food storage and use practices.

Demonstrates how to conserve land to protect water supply and other environmental items such as wildlife and open space.

Identifies with the historical development and present planning of a community for future growth in terms of healthful living.

Dear Donna,

I think you are lucky not to be a kid anymore. Ask your mother for a book about the facts of life. In the meantime, I will tell you some things you should know. You are hardly losing any blood at all....only three or four ounces. That's not very much, especially if you know there are at least 120 ounces in your whole body and your body keeps on making new blood. And anyway, it's not really like when you get a cut. It's much thicker. That's because mentrual flow is a combination of blood and soft tissue from the inside of your uterus. So stop worrying! Most of the girls here don't have cramps but here are some good exercises to make your cramps go away. They're from my sister Janie's booklet she got in high school. You can do them everyday and when you're menstruating (men stroo ate ing). (That's the right way to say it). Now that you've got your period, you better watch out about "odor" -- that's what my mother said.

Love,

Patty

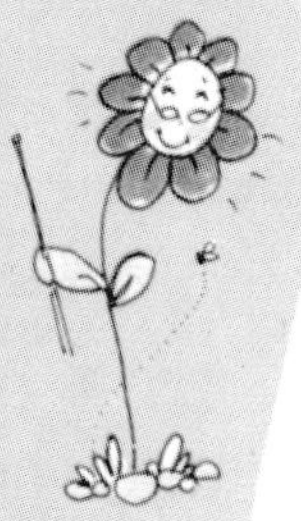

1. Stand with your face directly toward a wall. Your feet should be about 12 to 16 inches away from the wall. Raise both your elbows to the level of your shoulders and cross your arms. Lean forward so both elbows touch the wall and feel comfortable in this position. Next tilt your pelvis forward to touch the wall. While in this position keep your heels on the floor and your knees straight. Hold for one minute and return to original position.

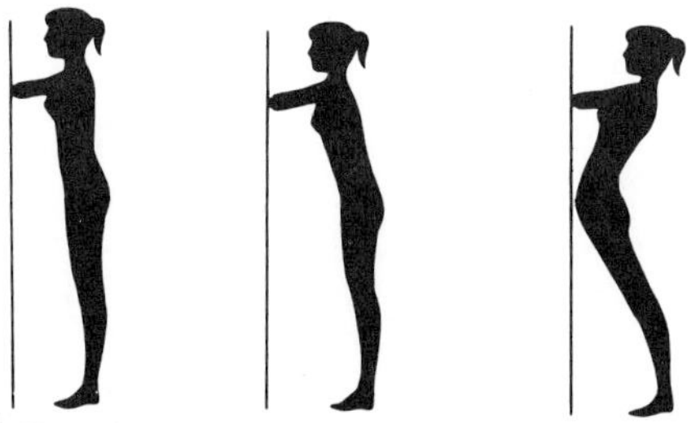

2. Lie on your back with knees bent, feet flat on floor and arms extended straight over head.

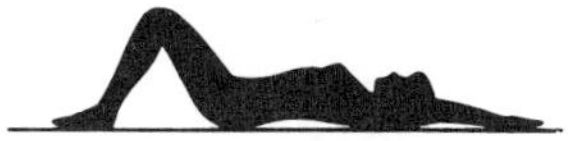

Swing your arms forward and at the same time push feet forward and move to sitting position.

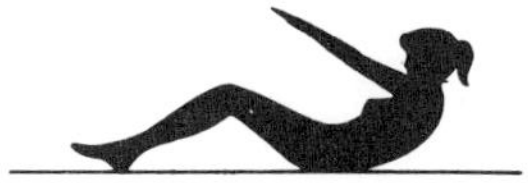

Reach forward and try to touch toes with fingers. Return to original position.

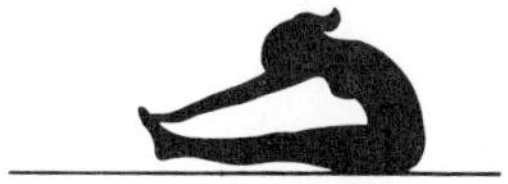

Figure 8–20   From the booklet, *Growing Up and Liking It*. (Courtesy Personal Products Company.)

Comments

INVITATION

I just stopped by to tell you
the lily on the seaward moor has opened.

I was out to watch dawn
wash in on the breakers,
and walking back, I saw—
something a little like leftover dawn,
a shade of shining in the wavy brush.
I was looking upon the lily.
An inward sun rose in me.

The lights I've seen today might well last
for all eternity, the way I feel.
I think the grave is not half so dark
since seeing such color
come out of the earth . . .
But I stopped by to tell you about the lily.
I could not bring it to you
without spoiling it for good.
Let me spoil you forever
by taking you to it.

—John Fandel

The "feeling" for preserving the environment that Fandel writes about is so artful and delicate that it can easily be missed by the bulk of mankind.[34] After all, hasn't the traditional American life style changed over the years from one of general conservatism and careful usage of all materials ("make it do" philosophy) to a technological and consumer appetite which gobbles more than half of the resources consumed in the world each year? It is only now that one asks . . . what can I do? And this, of course, is a difficult question since solutions to environmental problems are multi-disciplinary and often beyond the capacity of any individual. As reflected in the poem, one must become more concerned with the quality of his life rather than his pile of possessions—three-fourths of which he throws away each year.

Barry Commoner, in *The Closing Circle*, speaks to the heart of the issue when he says that we cannot deal adequately with the unwelcomed by-products of a complex, industrialized society as though they existed outside the total structure of that society. Our environmental ills are profoundly and intimately related to our most basic social, philosophical, and religious motivations. They reflect our concept of human purpose, our view of ourselves in relation to the world, and our view of our responsibility to ourselves and the generations that will come after us.

It is for this very reason that schoolchildren at an early age must begin to develop a lasting appreciation for their environment—an environment whose problems did not suddenly emerge, but

have resulted from the interaction of many complex forces. These forces—increasing population, technological advances in industry, the inability to satisfactorily absorb waste products, and an attitude of exploitative dominance of life space—have played a part in the current ecologic crisis. Complicating education in this area is the sheer magnitude of ecologically oriented materials available to students and teachers, as well as the political and racial overtones of environmental issues.[35]

Further complicating this area of education is the charge that many well-known environmentalists tend to be prophets of doom and have overdramatized the plundering of the planet. How indeed is the schoolteacher to know for certain that ". . . the human race is in danger of suffocating from overbreeding, of poisoning itself with pollution, of undermining its essential character by tampering with heredity, and of weakening the basic structure of society through too much prosperity"?[36] Does alarm provide the best atmosphere for finding rational solutions to worrisome problems? Was Aesop telling us something with his fable of the shepherd boy who cried wolf too often? How right in their forecasts are people such as Paul Ehrlich (*The Population Bomb*), Rachel Carson (*Silent Spring*), Barry Commoner (*Science and Survival*) and René Dubos (*Reason Awake*)? The answer to this question is that it took imagination, clear writing, an abundance of speechmaking, and staggering prediction figures to shake the average American out of his state of lethargy relative to his environment. Even though Commoner may have been in error when he said in 1963 that Lake Erie was so polluted that it was dead (it yielded 25,000 tons of fish in 1970), his

[34]Fandel, John, "Invitation," *Commonweal*, September 17, 1971, p. 17.
[35]See viewpoint of James Brown and Donald B. Stone, "Doomsday Prophets, Humanists and Responsible Educators," *School Health Review*, 3:6–8, July–August 1972.
[36]Maddox, John, "The Doomsday Syndrome," *Saturday Review*, October 21, 1972, p. 31.

admonitions and challenges to people to do something about pollution should make all Americans grateful to him. The danger now is that any exaggeration to stir people up, to get things done, may result in large numbers of people becoming anesthetized by overstatement, and the movement to measurably upgrade the environment will suffer a serious setback. It is important for teachers, therefore, to get their facts straight, to treat the subject soberly rather than fanatically, and involve students in small community projects with wide appeal.

By employing the phrase "environmental health" carefully much can be achieved. This may not be easy, because the phrase is somewhat of a misnomer; the problems of environmental health are not those stemming from a healthy environment. Rather, they are the problems arising from the deteriorating quality of the environment. Furthermore, the problems are not neatly packaged, but are involved with the transformation of the natural ecosystem to the human ecosystem. It takes a clever teacher to define and measure health in terms of an adap-

tive capacity toward environmental circumstances and hazards. With human adaptability the prime issue, health no longer is absence of all disease; instead it ". . . is a process of continuous adaptation to the myriad of microbes, irritants, pressures, and problems which daily challenge man."[37]

To make this topic more meaningful, one must do more than visit the local establishments such as bakeries, water works, and garbage disposal plants. There has to be some extensive thinking and action associated with the project. Very often a problematical situation calling for investigation and preplanning is necessary to arouse the class to see the value of a particular community health item. Certainly it is hardly a treat in many school systems today to be taken on a field trip to see the local organizations, but a sixth grade visit to a readily accessible mosquito breeding water hole

[37]See full review of this concept by Frederick Sargent II, "Man-Environment—Problems for Public Health," *American Journal of Public Health,* 62:628–633, May 1972.

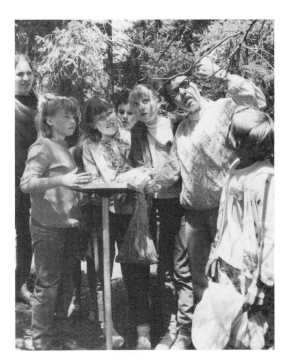

Figure 8–21 Ecology in the fourth grade environmental health program. (Courtesy Ellensburg Public Schools, Ellensburg, Washington.)

may challenge the class to do something about it. Such was the case in a Georgia community a few years ago. A project planned and initiated by schoolchildren blossomed into an endeavor by the whole community and greatly reduced the mosquito threat in the whole area. Even the pupil with the poorest memory would have trouble forgetting this kind of experience. And there are other activities along the same line. The report of a fifth grade committee on the cleanliness of rest rooms in local eating establishments would normally be received with a good amount of interest and enthusiasm, particularly if the report were to be followed up in some way. When it comes to garbage and refuse disposal, clean air, and water pollution, children have a real concern. They know first-hand when the

air is odorous, and they want safe water for drinking and clean water for their own boating and swimming. Thus, they are capable of getting the facts, telling the story, and influencing others to take action. Many up-to-date and informative teaching pamphlets are available each year from the U.S. Public Health Service and the U.S. Department of the Interior.

The Environmental Circle developed in New York State is an excellent teaching device, especially when the objective is to vividly demonstrate the association of land, water and air pollution. (See Fig. 8–22.) This circle can be enlarged and hung before a class for all to see. Helpful sources of scientific information, coupled with ideas for involving elementary students, may be found in magazines

ENVIRONMENTAL CIRCLE

SHOWING MANY KINDS OF POLLUTION AND THE EFFECT ON THE TOTAL ENVIRONMENT

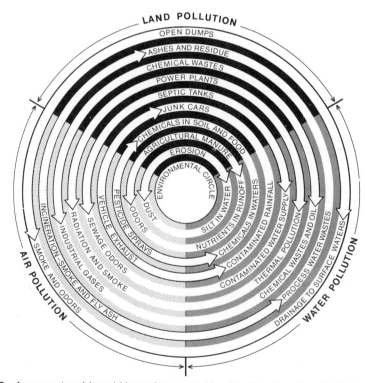

Figure 8–22 A proven teaching aid in environmental health. (Courtesy New York State Department of Environmental Conservation.)

such as *Consumer Reports*, *Today's Health*, and *Instructor*. In most areas there is an Audubon publication (such as *Massachusetts Audubon News*) which is rich in environmental and ecological items of use in the classroom. Now available throughout the several regions of the country is the *Environmental Newsletter*, published each month by the U.S. Environmental Protection Agency (free). The one from the New England Regional Office has been used widely in schools because it not only reports environmental happenings bearing on health, but it tells what groups of citizens and school children are doing to improve their immediate environment. The U.S. Public Health Service also has many materials. The film, *The Endless Chain* (Tribune Films, Inc.) is superb for bringing an intermediate class to face the ecological problems. The filmstrips, *Man and his Environment: a New Approach to Environmental Education* (American Association for Health, Physical Education and Recreation), and *Man's Natural Environment: Crisis Through Abuse* (Guidance Associates) can be very helpful in Grades 3–8. Of the several books dealing with this area the following should help the teacher put together interesting content and pupil activities:

Bernarde, Melvin A. *Our Precious Habitat*, New York: W. W. Norton and Co., 1970.
Commoner, Barry. *The Closing Circle*, New York: Knopf, 1971.
DeBell, Garrett. *The Environmental Handbook*, New York: Ballantine Books, 1970.
Dubos, René. *Man, Medicine and Environment*, New York: Praeger, 1968.
Graham, Frank. *Since Silent Spring*, Boston: Houghton Mifflin, 1970.
Michelson, Max. *The Environmental Revolution*, New York: McGraw-Hill, 1970.
Mitchell, John. *Ecotactics: The Sierra Handbook for Environmental Activities*, New York: Pocket Books, 1970.
Odum, H. T. *Environment, Power and Society*, New York: John Wiley, 1971.
Smolensky, Jack, and Haar, Franklin B. *Principles of Community Health*, Philadelphia: W. B. Saunders Co., 1972.
Environmental Study Guide, Grades 4–8, *All Around You*, U.S. Government Printing Office, Washington, D.C.

Ecological thinking, says Russell, "... suggests that most health-related is-

sues are not so much problems to solve as relationships to understand—some of which might be changed and others just lived with."[38] By the time a child is nine or ten he can be expected to respond. This viewpoint seems to tie in fairly well with the writers of the State of New York curriculum guides. The guides are worth reviewing, for they are particularly well organized. Content (topics) for the intermediate level is as follows:

I. The Environment and Health Status
   A. Explanation of relationship between man, environment and health
   B. History of environmental control
      1. Past
      2. Present
II. Man's Environment and Disease
   A. Explanation of the relationship
   B. History of relationship
III. Water
   A. Need for water
      1. Sources of water
      2. Uses of water
   B. Management for clean water
      1. Methods of management
      2. Role of government
         a. national
         b. state
         c. local
   C. Pollution of water
      1. Definition of water pollution
      2. Causes of water pollution
         a. communities
         b. industries
         c. improper use of land areas through highway construction, farming, forestry
      3. Effects of pollution

---

[38]Russell, Robert D. "Effects of Ecological Thinking on Health Education," *School Health Review*, 3:3–6, July–August 1972.

IV. Air
   A. Composition of air
   B. Need for air
   C. Pollution of air
      1. Definition of air pollution
      2. Causes of air pollution
         a. residential
         b. industrial
         c. automotive
         d. natural
         e. atmospheric conditions
      3. Harmful effects of air pollution
         a. health
         b. agriculture
         c. reduced visibility
   D. Control of air pollution
      1. Need for control
      2. Devices for control
         a. automotive
         b. industrial
      3. Measurements of pollution
         a. Ringelmann chart
         b. Dustfall
      4. Laws and regulations for air pollution control
         a. federal
         b. state
         c. local
   V. Food Protection
   A. Importance for health
   B. Food handling
      1. Definition of food handling
      2. Contamination problems
      3. Additive problems
   C. Supervision of food
      1. Agencies — laws
      2. The consumer
  VI. Water Treatment
   A. Improvement to health
   B. Sewage (liquid wastes)
   C. Refuse (solid wastes)
 VII. Insects and Rodents
   A. Rodents
   B. Insects
   C. Need for control
   D. Methods of control
   E. Responsibility for control
VIII. Maintaining a Healthful Environment

   A. In the home
      1. Purpose
      2. Responsibility
   B. In the community
      1. Purpose
      2. Service responsibility

Whether environmental health is taught indirectly or directly, it is a potential contributor to the basic understandings sought through such educational aims as self-realization and civic responsibility. One does not fully realize himself until he feels responsible for the welfare of others in his home town. And one does not come of age in this realization until he gains a certain satisfaction from actually participating in community projects.

Suggested Activities

Primary Level
   1. Write the following question on the board and ask for suggestions:
HOW CAN I MAKE MY TOWN A MORE PLEASANT PLACE IN WHICH TO LIVE?
Here are some of the expected answers:
   Do unto others as you would have them do unto you.
   Do not throw paper and other items out the window for someone else to pick up.
   Do not leave cans or bottles on the public beach or picnic area.
   Stay home when you have a cold.
   Use sprays such as DDT to help eliminate flies and other harmful insects.
   Help keep the house clean and sanitary.
   2. Ask the class to take home the following statement to think about overnight:
HEALTH IN OUR COMMUNITY IS THE RESULT OF THE WORK OF MANY PEOPLE.
Properly carried out, this may involve parents and others in the family and, therefore, become a far more valuable experience than it may appear to be on the surface (second and third grade).
   3. Call upon the local Audubon chapter for special programs and materials. The principles of ecology are well handled by this group; ways of develop-

ing observational skills will be brought out.

4. Through committee action, discover how fast the population is increasing or decreasing in the community. Build a simple line graph to cover a 20-year period. (Third grade.)

5. Raise the question: *How can some kinds of pollutants in the air be detected?* Fasten a sheet of white paper inside a shallow pan or spread a piece of glass with a thin coating of petrolatum. Place outside in different areas. Examine the surfaces now and then with a magnifying lens. Or, place white paper tissues outside in different places. Vary the length of time that the tissues are exposed to the air and *observe* their condition. Students will draw conclusions orally.

6. Show a large picture of a lake, reservoir, nearby stream, or river. Ask the class if they think it is safe to drink the water? Safe to swim in? Shortages of clean water affect the life of us all. Show the film, *Bulldozed America* (Carousel Films, Inc.).

7. Dramatize the effects of pollution; dramatization has more impact on children than talking about it. Start with two fish bowls with equal amounts of clean sand, washed pebbles, healthy greens, pure fresh water, four goldfish and a snail as a garbage-disposal scavenger, in each.

Both bowls will receive the same amount of light and warmth. Label one "Clean Environment" and the other "Polluted Environment." One team of students changes water daily, feeds fish, and keeps the "clean" bowl clean. The other team keeps a record of things put into "polluted" bowl: dirty nail, spit, dust, scrap of greasy bag, mud from shoe, dead leaf, cigar ashes, chewing gum, etc. Pupils note developing murky water and odor as well as lethargic fish with poor appetite. Clean "Polluted" bowl before fish die. (Second grade.)* *(See below)*

8. Talk about and illustrate with pictures and stick men drawings the various kinds of occupations in the community and how they have a bearing on one's health.

9. Plan together how elementary schoolchildren can promote good health in town or city. An idea or "think" session with teacher in background.

10. Ask the question: "How is the life of our town affected by the extremes of weather?" Post pictures collected by pupils depicting how the different plants and animals protect themselves against bad weather. Show the effects of unusual

*Activity reported by June Marie Schasre of Buffalo, N.Y., who used it with her second grade class.

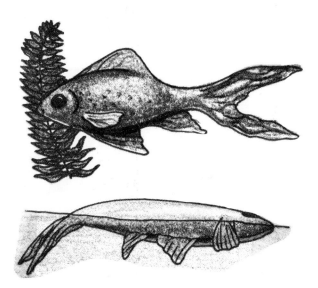

weather conditions. How do these things affect the fire departments, police departments, public works, doctors, and nurses?

11. Have a child who has recently been to a hospital tell the class something about life there. Look for misconceptions picked up from parents and others about the way hospitals function.

12. Visit a large grocery store. Prepare for this by having each pupil bring from home the name of one relatively inexpensive item to be purchased during the class visit. This will work with over 90 per cent of the pupils bringing the necessary money to purchase a particular food product. While at the store, ask the manager to show the class how perishable foods are stored and how cleanliness is practiced.

13. Investigate noise pollution. Experiment with different kinds of sound-absorbing materials. Line some cardboard boxes of the same size with various types of materials and place the same sound source, such as an alarm clock, inside each container in turn. What types of material reduce the sound most? Try acoustical tiles, bricks, cork sheets, fabrics, building insulation, glass plates, sheet metal, etc. Chart comparisons on a line graph. (Third grade.)

14. Bring a painted turtle to class. They balance our fresh water economy by eating 65 per cent pond weeds and many insects — and especially mosquito larvae.

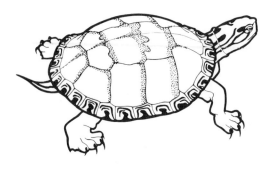

15. Reproduce the poster below for schoolwide distribution:

16. Clean up the classroom and follow this with voluntary statements from individual pupils on how they keep their homes and yards clean.

17. Secure copies of *Walter Waterdrop*, a coloring book from U.S. Environmental Protection Agency, Region VII, Kansas City, Mo. 44106 (1971). (First grade.)

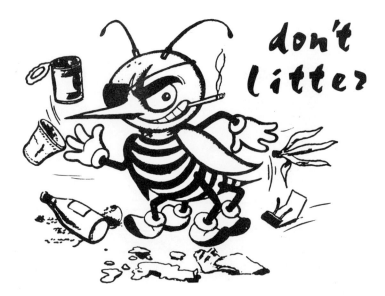

Intermediate Level

1. Receive a visitor from the local health department. Let this person tell about all the interesting jobs to be done. (Many people are available for this. In the small city there are only a few workers, but in a city like New York there are some five thousand workers in the health department.)

2. Build a series of eight or ten models depicting *What Our Community Should Do to Keep Everyone Healthy.* Assign several pupils to each model. When they are completed, exhibit them in the school library or other appropriate place. Following are some examples of models:

    a. *Maintain health records:* Show a clerk in an office pulling out a file drawer in a file cabinet.

    B. *Collect garbage:* Show a garbage man carrying a garbage can from a house to the truck.

    c. *Control communicable diseases:* Show several homes on a street. At the door of one home depict a man hanging a "Contagious Disease" sign on the front door.

    d. *Inspect restaurants and dairies:* Show a clean restaurant with people sitting and eating at tables, or show a scene depicting dishes being washed. A dairy barn scene would also be a good choice.

    e. *Keep drinking water safe:* Show a pumping station or model of a filter system. Or simply attach a real water faucet to a large piece of plywood with a model of a hand holding a glass just below it.

3. Have class *investigate* how much they know about their home sewage system. Where does their sewage go? Does the town or city have a sewage treatment plant? Does raw sewage or treated sewage empty into any stream or body of water? If so, what might the class do about it?

4. Take a field trip about town and view garbage and trash disposal, incinerators, kitchen grinders, and sanitary land fill. Show the relationship of all of this with pleasant looking areas on the outskirts of the community where there are no dumps with bad odors, flies, rats, or cockroaches.

5. Write a three paragraph statement on the news of a closed swimming area. What are the implications? (Fourth grade.)

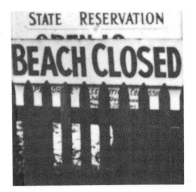

6. Prepare posters for placement in community stores, bus stations, banks, and business establishments. Some titles which suggest a picture are:

Do Not Jaywalk in (name of town)
This Community Is What You Make It!
Treat Others Courteously
Smile — Be Friendly and Say "Hello"
Don't Eat at Unclean Eating Places and They Will Be Forced to Clean Up

7. After some work on the topic of community health, ask the pupils to write some statements in support of the sentence:
THE WELFARE OF THE MAJORITY IS RELATED TO THE PRACTICES OF THE MINORITY.

8. Post the following news item; then begin planning the steps necessary to do the same thing in the local community:

NEWTON'S RECYCLING PROGRAM

A city-wide paper recycling program is underway in Newton, Mass.

The program will cost the city an estimated $30,000 per year but approximately one-third of the cost will be returned through the sale of the newsprint to a salvaging contractor.

The recycling effort is designed to prolong the life of the city's five year old incinerator and reduce the quantity of fly ash pollution.

Newton currently recycles glass and cans.

9. Using an appropriate dictionary, look up the meaning of words such as chlorine, fluorine, filter, pasteurized, disinfected, epidemic, swab, septic tank, reservoir, homogenized, bacteriology, abscess.

10. Divide the class into "Health Inspection Committees." Assign committee members according to personal choice. Permit the separate committees to survey the community and report back to class. Topics for survey may include:

Recreational opportunities for elementary age children
Cleanliness and handwashing facilities in city eating places

Cleanliness and handwashing facilities in the school
Safety hazards in and about the city
Cleanliness of city streets

11. Experiment with clean water and a closed water system—illustrating both evaporation and condensation. Show how temperature, light and turbidity influence water cycle. (See opp. page)

12. Set up water testing stations along a river or stream. Assign pupils to collect water samples. Then test for coliform bacteria per 100 ML, pH, NO_3, turbidity and color. (Sixth grade.)

13. Prepare a brochure for the start of a spring clean up campaign. Distribute the brochure.

14. Bring some mosquito wrigglers in water to class. Pour some oil on these and notice the results.

15. Investigate some of the new homes being built in the community. Make a list of the various inspections that a new house must pass and the reasons for these.

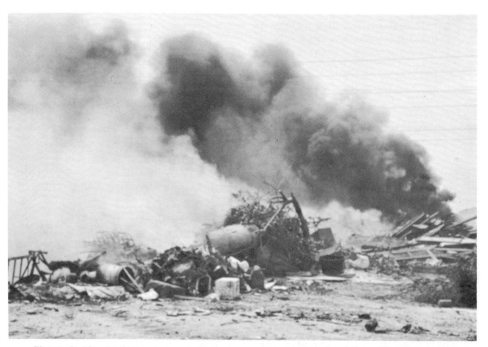

Figure 8–23 A trip to the local dump is an elementary school "must" experience.

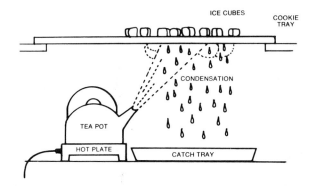

"THE

SPRING

OFFENSIVE"

YOU

CAN PLAY A PART

an admonition to recover the wastes in "gas, liquid and residue," thereby turning them into benefits to the environment and, above all, to the economy.

The revolutionary committees in villages and factories devote much attention to how wastes can be utilized. A recent issue of the *Peking Review* reports that a complex of factories in Shanghai collectively produced 200 suggestions for utilizing wastes, of which ninety were adopted. As a result, more than 200 tons of raw and other materials were recovered.

16. Investigate noise and hearing loss.[39] If possible, measure noise in decibels about the neighborhood.

17. Search for pollution activities in other lands (especially Europe). Start project by posting Chinese figures:

Everywhere in China these characters appear. They convey the equivalent of Keep America Beautiful, Conserve Resources, Prevent Pollution. Their literal meaning — *Three Wastes, Three Benefits* — allude to the natural triumvirate of land, water, and air, but to a Chinese, they are

三
废
变
三
利

[39] Helpful ideas may be found in "Noise — The Challenge of the Future," *Journal of School Health, 42*:172–176, March 1972.

18. Enlarge a county map. Appoint groups to fill in rivers, streams, forests, factories, and other environmental items. Conservation districts and flood plain lands may also be added.

11. ALCOHOL, TOBACCO, AND DRUGS

Behavioral Objectives

(Primary Level)

Describes all medicines as helpful items when illness occurs.

Explains that drugs correctly used help the body fight illness or relieve pain.

Explains that medicines incorrectly used can result in sickness, body damage, even death.

Demonstrates the dangers related to the home medicine cabinet.

Explains how to recognize glue, paint and other solvents that can affect health status.

Behavioral Objectives

(Intermediate Level)

Explains that tobacco and alcoholic beverages do not contribute to the development of growing boys and girls.

Identifies the factors that point for the need for moderation in adult smoking and drinking practices as one means of preventing heart, respiratory, digestive and mental illness.

Evaluates the use of sleep promoting and pain killing drugs, and the possible hazards involved.

Develops an explanation of the role of mental health as it bears on such things as excessive smoking, alcoholism, and drug addiction.

Investigates the several effects of narcotics in general and the laws governing their sale.

Portrays situations in which new drugs are discovered for the treatment of disease.

Comments

Since everything in the health area cannot be taught before the age of eight, the topics of alcohol, tobacco, and drugs are limited pretty much to the intermediate level where a concentration can be made at what would appear to be the "teachable moment." This does not rule out primary level discussions of helpful medicines, open medicine cabinets, aspirin control, stimulants, glue, paint, aerosol cans, and other items.

In some schools alcohol and tobacco are scheduled for discussion in the food unit; here they may be considered in terms of the effect on growth and efficiency of the human organism. There is nothing wrong with doing this, but there is evidence to indicate that this topic is big enough to warrant separate consideration. This is more than a growth problem for children; it is something that observing children know much about, and involves people from all walks of life and circumstances.

Actually, education about alcohol, tobacco, coffee, tea, and the like is not new. In 1882 Vermont passed active legislation adding temperance teaching to the public school curriculum with "... special prominence to the effects of alcoholic drinks, stimulants, and narcotics upon the human system."[40] Four years later 18 states and the District of Columbia had essentially the same requirements.

Alcohol and tobacco education have sometimes been labeled as controversial subjects. This is no longer true. Today, there is wide classroom discussion relative to the implications of drinking and smoking.

Alcohol Education. There is an increasing amount of evidence to suggest that alcoholic beverages are a part of the American culture. The Government-financed report, *Alcohol Problems: A Report to the Nation* (New York: Oxford University Press) recommends that a "deliberate effort" be made to make

---

[40]As quoted in J. E. Foster, "Scientific Temperance Instruction in the Schools," *Proceedings and Addresses.* National Education Association, 1886, Salem, 1887, p. 83.

drinking acceptable—if practiced in moderation—almost anywhere, including at church-sponsored functions. It is known that 75 per cent of all Americans drink, and that 40 per cent drink "regularly." The problem arises when drinking gets out of hand. One-third of all arrests in the United States are for public drunkenness. Thousands of persons with serious drinking problems are committed to mental institutions each year. Over half of the automobile drivers involved in fatal accidents have had high concentrations of alcohol in their systems. It is clear that the alcohol problems are more likely to be reduced through increased educational efforts—through prevention, not abstinence. Thus, the teacher's task is to bring out the factual information regarding excessive drinking and to stress responsible actions, rather than to moralize about the "evils of drink" to children whose parents probably enjoy the cocktail hour every evening.

The secret, of course, is to teach alcohol education at an early age (the maturity of the intermediate level pupil) in such a way that the readily normative drinking models, i.e., television, parents, and friends, are shown to be part of the American scene. Although research shows that the greater the number of drinking models, the more likely youngsters are to drink, it is still possible to point out that some things are saved until one is older—just as driving the family car is saved until later years. In the "permissive society," of course, it may always be difficult to say just when one is mature enough to learn to drink moderately. Moreover, alcohol research demonstrates again and again that the culture determines the practices—even at an early age. Socioeconomic status and childhood deprivations, therefore, may have more to do with early drinking patterns than what is taught in school.[41] In fact, there is a tendency to expect too much from alcohol education in the school setting. Although school efforts

help, the home and peer group influences ultimately will prove more important. Today, there appears to be no clear-cut level when adulthood begins—so children assume adult roles early. They copy adults at an earlier and earlier age. Often they seem to be trained for adulthood by exclusion from adulthood. Thus, by age 11 about 50 per cent of the boys have tasted their first drink.

Alcohol education must be acquired in relation to a particular situation; school activity must be related to life outside the school. Swimming can be dangerous, but it is taught in order to survive in the water. Drinking too can be dangerous, but it may be possible to teach how to drink safely—with personal and social responsibility. Or, as one educator put it, let us teach "survival in our cocktail culture." In this manner it may be possible in the years ahead to reduce the 6,500,000 figure of persons suffering from alcoholism.

The elementary school has a responsibility in this area chiefly because of pupil needs, that is, the "awakening interest." Fifth and sixth graders tend to become very curious about drinking. What does beer taste like? Will whiskey make you feel "funny"? How do people feel? Why do they lose control of their automobiles under the influence of alcohol? Do doctors use brandy or whiskey as a stimulant for sick people? These and a hundred similar questions are being asked today by children of this age level. Stimulants and narcotics are everywhere. Some children have been drinking tea and coffee for years. Many families have beer or wine with the evening meal. Cocktails are served in the home. People drink and drive without giving it more than a passing thought. Moreover, growing boys and girls are extremely observant of these things.

Because so many parents drink, the topic is a difficult one for the teacher to handle satisfactorily. She must not leave the impression that to take a drink is "criminal" or a mark of the "man about town." What she says must lead to abstinence during the growing years and moderation or temperance in the later years. Since a high percentage of adults

[41]Cahalan, Don and Room, Robin, *Problem Drinking Among American Men*, New Brunswick: Rutgers Center for Alcohol Studies, 1973.

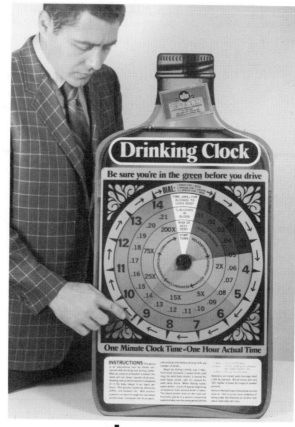

the Drinking Clock

The DRINKING CLOCK teaches what everyone must know about drinking and driving safety. This audio-visual aid is made from ¼ inch tempered masonite with a steel protected timer and is ideal for driver's education, health classes and law enforcement instruction.

The **classroom model** (17 x 34 inches) is intended for use in front of a room.

After an amount of alcohol is dialed on the clock, the hand points to the blood alcohol level, time required for alcohol to leave the body, minimum wait before driving, and increased risk of accident. The clock then runs down at the same rate at which the body metabolizes alcohol. With practice, a person learns to judge these same factors in any real situation.

Figure 8–24   An attractive teaching aid for alcohol education. (Courtesy Spenco Medical Corporation. P. O. Box 8113, Waco, Texas 76710.)

drink, one should not teach that anything short of total abstinence is reprehensible. Stress the harmful effects, but point out that some people use alcohol in moderation and without any complications. For this reason, the best education in this area will be one that encourages young people to develop insight into their feelings about themselves and others, and the role that alcohol may play in reducing sensitivity to standards of behavior consistent with their own family or group. Focusing on feelings and cultural drinking patterns in the intermediate and middle grades, when coupled with opportunities to discover the unhealthy and hazardous aspects of drinking, may help develop a higher level of appreciation for the school and teacher. Certainly, there is an abundance of data regarding beverage alcohol. It is time to transmit this information to the young in a more personalized fashion.

There are a number of fine sources of instructional materials relative to alcohol:

1. *American Medical Association,* 535 Dearborn Street, Chicago, Illinois 60610. (For information and lists of materials available).
2. *National Institute on Alcohol Abuse and Alcoholism,* 5600 Fishers Lane, Rockville, Maryland 20852 (For information and a comprehensive review of audiovisual materials). See "Alcohol: Questions and Answers."
3. *Rutgers Center of Alcohol Studies,* Rutgers—The State University, New Brunswick, New Jersey 08903.
4. *Alcoholics Anonymous,* Information Center, 337 East 33rd Street, New York, New York 10016.
5. *National Council on Alcoholism,* Inc., 2 Park Avenue, New York, New York, 10016. (A list of local affiliates can be provided and a list of materials is available.)
6. *Alcohol and Drug Problems Association of North America* (formerly North American Association of Alcoholism Programs), Education Department, 1130 Seventeenth Street, N.W., Washington, D.C. 20036. (A list of local affiliates can be provided.)
7. *Your State Department of Education.*
8. *Your State Department of Public Health* (or Department of Mental Health). Title of the department varies from state to state.
9. National Institute of Mental Health, HEW., Washington, D.C. See *Thinking About Drinking,* pub. no. 1683—Also, *Alcohol and Alcoholism.*
10. Licensed Beverage Industries, Inc., 485 Lexington Ave., New York, N.Y. 10017. (Free teaching materials for students stressing facts and moderation.)

Smoking Education. There is no question whether the young people who are now taking up smoking will suffer more illness and die earlier than those who do not. In fact, the earlier one begins to smoke, the greater the danger over a lifetime. According to the extensive research findings of the U.S. Public Health Service, approximately one million children now living in the United States will die prematurely of lung cancer alone.[42] Moreover, there are significant risks from smoking related to chronic bronchopulmonary disease, emphysema, peptic ulcers, cardiovascular disease, pregnancy problems, and skin aging.

The findings of a number of studies are in agreement that children start experimental smoking in the intermediate grades and develop into fairly regular smokers by the eighth or ninth grade. A Cincinnati, Ohio survey indicates that 22 per cent of schoolchildren start to smoke during the age bracket of ten years and younger; 60 per cent begin between 11 and 13.[43] The pupil is more likely to smoke if his parents or his older brothers and sisters smoke and if his friends smoke. If children have low goals, little ability, and little achievement, they tend to smoke earlier.

In a Seattle study of several thousand students, the majority of the boys began smoking cigarettes at age 12 or after, while the majority of the girls started at age 13 or after.[44] An interesting finding, and one of importance to elementary teachers, is that a comparison of those

---

[42]U.S. Department of Health, Education and Welfare. *The Health Consequences of Smoking,* Public Health Service No. 1696, Washington, D.C., 1964, 1967, 1969 and 1972.

[43]Streit, William K. "Students Express Views on Smoking," *Journal of School Health,* 37:153–154, March 1967.

[44]Harlin, Vivian Krause. "Response of School Children to a Questionnaire About Smoking," *American Journal of Public Health,* 62:566–574, April 1972.

still smoking with those who had given up the practice revealed that those still smoking represent a greater number of boys and girls *who began their smoking habit at the younger ages.* This ties in with Hammond's studies in which he showed that death rates are higher among current cigarette smokers who started at a young age than those who started later in life.

In a society in which cigarettes are advertised, sold and used everywhere and in which 40 per cent of the adults smoke or use some other kind of mood modifier, it is difficult to educate children to the extent that they will not start to smoke. There has been some reduction in adult smoking the last few years, and for awhile there was evidence to support the view that fewer children start to smoke when exposed to carefully planned educational programs.[45] Concentrated anti-smoking campaigns in Spokane, Washington and other sections of the country were successful. However, this has changed and there are currently more young people taking up smoking than before. The primary stumbling block to successful smoking education programs is youth's strong desire to conform and gain social confidence by doing what others do, or appear to do. And it depends upon who the "others" are. Having an older sibling who smokes appears to be the more important of all family variables. In the Columbus, Ohio study it was found that if a student has a best friend who smokes he or she is *nine times* more likely to smoke than are other students.[46] Moreover, where all of one's pals smoke, the probability is three to one that the respondent himself smokes. Where none of one's pals smoke, the chances are only one in a hundred that the respondent smokes. Of all the variables examined in this study, these two peer smoking behavior variables best differentiate smokers from non-smokers.

Other studies relating smoking to peer group attitudes and behavior point to the need to look beyond the classroom and into the community to observe the associations of youth. In the Indianapolis study of 49,034 schoolchildren, grades five through twelve, dozens of reasons were given for smoking and not smoking.[47] Although there were numerous reasons for smoking, such as "emotional improvement," "imitate adults," "eating substitute," and "to impress others," the big reason given was *peer influence.* This increased through the elementary school grades to a peak at the eighth grade, and declined thereafter to a low in the twelfth grade. This is a significant finding, for it means that somewhere in the 5th through 8th grade period is the prime time to get at the motivating forces and feelings that compel children to follow the gang, to do what they think everybody else does. If *status* is this important, then the teacher had better make arrangements to talk it over and get at the gut-level of feelings through small group discourse and study. The ten year old student is old enough to face this topic. Studies of young children indicate that they have feelings and have thought quite a bit about smoking. As non-smokers they are annoyed by second-hand tobacco smoke; but more than this the attitude they have toward their parent's smoking is generally one of worry and concern for their parents.[48]

In view of the above, what Daniel Horn has said is more meaningful than ever:

"The problem of staying off smoking is much more directly related to interpersonal relationships, the kind of world we live in,

[45]Davis, Roy L. "Progress and Problems in Smoking," *Journal of School Health, 37:*121–128, March 1967. See also J. L. Schwartz and M. Dubitzky, "Research in Student Smoking Habits and Smoking Control," *Journal of School Health, 37:*177–182, April 1967.

[46]Lanese, Richard R. et al. "Smoking Behavior: a Multivariate Conceptual Approach," *American Journal of Public Health, 62:*807–813, June 1972.

[47]Levitt, Eugene E. "Reasons for Smoking and Not Smoking Given by School Children," *Journal of School Health, 41:*101–107, February 1971.

[48]Cameron, Paul. "Second-Hand Tobacco Smoke: Children's Reactions," *Journal of School Health, 42:*280–284, May 1972.

environmental supports and personal values, than to specific knowledge about the effects of smoking on health."[49]

To implement this philosophy it will be necessary to break down some school organizations and permit interpersonal relationships to thrive. Using older students to work with younger students is one way. In Honolulu, secondary school pupils visit the fifth and sixth grade classes of elementary schools in the district and help the children become aware of the hazards of cigarette smoking by involving them in laboratory experiments, discussions and other stimulating activities.[50] *Facts on Smoking* sheets, questionnaires, and a smoke-solution apparatus were prepared. Most of the materials were contributed by the American Cancer Society. The upper-level students were told to use their own words, to take their time, and to relax when carrying on their dialogue. The natural casualness and individual sincerity was delightful to behold, and there was evidence that the elementary children were influenced by the older group. This youth to youth method of teaching was tried earlier with over 10,000 fifth and sixth grade pupils in Broome County, New York.[51] All settings were informal as teenagers worked with the elementary students. The reactions reported would encourage greater attention to this method of teaching:

From 5th and 6th Graders

"The high school boys are nearer to our age level and they know what it's like and they told it like it is."

From Principals to Youth

"Thanks for your interest in the boys and girls in our elementary schools."

"You should be aware that these kids really look up to you. You are heroes to them. They are impressed with what you say and do."

From Teenagers

"I quit smoking because I could not stand before the group of 5th and 6th graders and have them ask me if I smoked."

"We want this committee to continue."

Throughout the nation a tremendous effort has been made to improve smoking education programs. Practically every state department of education has developed special smoking and health curriculum guides, together with resource material kits. The same can be said for hundreds of large city school systems.

Helpful literature is extensive. Noteworthy curriculum guides may be obtained from states such as California, Pennsylvania, Washington, Massachusetts, New York, Arizona, Rhode Island, and Illinois. A wealth of curriculum materials are available from the American Cancer Society and the U.S. Public Health Service. The Children's Bureau in Washington distributes the pamphlet, *Why Nick the Cigarette Is Nobody's Friend*, for fourth and fifth graders and *A Light on the Subject of Smoking*, for sixth graders. The National Film Board of Canada distributes the Academy Award film, *The Drag* — a nine-minute animated film for young audiences. Elementary children seem to love the cartoon spoof film *The Huffless, Puffless Dragon*, put out by the American Cancer Society. Their filmstrip, *I'll Choose the High Road*, is also very

[49] Horn, Daniel. "Educational Aspects of Smoking Research," *School Health Review*, 2:12–15, November 1971.

[50] Arrigoni, Edward A. "Teenage Anti-Smoking Campaign in the Elementary Schools," *School Health Review*, 3:15–18, March-April 1972.

[51] McRae, Cameron F. and Nelson, Dorothy M. "Youth to Youth Communication on Smoking and Health," *Journal of School Health*, 41:445–449, October 1971.

good; and the filmstrip and discussion guide of the National Interagency Council on Smoking and Health is of real value to the teacher in this health education area.

A great variety of teaching ideas relative to discussion topics, classroom experiments, and other projects appear in the teaching guide, *Smoking and Health Unit* of the Spokane Public Schools.[52] Another source of ideas is the booklet, *Classroom-Tested Techniques for Teaching About Smoking*, distributed free by the National Clearinghouse for Smoking and Health, U.S. Public Health Service, 4040 N. Fairfax Drive, Arlington, Virginia 22203. Also available from the Clearinghouse is *Smoking and Health Experiments, Demonstrations and Exhibits*. Free copies of *What to Tell Your Parents About Smoking*, and other publications, are available from the American Heart Association. The publication, *What Educators Can Do About Cigarette Smoking* (1971), especially prepared for teachers, may be obtained from the American Association for Health, Physical Education and Recreation.

Drug Education

Early in 1973 a number of school health personnel began to wring their hands in despair over the ineffectiveness of so-called drug education programs. As deLone said earlier, "Drug-abuse education is booming today in schools across the country. But for most kids it's a bummer."[53] Millions of dollars of local and federal government funds are being spent for teaching materials—from attractive teaching kits with simulated drugs displayed to hundreds of films and filmstrips. Yet, the head of the U.S. Office of Education's drug-education division points out that there is little evidence to support the practice of

dispensing information by itself. It may even be counterproductive. In a New York City study there was found to be no evidence of any significant relationship between knowledge about drugs or awareness of the dangers of drugs and their actual use. The same findings have occurred in Harrisburg, Pennsylvania and Dallas, Texas.

What then can the schools do? Because drug abuse is so subtle and multidimensional, so tied up with the "rites of passage" of the young, the "instant gratification" philosophy in the culture, and peer group activity, it is difficult indeed to be certain that any one teaching technique will be measurably successful. One thing is for sure: the teacher must relate to the students and command their respect. Unfortunately, even in the elementary grades the "life-style" of the school as a rigid, conformity-bound institution is an anathema to potential drug abusers. And in many places their influence is modest in contrast to home, peers or neighborhood environment. But, if one will use the latter setting to get at student concerns, feelings, self-doubt, anxiety, loneliness, joy, belonging—the "here now" topics, something productive can emerge. Couple this with a total elementary school approach to the *cultural system* to discover how it fosters or perpetuates drug abuse. This may require institutional changes and be hard to accomplish in many schools. However, peer group programs and peer group efforts can be promoted far beyond anything taking place today. Informational programs researched, developed, and implemented by students, student-assisted counseling programs, student-produced plays and role-playing are all means of promoting peer group activity. This will call for great classroom and school flexibility, but it may lead to some personal decision making.

The program begins mildly in the primary grades. The concern is more with drug use than drug abuse. By this age children have seen much at home and on television having to do with the drug oriented society. Respect for drugs is taught well before the age at which chil-

---

[52]*Teaching Guide: Grades 5–12, Smoking and Health Unit*, September 1967. Publications Department, Spokane Public Schools, W. 825 Trent Ave., Spokane, Washington 99201 (price $2.50).

[53]deLone, Richard J. "The Ups and Downs of Drug-Abuse Education," *Saturday Review*, November 11, 1972.

dren might find themselves in a critical decision making position. Youngsters are capable of having a good twenty minute discussion on the role of the physician in assigning drugs to reduce disease, the role of the pharmacist, the importance of understanding information on labels, the safe storage of drugs in the home, how to make phone calls for emergency medical assistance, the effects of certain drugs on the senses and on performance ability, and the history of man's discovery of drugs such as aspirin, penicillin and antibiotics. At an early age one should learn that drugs are good in fighting disease — in preventing infections, in treating illness, in helping cold symptoms, in helping people sleep, in preventing discomfort and pain and in prolonging life.

The abuse factor is brought in at the intermediate level. The habit-forming tendency of drugs and their poisonous effects is a proper emphasis. So is the abuse of prescription drugs.

Children should know that alcohol is classified as a narcotic rather than a stimulant. They should appreciate the great need for sleeping pills, aspirin, and pain killing substances. Information about these items should relate to the medical, economic, and social effects when they are used correctly, and what is involved from both a personal and community viewpoint when they are misused.

There will be times when parents and educators wonder why it is necessary to give vivid instruction in the more potent narcotics. They will reason that it is enough merely to refer to tobacco and alcohol in the elementary school. Yet, more and more evidence is available to indicate that the 12 year old boy or girl is ready for this level of education about drugs.

Education pertaining to narcotics is part of the larger problem of health teaching. It relates to values in living, to confidence in oneself, to self-respect, and to the importance of developing personal traits and abilities which one is proud to possess. This is an opportune moment for young people to discover, perhaps anew, that psychological factors are vital in all health behavior — that happy, secure people have a kind of respect for themselves that does not need building up with narcotics or anything else.

Far and away the most helpful and complete manual for the teacher is the American School Health Association publication, *Teaching About Drugs: A Curriculum Guide, K-12*, second edition, 1972. (107 South Depeyster Street, Kent, Ohio 44240 — Price $4.00) Almost everything the teacher would want to know is here — colored photographs, descriptions, historical items, pharmaceutical information, glossary of slang terms, ways to identify drug abusers, teaching aids, and fully outlined programs. It is a superb publication with ideas that have been tried and proven. Intermediate grade content is set forth in clear detail with learning activities and resources under eight teaching objectives:

A. To know that drugs come from several sources. To appreciate their long history of use (definitions, sources of drugs, history, ongoing research).

B. To understand the difference between prescription and nonprescription medicines (legal considerations, following directions, destroying left-over prescriptions, types of medicines purchasable on prescription, how to use medicines).

C. To recognize that drugs as medicines have many uses, along with a potential for producing both good and bad effects (drugs as medicines — users, differing effects of medicines).

D. To know that many widely used substances contain drugs (coffee, cola, tobacco, alcohol).

E. To know that misused and abused medicines, drugs, and other agents may have serious effects on the individual (medicines are misused in various ways, dangers of misuse, abuse potential, brain and nervous system reactions, drugs abused for different reasons).

F. To identify common household products and to use them for their intended purposes (essential benefits of products, misused products, consequences of misuse).

G. To assume increasing responsibility for personal health (growing up is to become independent and responsible, early establishment of health practices, ways practices develop, avoiding drug use).

H. To understand and appreciate the relationship of drugs to total health (WHO definition and total health, relationship of medicines to health, potential of medicines).

In view of what has been said previously about the great amount of teaching material available for school use, the following resources have been very carefully reviewed and selected. (Other teaching materials appear in Chapter 10.)

Drug Education Curriculum Guide (1971) Lafayette Elementary School District, 3477 School Street, Lafayette, California 94549 (Price $6.50)

K-6 Drug Education Curriculum Guide (1971) Oakland City Unified School District, 1025 Second Avenue, Oakland, California 94606 (Price $2.10)

Values-Oriented Approach to Drug Abuse Prevention Education (1972) Orange County Superintendent of Schools, 1104 Civic Center Drive, West, Santa Ana, California 92701 (single copy free)

A Plan for Drug and Narcotics Education for Grades Four Through Twelve (1972) Vallejo City Unified School District, 211 Valle Vista, Vallejo, California 94590 (Price $5.00)

Common Sense Lives Here, A Community Guide To Drug Abuse Action National Coordinating Council on Drug Abuse Education and Information, Suite 212, 1211 Connecticut Avenue, N.W., Washington, D.C.

Drug Abuse Current Awareness System, National Clearinghouse For Drug Abuse Information, 5600 Fishers Lane, Rockville, Maryland 20852 (no charge)

Facts About Drugs (1972) David C. Cook Publishing Co., Elgin, Illinois 60120 (Manual of lessons to go with sixteen $12\frac{1}{4}'' \times 17''$ picture cards—See Fig. 8–25.)

What Will Happen If . . . a programmed instruction course on drugs (1972) National Institute of Mental Health, 5600 Fishers Lane, Rockville, Maryland 20852 (50¢)

A Guide to Drug Abuse Education and Information Materials (1973) National Institute of Mental Health, 5600 Fishers Lane, Rockville, Maryland 20852 (50¢)

Drug Abuse Curriculum Guide (1972) International Education and Training Inc., 1776 New Highway, Farmingdale, New York 11735 (unique teaching aids)

Tips on Drug Abuse Prevention (1973) National Institute of Mental Health, 5600 Fishers Lane, Rockville, Maryland 20852

About Drugs (Grades 4–5) (1972) Haskell L. Bowen and Les Landin, Fearon Publishers, Belmont, California 94002 (50¢)

To Parents/About Drugs (1971) Metropolitan Life Insurance Co., 1 Madison Ave., New York, New York (Free)

The Most Frequently Asked Questions About Drug Abuse (1972) Special Action Office For Drug Prevention, P. O. Box 1100, Washington, D.C. 20008 (Free) Also comes with a 3-record set of questions and answers.

Drug Abuse Education Slide Resource Kit (1971) National Audiovisual Center (GSA), Washington, D.C. 20409 ($55.00 complete kit)

K-6 Drug Education Program (1972) The Creative Learning Group, 145 Portland St., Cambridge, MA. 02139 (student booklets on a variety of drug topics—complete set $95.00)

The Drug Scene: Fact Not Fiction (1972) Encyclopaedia Britannica Educational Corporation, 425 North Michigan Ave., Chicago, Illinois 60611 (four supportive films with which young people will identify—*Weed, Acid, Ups/Downs,* and *Scag*)

Me, Myself—And Drugs (1972) Guidance Associates, Pleasantville, New York 10570 (3 part filmstrip $49.50)

The Problem of Drug Abuse (1971) Pharmaceutical Manufacturers Assoc., 1155 15th Street, N.W., Washington, D.C. 20005 (set of 78 colored slides describing the drugs being used in current cultures—$15.00 per set)

Drugs, Poisons and Little Children (K-3) (1972) Educational Activities, Freeport, N.Y. 11520 (a full color filmstrip that complements a larger series of filmstrips related to children—$12.95)

Drugs: A Primary Film (1972) Arthur Barr Productions, Inc., P. O. Box 7-C, Pasadena, California 91104 (A primary grade film which explores the use of drugs by the physician.)

Books

Teaching About Drugs, A Curriculum Guide K-12 (1972) American School Health Assoc., 107 Depeyster St., Kent, Ohio 44240.

Marihuana 1973 U.S. Dept. of Justice, Bureau of Narcotics and Dangerous Drugs, Washington, D.C.

Drug Education Content and Methods D. A. Girdano and D. D. Girdano, Reading, Massachusetts: Addison-Wesley Publishing Co., 1972.

Drugs and People by Donald A. Read, Boston: Allyn and Bacon, Inc. 1972.

Drugs, Society and Human Behavior by Oakley S. Ray, St. Louis: C. V. Mosby, 1972.

Suggested Activities (Intermediate Level)

1. Collect advertisements from magazines and newspapers having to do with the "benefits" of tea, coffee, cigarettes, cigars, pipe tobacco, beer, wine, cola drinks, and headache pills. Secure answers to such questions as:

    a. How much of this advertising is essentially true, and how much is misleading?

2. Over a period of one week, collect newspaper clippings that have to do solely with automobile accidents in which intoxication and drinking are involved. Post these on a frequently read bulletin board. Ask for questions. Questions will arise somewhat as follows:

    a. In how many feet can a driver of an automobile usually stop when traveling at 50 miles per hour (an emergency situation)? How much longer may it take when the driver has had a few drinks?

    b. What disposition is generally made of cases of drunken driving in the courts?

    c. How many automobile accidents involve intoxication?

3. Discuss the short film *Weed* (Marihuana). This may be obtained on loan from Encyclopaedia Britannica Films. Show also *The Tobacco Problem: What Do You Think?* This is exceptionally provocative.

4. While viewing TV or listening to radio, make a list of the number of times commercials encourage a person to modify (change) feelings or outlook on life through the use of a substance or product. Apply feelings to five ways to respond to smoking. (Fig. 8–26)

5. Invite a local druggist to appear in class and answer questions regarding habit-forming drugs, drug addiction, and the law on prescriptions. This is also a good time to discuss the sale of sleeping pills. Have the class prepare for such discussion by clipping from the newspaper items pertaining to deaths and near-deaths due to an overdose of sleeping pills.

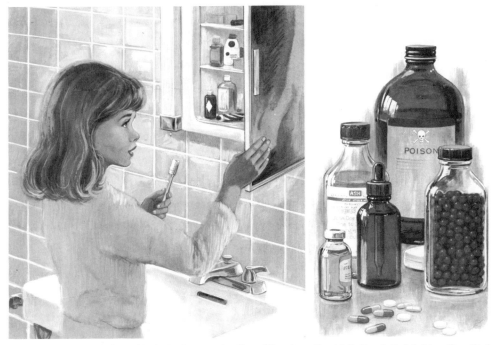

Figure 8–25 Teaching aids help focus attention. (Courtesy David C. Cook Publishing Co., Elgin, Illinois 60120.)

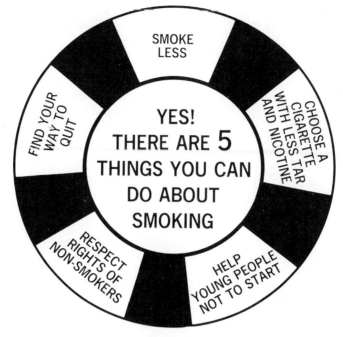

Figure 8–26

6. Dramatize the "smoker's cough." Act out three scenes. In scene No. 1, a chain-smoker is seen going about his daily activities. In scene No. 2, he is observed arising from his bed in the morning in a fit of coughing. In scene No. 3, his doctor is warning him to cut down his cigarette consumption because of the cough, its effect on appetite and consequent nutrition, its relationship to lon-gevity, its effect on the heart and blood pressure, its relationship to cancer and the respiratory system. Attract attention to topic by posting *Tar and Nicotine Content* chart. (U.S. Federal Trade Commission)(Fig. 8–27)

7. Engage a small panel of community "experts" on the topic of why people smoke. In this case the "experts" may be informed class members. One

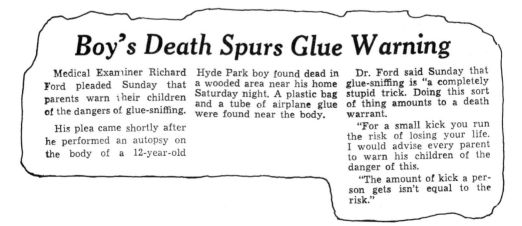

Boy's Death Spurs Glue Warning

Medical Examiner Richard Ford pleaded Sunday that parents warn their children of the dangers of glue-sniffing.

His plea came shortly after he performed an autopsy on the body of a 12-year-old Hyde Park boy found dead in a wooded area near his home Saturday night. A plastic bag and a tube of airplane glue were found near the body.

Dr. Ford said Sunday that glue-sniffing is "a completely stupid trick. Doing this sort of thing amounts to a death warrant.

"For a small kick you run the risk of losing your life. I would advise every parent to warn his children of the danger of this.

"The amount of kick a person gets isn't equal to the risk."

TAR AND NICOTINE CONTENT OF CIGARETTES
Federal Trade Commission, August 1971

(Tar content in this chart ranges from high of 33 mg/cig to 3 mg/cig, nicotine content from high of 2.4 mg/cig to low of 0.2 mg/cig.)

Brand	Type	Tar (mg/cig)	Nicotine (mg/cig)
Alpine	King, M	18	1.2
Belair	King M	17	1.3
	100 mm, M	19	1.4
Benson & Hedges	Reg (HP)	18	1.3
	King (HP)	20	1.4
	100 mm	21	1.4
	100 mm, M	21	1.4
Bull Durham	King	30	1.9
Camel	Reg., NF	25	1.5
	King	20	1.3
Carlton	Reg	3	0.2
	King	4	0.4
Chesterfield	Reg., NF	25	1.5
	King, NF	29	1.7
	King	19	1.2
	King, M	19	1.1
	101 mm	19	1.3
Domino	King, NF	27	1.4
	King	21	1.3
	King, M	20	1.3
Doral	King	14	0.9
	King, M	14	1.0
DuMaurier	King (HP)	18	1.2
Edgeworth Export	King (HP)	18	1.2
	100 mm	19	1.3
	100 mm, M	18	1.3
English Ovals	Reg. (HP)	25	1.8
	King (HP)	30	2.2
Eve	100 mm	17	1.2
	100 mm, M	17	1.1
Fatima	King (NF)	32	1.9
Frappe	King, M	10	0.3
Galaxy	King	20	1.4
Half & Half	King	24	1.7
Herbert Tareyton	King	29	1.8
Home Run	Reg., NF	19	1.3
Kent	Reg	10	0.6
	King(HP)	17	1.0
	King	17	1.0
	100 mm	19	1.2
	100 mm, M	19	1.1
King Sano	King	6	0.3
	King, M	6	0.2
Kool	Reg., NF, M	21	1.3
	King, M	18	1.4
	100 mm, M	19	1.4
L & M	Reg	16	1.0
	King (HP)	17	1.1
	King	19	1.3
	100 mm	19	1.3
	100 mm, M	19	1.2
Lark	King	17	1.0
	100 mm	18	1.2
Life	King	10	0.6
Lucky Strike	Reg., NF	29	1.7
Lucky Filters	King	22	1.6
	100 mm	22	1.6
Mapleton	Reg., NF	25	1.4
	King	23	1.1
Marlboro	King (HP)	19	1.3
	King	20	1.3
	King, M	18	1.1
	100 mm (HP)	21	1.5
	100 mm	22	1.5
Marvels	King, NF	23	0.8
	King	5	0.2
	King, M	4	0.2
Maryland	100 mm, M	20	1.3
Montclair	King, M	17	1.3
Multifilter	King (PB)	16	1.1
	King, M(PB)	12	0.9
New Leaf	King, M	19	1.3
Newport	King, M(HP)	19	1.1
	King, M	20	1.1
	100 mm, M	21	1.2
Oasis	King, M	18	1.1
Old Gold Straights	Reg., NF	22	1.2
	King, NF	28	1.5
Old Gold Filters	King	20	1.2
	100 mm	24	1.5
Pall Mall	King, NF	29	1.8
	95 mm (HP)	19	1.3
	95 mm, M (HP)	17	1.2
	100 mm	19	1.3
	100 mm, M	18	1.4
Parliament	King (HP)	16	1.0
	King	16	1.0
	100 mm	19	1.3
Peter Stuyvesant	King	19	1.4
	100 mm	20	1.5
Philip Morris	Reg., NF	24	1.5
Philip Morris Commander	King, NF	29	1.8
Picayune	Reg., NF	19	1.3
Piedmont	Reg., NF	24	1.3
Players	Reg., NF(HP)	33	2.4
Raleigh	King, NF	26	1.6
	King	17	1.2
	100 mm	18	1.3
Salem	King, M	19	1.3
	100 mm, M	20	1.3
Sano	Reg., NF	15	0.5
	Reg	4	0.2
Silva Thins	100 mm	16	1.1
	100 mm, M	16	1.1
Spring	100 mm, M	22	1.1
Tareyton	King	19	1.3
	100 mm	19	1.3
Tempo	King	12	0.9
Truc	King	12	0.6
	King, M	13	0.7
Vantage	King	12	0.8
Viceroy	King	17	1.2
	100 mm	18	1.3
Virginia Slims	100 mm	17	1.1
	100 mm, M	18	1.2
Vogue (Black)	King (HP)	27	0.9
Vogue (Colors)	King (HP)	18	0.7
Winston	King (HP)	20	1.3
	King	19	1.3
	100 mm	20	1.3
	100 mm, M	21	1.5

NF—Non-Filter (All other brands possess filters)
M—Menthol

PB—Plastic box
HP—Hard pack

Figure 8–27

may be designated as a community physician, another as a parent, and one or two others as active citizens. The panel should meet with the teacher before class in order to have several suggestions each as to why people smoke. (Examples: They enjoy it; they want to do what others do; it gives them something to do while waiting or talking; it is habit forming, and they feel a "need" for it; it keeps their weight down.) Moreover, how do you *feel* about the discussion? Would you say one of the following?:

> "SO WHAT?"
> "I DON'T KNOW"
> "I DON'T CARE"

8. Ask the direct question, "How many students have tried to smoke just for fun?" A few honest hands will be raised. Have these people tell how smoking affected them. It may have made them nauseated, even sick. Explain that medical authorities feel that smoking is of no benefit to anyone, but for growing boys and girls it is definitely harmful; one is not at one's best mentally, physically, or socially. In growing people it reduces the effectiveness of the muscle and nervous systems, may cause restlessness, dizziness, nausea, indigestion, increased heart beat, shortness of breath, and loss of appetite for good protein foods.

9. Write to the American Cancer Society for information on the effects of alcohol upon the length of life. Discuss the information received in class. Post information. Use clippings. Distribute American Cancer Society bookmarks (free).

10. Demonstrate the teaching device, The Mechanical Smoker. Available for $9.95 from Spenco Medical Corp., P. O. Box 8113, Waco, Texas, 76710. Let several pupils try it. The bulb draws nicotine from cigarette into plastic lung. (See Fig. 9–8.)

11. Consider alcohol as a beverage and its effect upon the body, mind, and society. Ask the question, "What are the common effects of alcohol on the individual and society?" Permit independent study Follow up with small group discussion

12 Call for a variety of words used to describe drunkenness: "high," "tight," "blind," "loaded," "on a binge," "happy," "plastered," "stoned," "tippler," "wino," "derelict," "bum," "common drunk," etc Discuss how these words make you *feel*. How really comic or tragic?

13. Experiment with water and alco-

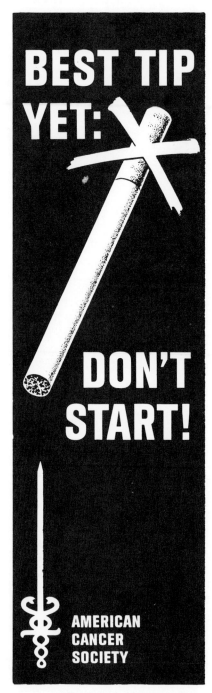

(Courtesy of The American Cancer Society.)

DRUG ABUSE PRODUCTS REFERENCE CHART

NAME	SLANG NAME	CHEMICAL OR OFFICIAL NAME	SOURCE	PHARMACOLOGIC CLASSIFICATION	MEDICAL USE	HOW TAKEN WHEN ABUSED	USUAL FORM OF PRODUCT	EFFECTS SOUGHT	LONG TERM POSSIBLE EFFECTS	PHYSICAL DEPENDENCE POTENTIAL	PSYCHOLOGICAL DEPENDENCE POTENTIAL	ORGANIC DAMAGE POTENTIAL
MORPHINE	WHITE STUFF M	MORPHINE SULPHATE	NATURAL (FROM OPIUM)	CENTRAL NERVOUS SYSTEM DEPRESSANT	PAIN RELIEF	SWALLOWED OR INJECTED	POWDER (WHITE) TABLET LIQUID	EUPHORIA, PREVENT WITHDRAWAL DISCOMFORT	ADDICTION, CONSTIPATION, LOSS OF APPETITE	YES	YES	YES, INDIRECTLY
HEROIN	H, HORSE, SCAT JUNK, SMACK, SCAG STUFF, HARRY	DIACETYL MORPHINE	SEMI-SYNTHETIC (FROM MORPHINE)	CNS DEPRESSANT	NONE, LEGALLY	INJECTED OR SNIFFED	POWDER (WHITE GRAY, BROWN)	EUPHORIA, PREVENT WITHDRAWAL DISCOMFORT	ADDICTION, CONSTIPATION, LOSS OF APPETITE	YES	YES	YES, INDIRECTLY
CODEINE	SCHOOLBOY	METHYLMORPHINE	NATURAL (FROM OPIUM); SEMI-SYNTHETIC (FROM MORPHINE)	CNS DEPRESSANT	EASE PAIN & COUGHING	SWALLOWED	TABLET, LIQUID (IN COUGH SYRUP)	EUPHORIA, PREVENT WITHDRAWAL DISCOMFORT	ADDICTION, CONSTIPATION, LOSS OF APPETITE	YES	YES	YES, INDIRECTLY
PAREGORIC		TINCTURE OF CAMPHORATED OPIUM	NATURAL AND SYNTHETIC	CNS DEPRESSANT	SEDATION, COUNTERACT DIARRHEA	SWALLOWED OR INJECTED	LIQUID	EUPHORIA, PREVENT WITHDRAWAL DISCOMFORT	ADDICTION, CONSTIPATION, LOSS OF APPETITE	YES	YES	YES, INDIRECTLY
MEPERIDINE		MEPERIDINE HYDROCHLORIDE	SYNTHETIC (MORPHINE-LIKE)	CNS DEPRESSANT	PAIN RELIEF	SWALLOWED OR INJECTED	TABLET LIQUID	EUPHORIA, PREVENT WITHDRAWAL DISCOMFORT	ADDICTION, CONSTIPATION, LOSS OF APPETITE	YES	YES	YES, INDIRECTLY
METHADONE	DOLLY	METHADONE HYDROCHLORIDE	SYNTHETIC (MORPHINE-LIKE)	CNS DEPRESSANT	PAIN RELIEF	SWALLOWED OR INJECTED	TABLET LIQUID	PREVENT WITHDRAWAL DISCOMFORT	ADDICTION, CONSTIPATION, LOSS OF APPETITE	YES	YES	YES, INDIRECTLY
COCAINE	CORRINE, COKE FLAKE, SNOW GOLD DUST, STAR DUST, BERNICE	METHYLESTER OF BENZOYLECGONINE	NATURAL (FROM COCA LEAVES)	STIMULANT, LOCAL OR TOPICAL ANESTHETIC	LOCAL OR TOPICAL ANESTHESIA	SNIFFED, INJECTED OR SWALLOWED	POWDER (WHITE) LIQUID	EXCITATION	DEPRESSION, CONVULSIONS	NO	YES	PROBABLE
MARIJUANA	POT, GRASS, TEA	CANNABIS SATIVA	NATURAL	HALLUCINOGEN	NONE	SMOKED OR SWALLOWED	PLANT PARTICLES (DARK GREEN OR BROWN)	EUPHORIA, RELAXATION, INCREASED PERCEPTION	USUALLY NONE; BRONCHITIS, CONJUNCTIVITIS, PSYCHOSIS POSSIBLE	NO	PROBABLE	NOT YET DETERMINED
HASHISH	HASH	CANNABIS SATIVA	NATURAL	HALLUCINOGEN	NONE	SMOKED OR SWALLOWED	SOLID, BROWN TO BLACK, RESIN	RELAXATION, EUPHORIA, INCREASED PERCEPTION	USUALLY NONE; CONJUNCTIVITIS, PSYCHOSIS POSSIBLE	NO	PROBABLE	NOT YET DETERMINED
BARBITURATES	BARBS, RED DEVILS, YELLOW JACKETS, PHENNIES, PEANUTS, BLUE HEAVENS, CANDY	PHENOBARBITAL, PENTOBARBITAL, SECOBARBITAL, AMOBARBITAL	SYNTHETIC	CNS DEPRESSANT	SEDATION, RELIEVE HIGH BLOOD PRESSURE, EPILEPSY	SWALLOWED OR INJECTED	TABLETS OR CAPSULES	ANXIETY REDUCTION, EUPHORIA	SEVERE WITHDRAWAL SYMPTOMS, POSSIBLE CONVULSIONS, TOXIC PSYCHOSIS	YES	YES	YES
AMPHETAMINES	BENNIES, DEXIES, HEARTS, PEP PILLS, SPEED, LID PROPPERS, WAKE-UPS	AMPHETAMINE DEXTROAMPHETAMINE METHAMPHETAMINE (DESOXYEPHEDRINE)	SYNTHETIC	CNS STIMULANT	CONTROL APPETITE, NARCOLEPSY, SOME CHILDHOOD BEHAVIORAL DISORDERS	SWALLOWED OR INJECTED	TABLETS CAPSULES LIQUID POWDER (WHITE)	ALERTNESS, ACTIVENESS	LOSS OF APPETITE, DELUSIONS, HALLUCINATIONS, TOXIC PSYCHOSIS	POSSIBLE	YES	PROBABLE
LSD	ACID, BIG D, SUGAR, TRIPS, CUBES	D-LYSERGIC ACID DIETHYLAMIDE	SEMI-SYNTHETIC (FROM ERGOT ALKALOIDS)	HALLUCINOGEN	EXPERIMENTAL RESEARCH ONLY	SWALLOWED	TABLETS CAPSULES LIQUID	INSIGHT, DISTORTION OF SENSES, EXHILARATION	MAY INTENSIFY EXISTING PSYCHOSIS, PANIC REACTIONS	NO	POSSIBLE	NOT YET DETERMINED
DOM	STP "SERENITY, TRANQUILITY, PEACE"	4-METHYL-2, 5-DIMETHOXY-ALPHA METHYL PHENETHYLAMINE	SYNTHETIC	HALLUCINOGEN	NONE	SWALLOWED	TABLETS CAPSULES LIQUID	STRONGER THAN LSD EFFECTS	?	NO	POSSIBLE	NOT YET DETERMINED
THC		TETRAHYDROCANNABINOL	NATURAL (FROM CANNABIS SATIVA) SYNTHETIC	HALLUCINOGEN	NONE	SMOKED OR SWALLOWED	IN MARIJUANA OR LIQUID	STRONGER THAN MARIJUANA EFFECTS	?	NO	POSSIBLE	NOT YET DETERMINED
DMT	BUSINESSMAN'S SPECIAL	DIMETHYL-TRYPTAMINE	SYNTHETIC	HALLUCINOGEN	NONE	INJECTED	LIQUID	SHORTER TERM THAN LSD EFFECTS	?	NO	POSSIBLE	NOT YET DETERMINED
PCP	HOG, PEACE PILL	PHENCYCLIDINE	SYNTHETIC	HALLUCINOGEN	VETERINARY ANESTHETIC	SWALLOWED	TABLETS CAPSULES	HARSHER THAN LSD	?	NO	POSSIBLE	NOT YET DETERMINED
MESCALINE	MESC	3,4,5-TRIMETH-OXYPHENETHYLAMINE	NATURAL (FROM PEYOTE CACTUS)	HALLUCINOGEN	NONE	SWALLOWED	TABLET CAPSULE	SAME AS LSD	?	NO	POSSIBLE	NOT YET DETERMINED
PSILOCYBIN		3/2-DIMETHYL AMINOETHYLINDOL 4-OLDIHYDROGEN PHOSPHATE	NATURAL (FROM PSILOCYBE FUNGUS ON A TYPE OF MUSHROOM)	HALLUCINOGEN	NONE	SWALLOWED	TABLET CAPSULE	SAME AS LSD	?	NO	POSSIBLE	NOT YET DETERMINED
ALCOHOL	BOOZE, JUICE SAUCE	ETHANOL ETHYL ALCOHOL	NATURAL (FROM GRAPES, GRAINS)	CNS DEPRESSANT	SOLVENT ANTISEPTIC, SEDATIVE	SWALLOWED, OR APPLIED TOPICALLY	LIQUID	SENSE ALTERATION, ANXIETY REDUCTION, SOCIABILITY	TOXIC PSYCHOSIS, ADDICTION, NEUROLOGIC DAMAGE	YES	YES	YES
TOBACCO	FAG, COFFIN NAIL	NICOTINA TABACUM	NATURAL	CNS TOXIN (NICOTINE)	EMETIC (NICOTINE)	SMOKED, SNIFFED CHEWED	SNUFF, PIPE, CUT PARTICLES CIGARETTES	CALMNESS, SOCIABILITY	LOSS OF APPETITE, ADDICTION, HABITUATION	POSSIBLE	YES	YES
GLUE		AROMATIC HYDRO-CARBONS	SYNTHETIC	CNS DEPRESSANT	NONE	INHALED	PLASTIC CEMENT	INTOXICATION	IMPAIRED PERCEPTION, COORDINATION, JUDGMENT	NO	YES	YES

Figure 8-28 Handy reference chart for teachers and students. (Courtesy American School Health Association and Pharmaceutical Manufacturers Association.)

hol, showing that even though the two look alike they affect substances differently. Place such items as raw liver, sugar lump, bread, and egg white in jars of alcohol; and put same kinds of items in jars of water. Note differences that occur. Live plants can also be used to show how alcohol does not contribute to growth.

14. Carry out a sociodrama in which a pupil must risk his popularity and reputation by not accepting an offer to smoke marihuana. Some pupils should accept and others decline.

15. Set up and conduct a mock trial, complete with defendant, lawyers, judge and jury. After searching the law, the pupils should be ready to justify use of a certain drug to judge and jury.

16 Create lists of telephone numbers needed fo emergencies. Take these home (primary level).

17 Look up the story of penicillin (Alexander Fleming). Do the same for quinine and malaria, and isoniazid and tuberculosis.

18. Role play the troubles an intoxicated person might have climbing the back steps and unlocking a door. Discuss what is incapacitating him.

19. Invite into class an athletic coach to talk about the relationship of smoking to athletic performance.

20. Visit the back of the drugstore and watch a registered pharmacist prepare a prescription. Note dangers and penalties of misusing potentially harmful substances.

21. Suggest several ways in which to face disappointments, stress, and unhappiness.

22. Present a panel of students with a moderator to discuss feelings and actions—when lonely, lose a contest, are unhappy, angry, afraid, jealous.

23. Discover and write out the meaning of a peer group. How does it bind a person? How does it relate to smoking? How do *you* feel about peer pressure?

24. Make up a display of such items as model airplane glue, paint thinner, and carbon tetrachloride. Permit everyone to take a light sniff and read the labels. Then discuss "glue-sniffing" and its rela-

tionship to death and permanent brain damage.

12. CONSUMER HEALTH

Behavioral Objectives

(Intermediate Level)

Describes the individual role of the consumer of healthful goods and materials.

Explains how truths must be separated from half truths in order to judge whether or not to purchase a health product.

Investigates the extent that superstitions and gullibility frequently prevent people from acting wisely in the selection and use of health products.

Relates how such items as clothing, food, and medical service vary in kind and quality and that the informed consumer, by his knowledge and actions, helps keep undesirable and unscientific products out of circulation.

Demonstrates how a careful consumer eventually helps to make a careful producer or manufacturer.

Appraises advertised health products: dentifrices, sports equipment, pain killers, cold tablets, cosmetics, vitamin pills, etc.

Supports the view that there is danger in self-treatment when ill—need to seek top professional care.

Comments

We cannot shield our children from the marketplace. We must prepare them for it. . . . Producers of toys, breakfast cereals, and other foods appeal to children . . . to pressure their parents into buying the advertiser's product . . . no consumer is fully protected unless he can recognize a charlatan when he sees one, unless he can discern the difference between puffery and fact in an advertisement, and unless he can use the information he is given to make the best buying decision for his needs.

Virginia Knauer,
Presidential Assistant for
Consumer Affairs

If this is the age of the consumer, as Virginia Knauer says it is, then the health teacher has a big job indeed. There is much to cover, from prescription drugs and medicines to foods and cosmetics. Almost every product has a health relationship. Over two million people are burned each year, many of them from flammable fabrics not satisfactorily regulated by government and industry. Worthless health products and remedies cost a billion dollars a year. A quarter of a billion dollars is spent by arthritic sufferers alone; and some fifty million dollars a year is taken from cancer patients and their families. So called "consumer steal" takes place daily because of misconceptions, misinformation and outright superstitions pertaining to diet, weight control programs, toothpaste hair preparations, deodorants, germ killers, etc. Perhaps it is not strange that in a six billion dollar a year cosmetic industry some 60,000 women develop reactions to cosmetics serious enough to consult skin specialists, and many more treat themselves.

In a society accustomed to seeking pleasure and relief through the use of drugs and other related products, it appears normal to be cajoled into popping a couple of pills into the mouth to get "fast, fast relief," "freedom," "pleasure," "sleep," "comfort," "relaxation," and "regularity." Through uncounted advertisements, children and adults are persuaded and conditioned not to accept any minor discomfort. And speed appears to be highly desirable as *Bufferin* is advertised to be "twice as fast as aspirin," *Anacin* goes to work "in 22 seconds after entering your bloodstream," and *Excedrin* would seem to rise above them all by being "an antidepressant to help restore your spirits."[54]

One frequently realizes that people hear only what other people want them to hear. Thus "educated" citizens are often ignorant. For example, in several communities in which the majority of the

voters are college graduates, the issue of fluoridation of the drinking water was voted down, yet fluoridation is by far the most effective means known to man for reducing tooth decay to a significant extent.

Misconceptions abound everywhere, particularly among children and youth. Here are just a few that fifth and sixth grade schoolchildren subscribe to:

Persons who have pimples usually have bad blood.

Taking vitamin pills will guarantee good health.

Hot food is more nutritious than cold food.

Most fat people are very healthy.

Tooth powders or pastes will always cure a person's bad breath.

It is all right to use sleeping pills without a doctor s advice.

Certain medicines will prevent the common cold.

The best doctors always promise to make people healthy

Cutting a person's hair makes it grow faster.

If you have any disease you'll always feel some pain.

A prospective mother can make the child more musical if she listens to good music.

According to the Federal Food and Drug Administration's bureau of enforcement, the most effective tool in combating quacks is publicity, particularly exposure in courts. Collecting newspaper clippings exposing quacks and false health claims is a practical project for consumer health classes. The class should know that any time the Federal government is aware that the consumer is being misled into believing that certain foods and products will prevent a disease that is difficult to treat, they will take regulatory action

Government regulations, a conscience in the manufacturing world, and such things as better labelling practices all help the consumer, but ultimately the most effective means of creating a more enlightened consumer is an education

[54]See especially the illuminating report, "Aspirin and Its Competitors," *Consumer Reports*, August 1972, p. 540.

dealing with scientific inquiry, discovery, and a sophisticated concern for what is being purchased.

At what age do children become aware of the truths and half-truths in the world in which they live? When is the "teachable moment" for discussing the validity of a multitude of health claims—claims made by the wise and honest as well as the charlatans and quacks? How can we help the student learn that consumer health means to buy wisely from the standpoint of health and safety? This kind of education begins with observant eyes and ears, awakening minds, and the simple but sharp questions of nine and ten year olds. They read the ads, hear the radio and television commercials, and wonder whether one health product really *is* better than another. Moreover, those students who *inquire* during the early years are more apt to be the ones demanding evidence in their later school years. Such inquiry can be nurtured through the presentation of relevant learning experiences. In the final analysis, relevance is one's personal answer to the question "So what?".

According to the American Medical Association, by the time a pupil graduates from the elementary school he should be able to defend at least five concepts:[55]

1. Self-medication should be avoided.
2. It is important to seek sound advice concerning health care.
3. There are no special health foods.
4. There are many kinds of "doctors" who will treat us when we are ill, but some who claim to be able to treat us are not qualified or adequately prepared.
5. Diagnosis of health problems should be made by a medically trained physician and medication should be taken under the direction of a physician.

Concepts and activities go together. For planning purposes, here are a few

possibilities for the upper elementary grades:

1. *Consumers influence the price and quality of health products.*

Both tooth powder and toothpaste used to be widely available Consumers preferred pastes, so many tooth powders disappeared from the market. Consult newspapers for comparative prices of dentifrices. Do the same for soaps and mouthwashes.

2. *Consumers face individual health problems. Choosing a physician and having an examination are two examples.*

Have the school nurse discuss physical examinations and the danger of self-treatment. Discuss the qualifications of a physician.

3. *Superstitions may influence what a person buys and does.*

Build a list of health superstitions and misconceptions. Examples: "An apple a day keeps the doctor away." "Carry a horse chestnut to ward off rheumatism."

4. *Not all doctors are physicians.*

Formulate a list of the various kinds of doctors and indicate the specialty of each.

5. *Changes in medicine are happening so rapidly that it is impossible for most people to be aware of the latest happenings.*

Ask each student to name a remarkable medical breakthrough in the past several years.

6. *Prescription medicines are those used safely and effectively only under a physician's or dentist's supervision.*

Examine some prescription labels. Note date and directions.

7. *The main purpose of health advertising is to sell products and services.*

Discuss the meaning of the word *ethical.* What does "fairness in advertising" mean to students?

8. *Advertising labels should be correct; they must not be false or misleading.*

Examine ads and labels. Do the names of famous people influence persons to buy a product?

9. *Advertisements sometimes encourage the consumer to buy things he doesn't really need.*

---

[55] *Defenses Against Quackery:* A Resource for Teacher Concepts and a Sample Teaching Unit for the Elementary School (1–6), Dept. of Health Education, American Medical Association.

What is "emotional buying"? What is the influence of such expressions as *low calorie, less tar?*

10. *The Underwriters Laboratories (UL) examine and test devices, materials, and apparatus used by the public.*

Compile a list of electrical devices that show the UL label.

11. *The Department of Agriculture inspects and grades meats and poultry.*

Interview some butchers to discover how they aid in safeguarding meat.

12. *Quacks invent nonscientific machines to exploit the gullibility of people.*

Discuss vibrators, spot reducers to remove weight, cancer-cure machines.

The long list of "watchdog" duties carried on by such consumer protection agencies as the Food and Drug Administration, the Federal Trade Commission,

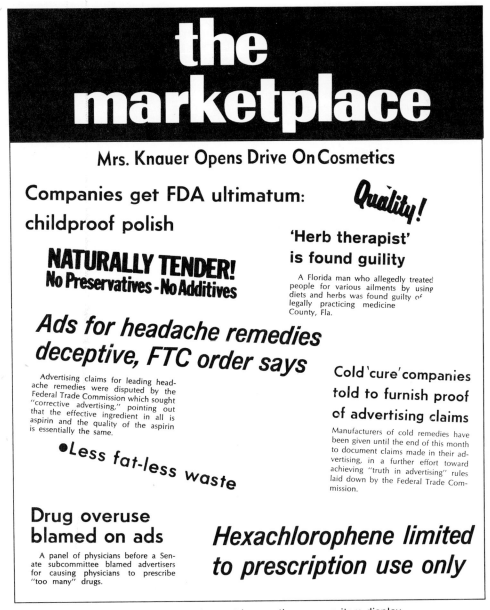

Figure 8–29 Awaken interest by creating a news item display.

and the U.S. Post Office Department can be brought to the attention of schoolchildren by obtaining excellent literature from these respective Washington agencies. Extensive lists of consumer health publications are available Every topic has been explored. For example, if questions arise relative to cosmetics, then *Cosmetics Facts for Consumers* (FDA Publication No. 26) is most appropriate

The FDA has *Consumer Protection* packets consisting of booklets, leaflets, and teaching suggestions suitable for use in health, science, and home economics classes. These packets (Packet A: *Foods;* Packet B: *Drugs and Cosmetics*) sell for $1.50 in the U.S. Government Printing Office.

A principal reference source is the *Suggested Guidelines for Consumer Education, Kindergarten through Twelfth Grades*, developed by The President's Committee on Consumer Interests, and available from the Superintendent of Documents for sixty-five cents. It contains a general section on methods of implementation including discussions of the individual teacher approach, the team approach, the interdisciplinary approach, and the systems approach. Another publication, *Consumer Education in an Age of Adaptation,* has a number of good teaching activities plus devices for identifying and evaluating students. (Consumer Information Services, Dept.

203, Public Relations, Sears, Roebuck and Company.)

Suggested Activities

1. Identify doctors who take care of special health problems such as eyes, feet, and teeth; also, medical specialists such as pediatricians, obstetricians, and psychiatrists. Why are there so many different kinds of specialists?

2. Americans spend over 30 billion dollars for medical care each year. The hospitals' share of this figure has more than doubled since 1929. Appoint class committees to find out why.

3. Give an overnight assignment requesting the class to make up a list of superstitions about health and disease Suggest that they check with their parents and others in their neighborhood so that their list will be as long as possible. Make a combined list of these findings the next day. Add to the list a number of superstitions such as the following:

Onions worn around the neck prevent disease
Aluminum cooking utensils cause cancer.
Wearing an iron ring prevents backache (rheumatism too).
Toads cause warts.
Wearing rubbers indoors will injure the eyes.

Per Person Annual Expenditures

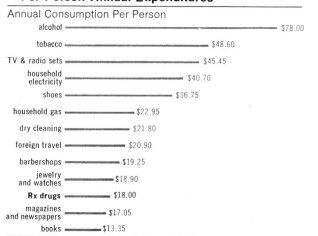

Annual Consumption Per Person

alcohol	$78.00
tobacco	$48.60
TV & radio sets	$45.45
household electricity	$40.70
shoes	$36.75
household gas	$22.95
dry cleaning	$21.80
foreign travel	$20.90
barbershops	$19.25
jewelry and watches	$18.90
Rx drugs	$18.00
magazines and newspapers	$17.05
books	$13.35

An apple a day keeps the doctor away

People were healthier in the "good old days."

When your time comes you will die, no matter how you live.

4. Collect a variety of labels from cans and bottles and advertisements from the newspapers and magazines for class discussion. Post some of them.

5. Study the bar graph on p. 270 and note the comparisons. Set up problem-solving groups to find out why. Report back to class group by group.

6. Post on the classroom bulletin board a list of community sources where reliable health information may be obtained. Follow this up with a committee visit to each of the sources. This will involve most of the class if properly organized.

7. Bring in an outside speaker to show how the consumer is being protected (a county health agent, local physician or health officer, or Food and Drug Administration official). Prepare questions ahead of time to ask the visitor.

8. At one time the Federal Trade Commission had complaints pending against the manufacturers of eight, over-the-counter analgesics: *Bayer Aspirin, Bufferin, Anacin, Arthritis Pain Formula, Excedrin, Excedrin P.M., Cope,* and *Vanquish* for false or misleading advertising. Discover why. (At least one source is *Consumer Reports* for August, 1972.)

9. Investigate health insurance. Send pupils to insurance agencies in an independent study effort. (Obtain copies of *Money Management: Your Health and Recreation Dollar*, Household Finance Corporation.)

10. Identify methods used to sell goods and services; promotion gimmicks, trading stamps, coupons. Discriminate between informational and motivational advertising. Collect leaflets and labels.

QUESTIONS FOR DISCUSSION

1. The nature of the modern school is such that an imaginative teacher may set up almost any activity for her class to engage in. To insure that only the proper activities are taught, what should the teacher use as her guide?

2. What seem to be the two or three significant differences between health emphasis in the primary grades and health emphasis in the intermediate grades?

3. How can proper progression in a health topic between grades be assured? Especially in a school where there is no supervisor or health consultant?

4. What are the several ways in which materials and teaching aids may be selected when implementing a major health topic?

5. Prepare teaching outlines for the study of health topics using suggested teaching activities other than those appearing in this chapter.

SUGGESTED ACTIVITIES

1. Examine the health curriculum materials used in a particular elementary school. *How* are they employed? *How involved* are students? Suggest examples of both good and poor teaching practices, if possible, to fairly appraise a local situation. Also, comment on the difficulty of doing a good evaluation here.

2. Carefully examine several curriculum guides pertaining to elementary school health education. (These are generally found in the college or university library with other professional education materials.) How are the specific objectives or purposes set up? Are they arranged in terms of concepts? Competencies? Outcomes? Goals? Behavioral objectives? See if you can discover the rationale behind the terms used.

3. Review the research relative to smoking education. Write a short paper setting forth some of the evidences of success and failure in the smoking education programs nationally.

4. In a sense, Consumer Health embraces all major health teaching topics. After briefly reviewing each of these topics, formulate a list of what might be called "common abuses," that is, a listing of ways in which the consumer may be put at a disadvantage through half-truth advertising and questionable products.

SELECTED REFERENCES

Bobbitt, Blanche G., and Lawrence, Trudys. "Enrichment Activities in Health Education for Intellectually Gifted Pupils, Grades One to Nine." *Journal of School Health, 36*:223–234, May 1966.

Fodor, John T., and Dalis, Gus T. *Health Instruction: Theory and Application.* Philadelphia: Lea and Febiger, 1966, Chapter 6.

Fodor, John T. "A Conceptual Approach to Curriculum Development in Venereal Disease Education." *Journal of School Health, 43*:303–308, May 1973.

Fulton, Gene B. and Fassbender, William V. *Health Education in the Elementary School.* Pacific Palisades, California: Goodyear Publishing Co., 1972.

Griffin, Mariellen. "Techniques of Relating Health Instruction to the Real World." *School Health Review, 3*:18–20, March-April 1972.

Grout, Ruth E. *Health Teaching in Schools,* 5th ed. Philadelphia: W. B. Saunders Company, 1968, Chapter 6.

Harrelson, Orvis A. "Nutrition Education Through Cooking." *Instructor, 82*:58–59, February 1973.

Irwin, Leslie, Cornacchia, Harold, and Staton, Wesley. *Health in Elementary Schools,* 2nd ed. St. Louis: C. V. Mosby Co., 1970.

Martin, Ethel A. *Roberts' Nutrition Work with Children.* Chicago: University of Chicago Press, 1972.

Oberteuffer, Delbert, Harrelson, Orvis A., and Pollack, Marion B. *School Health Education,* 5th ed. New York: Harper and Row, 1972, Chapter 2.

Ragan, William B. and Shepherd, Gene D. *Modern Elementary Curriculum.* New York: Holt, Rinehart, & Winston, Inc., 1971, Chapters 7 and 14.

Smith, Ralph Lee. *At Your Own Risk: The Case Against Chiropractic.* New York: Crowell, 1970.

Turner, C. E., Sellery, C., and Smith, Sara Loise. *School Health and Health Education,* 6th ed. St. Louis: C. V. Mosby Co., 1970.

VanTil, William. *Curriculum: Quest for Relevance.* Boston: Houghton Mifflin Co., 1971, Chapter 30.

Willgoose, Carl E. "Mental Health At An Early Age." *Instructor, 81*:58–59, October 1971.

9 METHODS AND TEACHING AIDS IN HEALTH INSTRUCTION

All too often we are giving young people cut flowers when we should be teaching them to grow their own plants. We are stuffing their heads with products of earlier innovation rather than teaching them to innovate.[1]

—John Gardner

The biggest shortcoming in teaching today is in not providing a setting for decision making. In examining the "setting" at least two assumptions have been in error much of the time. One is that if children are provided with basic information, the cognitive learnings, the resulting amount of understanding will serve them well and be realized through a change in their everyday behavior. This just isn't true for most boys and girls. It has been a simple solution to educational needs for a long while. And as H. L. Mencken once said: "There is a solution to every problem: simple, quick, and wrong."

The other problem of "setting" which limits personal commitment and decision making is socioeconomic inequality. James Colemen, after studying the ghetto areas and the dehumanized and disadvantaged families, gave construc-tive advice when he warned that it is a mistake to expect schools to work on their own. They can reinforce the values of the culture around them. But where those values are negative, teachers can do little to soften the tragic consequences. More recently, Harvard's Christopher Jencks has said essentially the same thing.[2] Also related is that the day-to-day internal environment of the school and community is highly variable, and a quality education can only be obtained if both students and teachers find the school and community a satisfactory place in which to be. Any serious discussion of teaching methods and teaching aids, therefore, must acknowledge that the school and its immediate environment have to be attractive to children and generate a response in terms of feelings and actions. John Gardner would

---

[1]Gardner, John. *Self-Renewal.* New York: Harper and Row, 1965, p. 21.

[2]Jencks, Christopher and Riesman, David. *Inequality: A Reassessment of the Effect of Family and Schooling in America.* New York: Basic Books, 1972.

ask for nothing less than these prerequisites to decision making.

THE MEANING OF METHOD

The word "method" has a number of implications for people in education. In a sense, it is the very body of educational endeavor, for it involves more than objectives and curriculum. It involves the effectiveness of the program — a program in which curriculum and method cannot be divorced.

Educational method is as much the concern of the instructor as is the mastery of the subject matter used in teaching. Familiarity with this one item makes the teacher an educationalist, rather than simply a specialist in sociology, biology, or mathematics. In fact, it is sound methodology coupled with an understanding of subject matter and children that makes the well-rounded instructor.

Historically, teaching has always been considered an art. Art and science are different and their methods contrast. Science is analytical; it breaks things up, seeks detail, and looks for causes. Art, on the other hand, is engaged in giving *meaning to experience*; it puts things together — synthesis rather than analysis. Fauré in his monumental history of art reminds us that, "Science relates fact to fact; art relates fact to life." Both science and art are regularly employed by the instructor who knows what to teach and how to teach it. The *how* is important. It is the means selected to achieve objectives.

All methods need examination because what works with one child or group may not work as well with another child or group as long as there are bona fide individual differences; "what is one man's meat is another man's poison." Sometimes formal methods operate for the welfare of the pupils; at other times informal methods seem better. There are so many specific and worthwhile objectives in elementary school health education that it is reasonable to expect a

number of methods to prove successful, depending on the local situation.

METHODOLOGY AND TEACHING AIDS

Within the limits of their capacities, children can be motivated to learn. Obviously, whatever holds and attracts attention is going to determine action; William James said as much decades ago. Whether attention is held by a particular teaching procedure, such as a warm discussion, or an aid to instruction, such as a model or filmstrip, makes little difference. Both the method and the teaching aid get at the *how* of teaching, the concern of this chapter. Therefore, in this book methods are not divorced from materials, with one chapter following the other as though the topics were somehow disconnected. Methodology — the way instructional materials are used — will be discussed later on. If the teaching aid is employed in such a way that it does what Jean Piaget would have it do — namely, help the student to become the principal agent of his own education — then it is a most effective addition to methods employed.

THE FOUNDATION OF METHOD

The chief concern of methods in education is to *involve* children in the learning process. Where such involvement is missing, the school is as Silberman well described it — a grim, joyless place where there is little pleasure in creating and little sense of self. In too many schools there is no fun and individual spontaneity is so low that few pupils ask *why* about what they are doing. Erik Erikson labelled such a condition very well when he said that ". . . the most deadly of all possible sins is the mutilation of a child's spirit." However, lest one become pessimistic and depressed, it should be pointed out that schools *can* and *are* organized to facilitate spirited learning.

Increasingly, schools are being organized to encourage students to be creative, to question, and to express their feelings. Teaching schedules have been made flexible; the staff has been differentiated and team teaching practices have been implemented so that teachers with particular strengths can be used efficiently; children are free to move about and talk quietly about what they are doing; instruction is individually prescribed; and numerous ideas are being tried in and around the classroom that were never considered in the past.

Perhaps more important than anything else, in recent years, has been the wholesome attention given to behavior modification. The consideration given to the affective and action domains has been most helpful. The goal is to help students learn and accept relevant facts and ideas which will lead to rational decisions, and help modify their behavior in line with such decisions. As Godfrey Hochbaum points out, this behavior change or modification is a process — not merely a teaching method, but something that takes place *within* the individual;[3] it is not something done to the individual. Behavior modification occurs when an individual reaches an intellectual and "gut-level" state where he is knowingly dissatisfied with his present behavior, searches for and finds a new behavior that appears to be more satisfying to him, and then, says Hochbaum, if he is able, he changes his behavior accordingly. The big teaching job is to bring pupils to the state of dissatisfaction where they are aware of their condition. This is when real education begins. It is somewhat like getting the heavy drinker to admit he has a problem. Then he can be helped. Heretofore he couldn't be reached.

SUCCESSFUL HEALTH TEACHING

Many who have taught in the elementary and middle schools for a long period of time have found that health and health-related subjects can be made very interesting. Bensley finds that effective health instruction requires four conditions:[4]

One: *Learning must be enjoyable.*
Two: *Students must become emotionally involved in the learning process.*
Three: *Students should be granted a degree of academic freedom to explore their own health needs and interests.*
Four: *The teacher needs to know his students.*

In health teaching, the method selected should concentrate more on the *why* than on the how. This will get one away from what J. B. Priestly calls "a narrow world of how-the-trick-is-done" to a thoughtful understanding of relationships. In this connection, good teaching brings at least nine variables together so that they bear on one another:

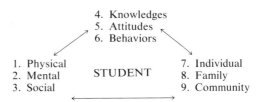

One reason certain health topics have been considered by many pupils to be dull and boring is that they have not been related to the day-to-day experiences of the class. Taught on a strictly cognitive level, the story of human blood could be dry indeed. But related to the social consequences in the larger community it can come alive. Blood is quite different when considered as part of an automobile accident — with the police department, curious onlookers, ambulance service, emergency hospital activity, and the family feelings for the victim all brought to bear on the situation.

The work of Mager in *Developing Attitudes Toward Learning* and Krathwohl and Bloom in the *Taxonomy Of Educa-*

[3]Hochbaum, Godfrey. "Behavior Modification," *School Health Review*, 2:5–10, September 1971.

[4]Bensley, Loren B. "Ideas for Successful Health Teaching," *School Health Review*, 3:37–38, May-June 1972.

tional Objectives has been most helpful in focusing attention on student experiences as a way of improving teaching methods. By getting at the development and measurement of behavioral objectives they demonstrated the need to alter methodology. In short, one cannot expect to reach the behavior/action domain without involvement to a greater or lesser degree with cognitive and affective learning. This was noted in the previous chapter in the discussion of drug education when it was pointed out that "life-style" talk and "here-now" views had to be aired and felt in the peer group setting if any behavior change was contemplated. If peer influence and a pupil's idea of status are important in the smoking program, for instance, and call for understanding and appreciation, then they are just as important in other major health areas as a prerequisite to learning and decision making.

As health teaching activities are organized and developed, it makes sense to couple expected behavior outcomes with specific methods and teaching aids. If the objective is to have third grade pupils brush their teeth in a proper and effective fashion, then the question of which method to choose arises. Talking about the subject does little good. Showing a film seldom causes more than a brief pause to think about brushing in a particular way. Even a teacher demonstration appears futile. On the other hand, a classroom toothbrushing drill with real materials is novel and practical enough to have some carry-over value —particularly if there is less drill and more fun involved. Thus, the expected outcome determines the method. The behavioral statements, of varying degrees of specificity, shown below, are used to clarify objectives, but might be achieved by employing one method rather than another.

It is easy to see that effective health teaching in any one health area may well involve several methods, particularly in a school that encourages creativity, has a flexible attitude toward instruction, and has on hand a number of teaching aids. Different children can work on different aspects of the health topic and use different methods. Variety is more than the

Behavioral Statement	**Possible Method of Achievement**
1. Administer artificial respiration in an effective manner	Slow motion loop film review coupled with paired teams for practice
2. Read an oral thermometer correctly to the nearest tenth of a degree	Experiment or demonstration
3. Run a fifty yard dash in eight seconds	Experiment or discovery approach
4. Analyze the labels from several cereal packages in terms of nutritive value	Small group investigation
5. Illustrate several ways in which sources of drinking water become polluted	Field trip
6. Demonstrate safety on the playground	Role playing or group demonstration
7. Construct a diagram illustrating the effect of tobacco smoke, tar and nicotine on human lung tissue	Contract or problem-solving
8. Prepare twenty true-false questions relative to the use of prescription drugs	Library or independent study

spice of life. It is also the spice of teaching and learning. Variety bolsters interest and acts as a motivating technique. When all health topics are taught in a similar manner, it is difficult to maintain the interest of the class, for the element of surprise and anticipation is missing. Even a little bit of that which one pupil loves the most continues to remain high in his esteem when it is used sparingly.

Experimentation in method is to be encouraged. Varying the health teaching method is an effective way of determining how the class responds to a number of sound approaches. From this kind of experimentation successful methods are developed for the teaching of a particular health topic. One can begin to answer specific questions such as, How best to teach alcohol and narcotics? Will a white rat experiment actually put over the true meaning of vitamins? Shall I plan a demonstration? What can my pupils discover?

Conscientious teachers are generally interested in the improved method. It is sometimes believed — and always hoped for — that the discovery of a new and better method automatically results in a sudden rush to accept it. The history of education, which is not at all subtle, points out that this is far from being true. Once a new method is discovered and described, the most difficult job, that of gaining acceptance, is still undone.

The lack of immediate acceptance of a desirable method has its basis in an element of human inertia or resistance to change. People fail to appreciate that some change is inevitable. Also, some methods are more difficult to use than others. Arranging a discovery experience is frequently more time-consuming than preparing a lecture.

The versatile teacher who has several ways of approaching health topics does more than successfully teach the topic; she actually promotes a mentally hygienic situation in the classroom, for children appreciate something different, and they tend to show more real enthusiasm and genuine happiness when their teacher is flexible.

EXAMPLE AS METHOD

In addition to the specific methods employed by the teacher, the very example set by her is in itself an educational method.

I

I'd rather see a sermon
  Than hear one any day;
I'd rather one should walk with me
  Than merely show the way.
The eye's a better pupil,
  And more willing than the ear;
Fine counsel is confusing,
  But example's always clear.

II

I soon can learn to do it,
  If you'll let me see it done;
I can see your hands in action,
  But your tongue too fast may run.
And the lectures you deliver
  May be very fine and true,
But I'd rather get my lesson
  By observing what you do.
For I may misunderstand you
  And the high advice you give,
But there's no misunderstanding
  How you act and how you live!

—Anonymous

We who work with youth do not need superagencies and complicated programs; we need a re-emphasis of the simple truth that the kind of people we are is infinitely more important than programs. If we give youth an example of fit living, they will want to be fit themselves. Here is the challenge:

He who would kindle another must himself be aglow.

—Drinkwater

GROWTH THROUGH PARTICIPATION

It is safe to say that where participation is the fullest and mere spectatorship is at a minimum, effective learning tends to be at its best. Will Durant sums this viewpoint up very nicely when he says, "The wisest of our children will not be those who merely enjoy the spectacle; it will be those who climb out of the pit upon the stage and lose themselves in action." To lose oneself in action has powerful implications. It means that the activity is total and the individual is completely wrapped up in the subject. It is a rare state, indeed, and one that most teachers hope to witness more often in their teaching careers. It is not a strange state because one cannot set a limit to which children will go to pursue the things they are truly interested in. Methods that promote experiences which fire the curiosity of youth are priceless. For curiosity, says Alexis Carrel, "is a necessity of nature, a blind impulse that obeys no rule."

CONCEPTS AND DISCOVERY

Good teaching invariably concerns itself with conceptual understanding, for concepts are the ingredients for thinking. In fact, thinking actually is the process of organizing and storing concepts. In this respect, Bruner has pointed out the importance of establishing these "structures" of knowledge so that the student can find *meaningful relationships* among comprehensive ideas, rather than having to struggle with countless facts in isolation.

Simply stated, therefore, a concept is an understanding of something—a way of making meaning of things. Woodruff speaks in part of the concept activity as starting with perception, moving to register an experience, forming concepts through thinking, making a decision (choosing), and drawing conclusions.[5] Significantly, it is the *experience* itself which seems to count as the greatest single factor in conceptual learning, far outweighing mental age or vocabulary strength.

It is at this very point that the discovery idea becomes germane. Concepts are more easily formed when the student's learning is a product of his own curiosity

and thinking and of his manipulation of basic facts. What he alone discovers means something.

Brecht, the playwright, substantiates this method in *Galileo*. In the opening scene he shows the great Italian scientist, Galileo Galilei, in the early 1600's teaching a young boy the particulars of the movement of the earth about the sun. As he initiates the lesson there is no lecturing, no explanation; instead, Galileo asks the lad to examine his device for showing the way the planets move about the sun. "What do you see?" says the great man. "Count the bands. How many are there?" When doubting Thomases and scientists came to visit him, he taught the same way. When each would gaze into the crude telescope, Galileo would ask, "What do you see? Describe to me what you see." This not only awakened interest, but it tied the observer securely to the topic because his own *trusted senses* were involved. What he saw was real to him; it was not something someone described to him in mere words and phrases. It became a part of him and was not lightly considered and soon forgotten.

It is exactly this kind of teaching methodology that is sought by Bruner when he speaks of organizing the perceptual field around the person as center. Moreover, says Bruner, "The importance of early experience is only dimly sensed today. The evidence from animal studies indicates that virtually irreversible deficits can be produced in mammals by depriving them of opportunities that challenge their nascent capacities."[6]

VALUE CLARIFICATION AND HEALTH TEACHING

Believing that lasting decisions can be achieved when individuals are aware of their values, Raths, Harmin and Simon set out to make the study of human val-

[5]Woodruff, Asahel D. "The Use of Concepts in Teaching and Learning," *Journal of Teacher Education*, March 1964, pp. 81–97.

[6]Bruner, Jerome S. "Education As Social Invention," *Saturday Review*, February 19, 1966, p. 70.

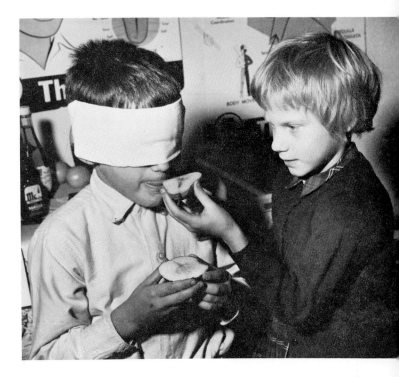

Figure 9–1 The discovery method leads to concept formation. (Courtesy Mrs. R. G. Holmes, Greenacres School, Scarsdale, N.Y.)

ues a practical activity, and one that would advance educational methodology.[7] They considered the several ways in which values can be transmitted and came to the conclusion that thoughts and accomplishments must somehow be linked together.

In the clarifying approach to values it is acknowledged that the values held by an individual at any time are relative, personal and situational. Also, there is no attempt to transmit the "right" values, but to assist a student in the clarification of his own values so that he can adjust to his world, and play an intelligent role in influencing it.

In addition to teaching in such a way that the student will discover values

there is the task of helping him learn skills to enable him to continue the clarifying value approach throughout his life — values that can be applied personally and socially. The methodology for this approach to learning involves working with children to sensitize them to value issues, to give them experiences in thinking critically, to share perceptions with others, to learn cooperative problem-solving skills, and to help them learn to apply value skills in their own lives.

The several broad value skills that can be advanced through classroom techniques are:[8]

Choosing
1. Seeking alternatives when faced with a choice
2. Looking ahead to probable consequences before choosing
3. Making choices on one's own, without depending on others

[7]Raths, Louis E., Harmin, Merrill, and Simon, Sidney B. *Values and Teaching: Working with Values in the Classroom.* Columbus, Ohio: Charles E. Merrill Publishing Co., 1966. See also the later work by Raths, *Teaching for Learning.* Columbus, Ohio: Charles E. Merrill Publishing Co., 1969. Also, see the chapter on values by Harmin and Simon in Dwight W. Allen and Eli Seifman (Eds.). *The Teacher's Handbook*, Glenview, Illinois: Scott, Foresman and Co., 1971.

[8]Raths, Louis E. *Teaching for Learning.* Columbus, Ohio: Charles E. Merrill Publishing Co., 1966.

Prizing

4. Being aware of one's own preferences and valuations
5. Being willing to affirm one's choices and preferences publicly

Acting

6. Acting in ways that are consistent with choices and preferences
7. Acting in those ways repeatedly with a pattern to one's life

Note that these seven skills are *progressive*. Activity begins with appraising the situation and noting alternatives. From this develops an affirmation of choice. The decision has been made, and from this evolves the behavior change—a change that one is committed to and makes room for in his style of living.

Sometime ago Albert Einstein characterized this age as "a perfection of means and a confusion of goals." This might well apply to many children who are not at all clear about what their lives are for. Many have never explored alternatives to any degree. Thus children are seen at times in many expressions of weakness—apathetic, flighty, inconsistent, or uncertain—or as drifters, overconformers, overdissenters, or role players. One thing uniting them all is that they have not found themselves. To expect them to enter the game of living and find health practices vital is a great deal to expect. But there is hope if the teacher can present alternative health situations and encourage children to make choices, and to make them freely. This is where the valuing process begins.

Arriving at values through traditional means is not without useful effect. Thus the employment of logical arguments, persuasion, setting an example, establishing regulations and appealing to conscience are all useful approaches. Where value clarifying differs is in the *method of responding to things a student says or does*. If, for example, in a lesson on vision, a fifth grade boy were to say, "I'm getting some eyeglasses this weekend," how might a teacher respond? Possibly,

"Isn't that wonderful," or "I hope you'll like them."

From these responses it is not likely that there will be very much clarifying thought by the student. If the teacher had responded by saying, "Getting some glasses are you? Do you think you'll like them?" Opportunity for a clarifying response is now possible. The student might say, "No, now that you ask, I'm not too happy about wearing glasses. I know a boy who has to wear them and some kids laugh at him." If there is time to pursue this issue further more clarification should occur, and it is likely the student will develop an alternative feeling about wearing glasses—particularly if the total discussion has been open, non-threatening, and avoids moralizing. In short, teaching health in a way that relates to student feelings, attitudes, aspirations, beliefs, and worries is a method with potential for reaching every child. Questions, of course, have to be phrased in keeping with the Raths-Harmin-Simon seven essential and progressive value skills. For example, in advancing the values of non-smoking in an intermediate level class where several children have tried smoking, questions might develop. See chart at top of opposite page.

Since it is frequently difficult in the large classes to work efficiently with individuals, Raths, Harmin, and Simon suggest that the teacher prepare a *value sheet* to be used with groups. This may consist of a provocative statement followed by a number of questions, and duplicated on a sheet of paper so that all classmembers have a copy. In this fashion a particular health issue may be raised that has value implications for the students. Following a brief period of thinking about the statement, the students may enter into discussion, or each may prepare answers to the questions. The value sheets can have statements that are controversial, dealing with such topics as the legalization of marihuana, lowering the drinking age, the use of shoulder straps as well as seat belts, etc. Or, they can be simple and deal with four or five questions such as shown on opposite page in the area of mental health:

1. Choosing freely
   a. Do your parents know that you have tried smoking?
   b. Where did you first get the idea that smoking might be fun?
   c. Do your friends feel the way you do?
2. Choosing from alternatives
   a. Was there more than one reason for starting to smoke?
   b. Did anyone help you with your decision?
   c. Did you consider not trying a cigarette? What went into your final decision?
3. Choosing thoughtfully and reflectively
   a. Have you thought about the Surgeon General's Report on the consequences of smoking cigarettes? Does it bother you that people who smoke have more heart and lung difficulties?
   b. Can you explain how you might grow up smoking more than you do now and not suffer any illness from smoking?
   c. Where will your choice to smoke take you? Do you have some feelings about having made this choice?
4. Prizing and Cherishing
   a. Would your life be different *without* tobacco? Would it be different *with it*?
   b. Are you glad you smoke? Do you feel bad about it sometimes?

Do you really prize cigarettes?
   c. Would you want your good friends or your younger brother or sister to start to smoke?
5. Affirming
   a. Would you be willing to give a short talk to a class of third grade children about the hazards of tobacco smoking?
   b. How do you think you can go about telling others that smoking leads to all kinds of health difficulties?
6. Acting upon choices
   a. What will you do first to help others not to start smoking?
   b. What will some of your friends say if you try to get others to give up cigarettes? Have you thought about this? Have you done much reading on this topic?
   c. Are you making plans to meet with younger children who might take up cigarettes for fun or experimentation?
7. Repeating
   a. What have you done so far to help others? How often?
   b. Have you plans for getting some of your good pals involved in helping you with younger children in your neighborhood?
   c. Are you glad you gave up smoking and are helping others to do the same? Would you do it again?

Value Sheet For Mental Health

Fair Play

1. Does fair play mean anything to you? Explain.
2. When you play a game with your friends what is it that you do that is an indication of fair play?
3. Just what is sportsmanship? How would you describe it?
4. Is sportsmanship necessary in games and sports? What have you read or heard about justice, equal-

ity and fair play? Is there fair play in the world of business? In sports?
5. How do you feel when you are fair with people? Are people who treat others fairly in a good state of mental health?
6. Do you plan to make any changes in your manner of working with people? If not, write "no changes."

Although there are numerous ways of provoking a discussion of health values, Simon likes the method of getting at value clarification through *weekly reaction sheets*. Each week for four or five weeks the student is confronted with a series of questions for which he must write out answers. Basically the sheets ask the point blank question: did you act on any of your values this week? What did you do? Looking at how people live their lives in a systematic, non-moralizing fashion works to bring health issues to the forefront. Simon asks soul-searching questions.[9] They can be applied to any intermediate and middle school health topic. Note how they progress to the action level:

1. What was the highpoint of your week?

2. With whom were you in emphatic disagreement or agreement this week?

3. Do you have any gripes about your educational program?

4. Did you work on any plans this week for some future adventure you are planning to have?

5. In what way could the week have been better?

6. Did you make any changes in your life this week?

7. What did you procrastinate about? Do you know?

8. Did you *act* on any of your values this week?

Answers to these questions serve to focus both student and teacher attention on value indicators such as purposes, aspirations, attitudes, interests, feelings, beliefs, problems and obstacles.

IMPROVED HEALTH EDUCATION METHODS

The health-educated person is one who translates the understandings, attitudes, and skills learned in the classroom into his daily life. He is more than health-

informed, chiefly because the teaching methods employed by his teachers encouraged him to practice desirable health behavior through many first-hand experiences. Method has made the difference, and method continues to make a difference when some of the following points are kept in mind:

1. *Present day concepts of method are far removed from the days of the teacher-dominated classroom.* The emphasis upon the teaching of health facts and memorization of body parts has given way to an emphasis upon understandings which will improve living. Says Allan Cohen, a clinical psychologist from the University of California, "Treat kids as humans in discussion groups." Present objective evidence, and not just from textbooks. Focus on the person. Discuss social responsibility for youth by youth. Moreover, teach children to accept themselves for what they are, and for what they can be. They need high expectations from others which will inspire them to be the best they can be. Said Goethe:

> If you treat an individual as he is, he will remain as he is, but if you treat him as if he were what he ought to be and could be, he will become what he ought to be and could be.

2. *Cooperative planning of the health lesson is time-consuming, but it is well worth the effort.* Even in the kindergarten the children can and should begin to plan some of their activities. Cooperative planning for projects, units of work, parties, trips, and other classroom activities helps develop a sense of social responsibility, for children are concerned with the success of those activities which they themselves have planned. Such activities tend to create a favorable state of mental health and very often promote high morale and class spirit.

3. *Health instruction lends itself most favorably to creative activity on the part of elementary education pupils.* Learning has to be personal if it is to be used. When a pupil feels intimately involved in the learning situation, he will begin to

---

[9]Simon, Sidney B. "Promoting the Search for Values," *School Health Review*, 2:21–25, February 1971.

want to use the ideas that are there for him. In this respect, there is hardly anything more personal than one's creative activity, but to be creative requires a definite setting, an atmosphere within the classroom conducive to freedom of expression. Practically all courses of study that border on some form of science present a number of opportunities for creativity. Health is no exception. Children need to be creative, but some teachers never quite see it because they cannot subordinate their adult needs or desires to those of the child.[10]

Children are creative in different degrees in different media. They may paint, draw, engage in dramatic play, express themselves through pantomime or impersonation or with puppets or other dramatic forms, may develop rhythms or dances, write music to be sung or played, or make a simple musical instrument, model with clay, weave, cook, sew, build with blocks, and write stories or poems. These and many other related forms of expression are natural to children. A number of these experiences, when carried on during health instruction, may be drawn together in such a way as to supplement each other and enrich the whole school program.

4. *Health is taught accurately and from a positive viewpoint.* Well-being is emphasized rather than ill health. Health is associated with happy people and more productive living.

Good health instruction teaches children how to evaluate health information and obtain reputable advice. Self-diagnosis and self-medication are discouraged.

5. *Stress immediate health goals rather than long-term ones.* One should say, for instance, "Our teeth will be white and beautiful when we brush them," instead of "if you brush your teeth you won't get cavities."

6. *In teaching health, certain learning practices and experiences are to be avoided.* Not only are some activities

ineffective, but they may be actually harmful. Avoid such things as the following:

Awarding artificial prizes for good habits of attendance in school, or promoting "healthiest child" contests.

Scheduling health education on rainy days as a substitute for physical activity, thereby punishing the pupils because it rained.

Making children overly health conscious. There are already too many neurotic adults filled with fears and worries about their health.

Using one pupil in the class as an example of a defect.

Over-using parodies or nursery rhymes and songs.

Preaching good health and promising a long life. It is better to practice healthful living oneself and be the example of the moment.

7. *In health teaching, the wise teacher uses the classroom only as a useful adjunct or tool in learning.* Simply stated, the classroom has its limitations. It might at times be referred to as an educational roadblock, because it often places a barrier between student and teacher and frequently removes the world of books, ideas, and words from the real world. Fortunately, in many places, classrooms have changed. Freedom to learn is reflected in flexibility of various kinds of "furniture." Differentiated staffing benefits children by the variety of adults with whom they come in contact. And the library common where children relax and read in attractive surroundings is seen more often.

Most children live in communities large enough to provide an excellent laboratory setting in which to seek the solutions to problems initiated in the classroom. The manner in which one seeks the solution is the meat of the experience. Cantril says that the very process of seeking the solution may be more satisfying than the end goal achieved.[11] He is referring here to the

[10]Lowenfield, Viktor. *Creative and Mental Growth.* New York: The Macmillan Co., 1956, p. 9.

[11]Cantril, Hadley. *The Why of Man's Experience.* New York: The Macmillan Co., 1950, p. 202.

value placed on the process of seeking and striving, the satisfactions derived from trying to determine direction or achieve a solution. It is what children mean when they exclaim, "Golly, that was fun!" or "I certainly enjoyed that game," and secretly regret that the game is over, no matter who won.

8. *Instruction in anatomy and physiology as a means of health education has its limitations.* The emphasis is controlled, for there is a tendency for pupils who have been taught with a maximum stress on anatomy and physiology to have less of an understanding of the basic health concepts than pupils taught with a minimum emphasis on these two helping sciences. This is not to say that one should omit reference to body structure and function. It is just a word of caution to those teachers who may find themselves teaching the names of bones and organs, and other similar facts and figures, without proper concern for the use of such knowledge by the students. Several pupil-interest surveys have revealed that some of the health studies of body functions have been "dry" indeed. And one of the dryest is the lesson on the circulation of the blood. With a little preplanning by teachers and pupils, such a topic may be taught in a way to satisfy the inherent curiosity of most of the class.

9. *Health facts brought out in the various methods of teaching are related to life situations.* This is a rewording of the old statement that knowledge is power, but it is not necessarily so without understanding. Facts are facts, and they may be learned as such, but attitudes and habits do not change unless teaching methods provide for changes. Edna St. Vincent Millay wrote a poem, *Huntsman, What Quarry?* It clearly expresses the need for something more than facts.

> Upon this gifted age, in its dark hours, rains from the sky a meteoric shower of facts . . . . they lie unquestioned, uncombined. Wisdom enough to leech us of our ill is daily spun, but there exists no loom to weave it into fabric.

10. *Materials strengthen methods.* Teaching aids exist to facilitate the method. Because of them the method should be more meaningful. In the large 15″ × 20″ study print (Figure 9–2) the teacher employs this display aid to focus on germs. Cleaning tools are brought to class and demonstrated. A "mess" is made in one part of the classroom. Volunteers clean it up. Then drawings are shown of germs, rats, flies, and other things that thrive on dirt. The concept that germs live in dirt is put accross.

TEACHING PRACTICES APPLIED TO HEALTH EDUCATION

In their book, *No G.O.D.s In The Classroom*, Mallan and Hersh talk at length about teaching, and point out that there is no one way, magical or otherwise, to make it easy. They go on to define teaching as doing — planning, selecting, evaluating, communicating, adapting. Beyond this, say the authors, teaching is part of the decision making process as one appraises the influences from the teaching act. Moreover, ". . . it is a 'systems' approach deliberately designed to change human behavior. The teacher designs the 'system' and administers all the interacting 'subsystems' or parts. (It is perhaps the most complex undertaking known to man.)"[12] This is particularly so in the health teaching area as one responds to the answers from three questions:

1. What can students learn largely by themselves?

2. What can students learn from explanation largely by others?

3. What learning requires personal interaction among students and teacher?

The clever teacher may be able to apply almost any teaching method to health instruction. The following paragraphs explain the more common teaching techniques or practices with some

---

[12]Mallan, John T., and Hersh, Richard. *No G.O.D.s In The Classroom,* Philadelphia: W. B. Saunders Company, 1972, p. 21.

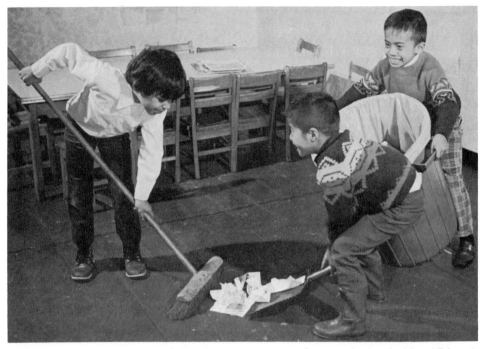

Figure 9–2 Good teaching promotes involvement with fun. (Courtesy Society for Visual Education, Inc. Print SP 178 from picture-story print set.)

comments relative to suitability for health teaching.

Lecture. Despite the admonitions of some people, there is little cause to condemn the lecture method. Properly applied in the grades, it can be used to bring basic health facts to the pupils, a necessary foundation for more work to follow. It need not be dry, authoritative, uninteresting, and unstimulating—criticisms sometimes launched by students.

With the short span of interest evidenced at the elementary level, the lecture by the teacher should probably be

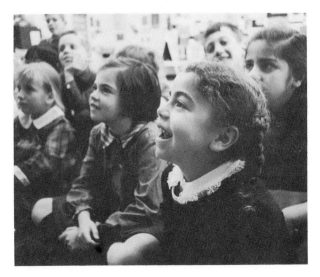

Figure 9–3 When interest is high the method is sound. (Courtesy National Education Association and Joe DiDio.)

given in the form of a chat or story, informal and yet precise. The danger is for the teacher to get too wrapped up in the topic and to overtalk to some degree. Frequent repetition can produce hostility toward the communicator, greater rigidity in existing attitudes, and forgetting or distortion of previously received information. No wonder children who have heard the toothbrushing lecture so often sometimes refuse to brush their teeth at all.

The health lecture must be arranged carefully with the teacher using appropriate instructional aids to put across significant points. Health teaching must not fall back upon mere luck and chance, magic, exhortations, and preaching. Facts relative to vitamins or the physiological effects of alcohol on the body may be given orally, but they will probably be better retained and recalled if they evolve from student explorations and questioning.

Class Discussion. A short lecture followed by preplanned discussion can be very effective in initiating a health unit. Discussing health information previously presented by the teacher gives meaning to the facts. Ideas are spread about through conversation. Conversation connotes reciprocity, not monopoly. "Discourse," says Pope, "is the sweeter banquet of the mind."

While there are many areas of the health curriculum which require careful planning and preparation, it is nevertheless possible for a planned unit to have an unplanned beginning. The following lesson was the introduction for a unit on poison prevention in the first grade class of Anne Cornetta of Woburn, Massachusetts:

"We were discussing possible ways of helping mother around the house, with the hopes of deciding a few practical tasks which would be feasible for six-year-olds to carry out. One child announced that he could wash and wax the floors because he knew just where mother kept all her cleaning supplies—in the cabinets under the sink. A few others chimed in that they could do this, too, but some could not—their mothers kept these things on a high shelf where they could not reach them. It seemed best to abandon the discussion of helping mother, since the children seemed much more concerned with the reasons why cleaning fluids etc., should be out of reach; that even though they themselves were old enough to know better, little brother or sister or a visiting baby might get into them. The high interest expressed by the children prompted the development of a unit on this subject. To maintain this interest the following home assignment was given, watch the baby to see what he does when he is handed a small object (or almost anything). The next day someone had a report—he put it in his mouth! We then went on to name and list various things we must be careful of, illustrate and cut them out for display on the bulletin board. . . ."

There are a number of techniques which may be used to make the discussion more effective:

1. An overnight assignment, which requires some study or searching for ideas at home, will provoke a number of good questions the next day in class.

2. A list of questions, raised in earlier sessions and distributed prior to the discussion, helps the student who is a poor thinker. In studying teeth in the third grade, for example, questions such as these tend to generate personal curiosity:

How many teeth do I have?
When will I have all of my permanent teeth?
Will baking soda and salt clean my teeth?

3. A cloister discussion or "buzz session" where the class is divided into small groups is often productive.

4. The "show and tell" technique promotes wide discussion, especially when "show" items are carefully chosen. (See Fig. 9–4.)

The discussion also provides a chance for pupils to share their problems in class. Some things are elicited in discussion which may be the basis for trouble in later life. Children will often talk about their fear of the dark, the problems they have with younger brothers or sisters, or the fact that someone does not like them.

Psychologist Kurt Lewin has experimented with group discussion—decision technique in influencing attitudes and behavior. In essence it allows no one to tell a group what to do; a trained person leads discussions so that decisions come from the group itself. Similarly, in health, a person may be influenced more by his

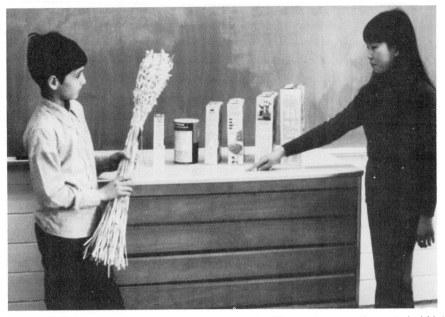

Figure 9–4 Studying cereals in class. The "show and tell" technique continues to hold interest. (Courtesy Cereal Institute, Inc.)

own decision than by one he is asked or forced to accept.

In a large regional elementary school, Sally Kaiser discovered that her sixth grade students would discuss mental health and make decisions more realistically when the following "Where Am I Going?" diagram was put on the board for all to see:

In another school, the intermediate level of health instruction was measurably enriched and improved through the addition of the *Fishbowl* Technique:

1. Divide class by having them count off in 4's.
2. Arrange 1's and 2's in one part of the room; 3's and 4's should be in another part of the room.

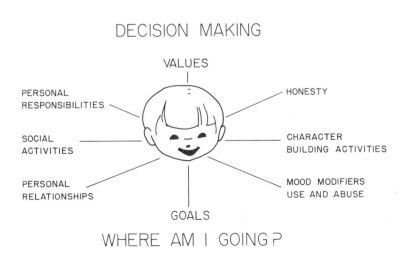

DECISION MAKING

VALUES

PERSONAL RESPONSIBILITIES

HONESTY

SOCIAL ACTIVITIES

CHARACTER BUILDING ACTIVITIES

PERSONAL RELATIONSHIPS

MOOD MODIFIERS USE AND ABUSE

GOALS

WHERE AM I GOING?

3. Assign a leader and health subject. The 1's are talkers; 2's are observers.
4. *Observers* are not permitted to participate in discussion. They watch to see that talkers are adding to group and not fooling around.
5. *Talkers* explore the subject together.
6. *Leaders* assume responsibility for getting everyone to talk—or listen.
7. After a set period the roles of talkers and observers are reversed.
8. Following the discussion, talkers and observers each tell the other "how he did" when he was the talker.
9. Class unites to have a larger discussion with all information reinforced by the teacher.

Fishbowl set up, an inner and outer group:

O = observer
X = talker

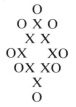

```
        O
      O X O
       X X
     OX    XO
     OX XO
        X
        O
```

10. An example of a Fishbowl discussion topic:

Your older brother (eighth grade) smokes. He brags to you how good it is and how all his friends smoke too. How does this affect you? What do you do?

Question-Answer. This is very much related to the class discussion method of teaching. Here the pupils ask questions and receive answers. The secret in using this technique is to anticipate the questions the class will ask and have vital answers ready. This may be accomplished by first initiating a certain health topic and then asking the class to prepare several questions on the topic. Once motivated, pupils will come up with a number of pertinent questions; when the pupils cannot suggest proper answers, the teacher is called upon to speak. A fifth grade class, for example, may proceed with specific questions and answers on the common cold.

Textbooks. Textbooks may be used so that they are classified as aids in the health instruction program. They may also be used as an effective method of health teaching.

Children cannot learn everything by experimenting or by first-hand experiences. Much is learned from reading textbooks, supplementary books, bulletins, magazines, and newspapers. Reading is sometimes condemned as a poor way to learn about health. It is often used so much that the health course degenerates into a course of reading about health. This criticism is leveled not against textbooks and reading as a method of learning, but against the *way* in which reading is used. It must not be a cut and dried approach where the teacher says, "Today we are going to study hearing. Open your books to page

Question	Answer
1. Do we know what causes a cold?	1. A virus is believed to be the culprit. Or, perhaps, several viruses.
2. Is cold weather a cause of colds?	2. No. Cold weather can't cause a common cold, but it may lower your resistance to one or aggravate an existing cold.
3. How about drafts and dampness? Won't they cause colds?	3. No. If there is no virus around, or if you are in a period of relative immunity, you could stand in ice water or in a draft for hours at a time without catching a cold.
4. What lowers resistance to a cold?	4. Poor nutrition and fatigue are believed to play a part. That's why it is wise to eat sensibly and get plenty of rest during the common-cold season.

36, read the first four pages, and tell me what you have read." It is this kind of procedure that makes children dislike health education.

In the small elementary school where the teacher may not have enough time to prepare all of her own study materials, the textbook can be quite helpful. It should not be a crutch on the one hand or the bible of the health class on the other. It is simply used as a common tool for all children. In the case of the example of a class about to study hearing, it would be better to engage in some exploratory activity before using the textbook. Children might be asked to bring things to class which make a sound. The next day all kinds of sounds could be demonstrated in class. A violin, a flute, a drum, a ticking watch, a whisper, all stimulate interest in how the ear actually hears sounds. Someone may say, "When I had a cold I couldn't hear very well. Why didn't the sound get into my ear?" This may be the opportune time to delve into the textbook, especially if it has a particularly good picture of the ear structure.

Textbooks, therefore, are useful as guides, and reading is an important tool in learning about health. The reading is done with a specific purpose—to solve a problem, to secure more information, to learn how to do an experiment, or to answer a question. Moreover, health stories can provide informational material which will arouse pupil interest in studying a topic. Most textbook publishers today think of the textbook as a focal point for learning, and made available with it are a number of other learning materials.

For a discussion of criteria for selecting textbooks and other printed materials see page 321.

Library. Because reading is more effective when it is done from several sources, the library method of teaching health holds considerable merit. Sources which supplement one another provide more information and present different points of view. It cannot be overstressed that the study of health should develop a scientific attitude in children. This means that pupils need to be open-minded, seek reliable sources for evidence, be curious, and know that there is a cause for everything. It means that pupils need a chance to appraise many health situations by experimenting and reading widely.

The library is well suited for note taking which can be a part of health research needed in problem-solving, independent study, and other learning practices. With the help of the librarian, properly selected reading materials are made available, and pupils find things from books that simply cannot be discovered through observing, interviewing, and experimenting.

The elementary school library plays an important role in the entire school health program. Children need to be able to use it freely as a source of books, pamphlets, magazines, recordings, films, slides, maps, globes, reference books, atlases, dictionaries, and audio-visual projectors. The attitude of the classroom teacher toward the library usually determines how functional the library method of teaching about health becomes. The cooperative efforts of the teacher and librarian in setting up a health exhibit in the library or classroom often produce considerable pupil interest.

Problem Solving. No pupil ever becomes an improved problem solver by filling in the blanks in a workbook, by looking up the definition of something, or by just living in the same room with a cage full of white rats and a set of health textbooks. Here the ancient laws of use and disuse apply. One is better able to solve problems when he has solved previous problems—problems which mean something to him.

The older approach to teaching was to get students to master subject matter by relating it to real external life, thus demonstrating its utility. It was direct teaching. Jerrold Zacharias and others put the focus on indirect teaching—which refers to the teaching of styles and ways of thinking, as against teaching the myriad of facts that such thought deals with. Now, children are encouraged to solve problems in their preferred ways, to use their best abilities, and to employ what they have already learned as tools in their problem-solving.[13]

Solving problems is not something that takes place easily. Children have to want to find answers. They have to *discover* the problem first. They have to be disturbed, even frustrated, before they have the urge to set forth in search of health information. Motivation is involved here. In one school class the children, as they approached the end of the school day, were talking about eyesight. One boy asked the teacher to tell him how many people wear eyeglasses. Someone else wondered how many schoolchildren wore them. An overnight assignment was then made; the children were charged with "counting noses" and finding out how many people wore eyeglasses in their neighborhoods. Such near-at-hand problem-solving activity did much to provoke class discussion the following day.

In a southern school the dietitian was invited to tell about her duties to a fourth grade class. She indicated that she was distressed at the amount of food being left on the children's plates following the noon-hour lunch period. After some discussion, the class agreed that this was a problem and that they would accept the challenge to solve it. They formulated a plan of attack, divided into small groups, and made an on-the-spot survey of the school lunchroom during the eating period. Upon returning to class and talking over the problem, it was decided that one way to solve the problem might be to organize a "Clean Plate Club." The dietitian decided to give it a try. She had buttons made, such as political candidates use, bearing the words CLEAN PLATE CLUB. All elementary teachers were given the number of buttons needed each day. Each day some buttons were recalled as occasions arose. Most teachers ate with their children and found it easy to observe the plate of each child. The pupils were so eager to wear the buttons that they made a real effort to eat all their food, even the food that they normally disliked. The original fourth grade problem solvers appraised the button situation and concluded, along with the dietitian, that they had successfully solved the problem. They had exercised the strength to act. This strength is what Rollo May calls "the power to do the valuing"—the courage to decide and act for oneself, which is the moving force of human growth. Kierkegaard calls it "the alarming possibility of being able." It can only come from within the person. The "too active" teacher, says Russell, is the one who is so structured that little is left to the students—it is a case of "teacher says," "teacher assigns," "teacher shows," "teacher questions," etc., and the pupil's opportunity to make choices for himself is limited.[14]

Important health problems are usually made known with the help of the teacher. She often leads the way in discovering such items as community health hazards, causes of accidents and illnesses in school, causes of school absences, difficulties in eating, and personal unhappiness.

Problems are solved when children recognize the problems, gather pertinent data, verify and interpret the data, and present conclusions. Data may be gathered by reading, looking at pictures, viewing a film, taking a trip, experimenting, listening to a transcription, asking someone who is an authority, making a survey, and discussing the way we feel about a situation. Conclusions should be made in a general way so that they represent at least one solution to the problem.

Experiment. In many ways the experimental method of teaching health is related to problem solving. It is more formal, but it is founded on the same kind of pupil interest and is successful when there is a burning curiosity to *find out* why we act as we do, or what makes us "tick."

This method is especially stimulating

[13]Torrance, E. Paul, and Myers, R. E. *Creative Learning and Teaching*, New York: Dodd, Mead & Co., Inc., 1970.

[14]Russell, William. "A Method for Accommodating the Will—a New View," *Journal of Education, 154*:15–20, December 1971.

to upper grade schoolchildren who are entering the adventuresome period where they rise quickly to almost any challenge to discover and explore. This is the period that Charles Kettering spoke of when he expressed his views on his own aspirations at an early age. He was always intrigued with the "why." He wanted to know "why" the black cow could eat green grass and give pure white milk. It drove him to experiment in chemistry and biology and became a moving force in initiating his famous career.

True conviction comes from testing and trying things out by oneself. Sometimes simple classroom or laboratory experiments involving the principles of food decay, moisture, or cleanliness carry more conviction than many of the elaborately printed materials and expensive films one may obtain on the topic. The really effective experimental method requires a thorough organization. This is just as true with second graders as it is with secondary school pupils. Some of the points to keep in mind when setting up a health experiment are as follows:

1. Keep the experiment simple. Simple homemade equipment is often more satisfactory than the more elaborate kind.

2. Perform experiments or have them performed in such a manner as to cause children to think. Do not tell the answers or have the pupils read them. Permit them to experiment and find out.

3. Plan experiments carefully and let the pupils do much of the planning. If the plan fails, the pupils have some basis for deciding why it did not work since they were the ones who made the plan.

4. Warn pupils not to make sweeping generalizations from one small experiment. Most pupil experiments do not *prove* anything. They merely help pupils answer a question or understand an idea.

5. Permit pupils to perform the experiment themselves. They should work in groups if sufficient materials are available; otherwise the experiment should be carried out where all can see it.

6. Encourage children to originate experiments in order to solve a problem. If one pupil asks the teacher what would happen if the body did not get enough calcium, with a little encouragement another pupil might suggest an animal feeding experiment (Figures 9–5, 9–6, 9–7).

7. The basic purpose for performing

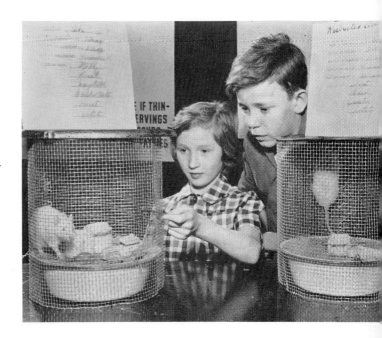

Figure 9–5 Rat feeding experiment. (Courtesy National Dairy Council.)

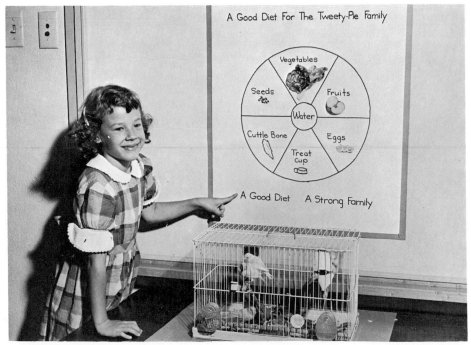

Figure 9–6 Bird feeding experiment. (Courtesy *Health Education Journal*, Los Angeles City Schools.)

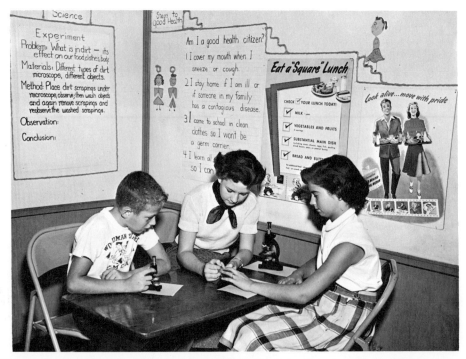

Figure 9–7 Examining fingernail dirt under the microscope. (Courtesy *Health Education Journal*, Los Angeles City Schools.)

an experiment is something much broader than just to answer the question raised. An experiment, to be worthwhile, should answer questions about things children see in the world about them. Too often this application to real-life situations is overlooked.

8. It is not necessary to have records of all experiments performed in the elementary school. The teacher may be guided by the idea, "Is there any reason for writing anything about this experiment?"

Children can experiment at every age. Even second graders can study moisture as it relates to colds and sore throats by holding a damp cloth over a heater and observing what happens. Third graders can watch mold appear on a crust of bread and draw valid conclusions without going into any further experimentation. Some of the health experiments that have proven especially valuable over the years include:

Animal feeding experiments to measure the effect of certain foods on growth.

Individual height-weight measurements.

Decay of foods under different situations.

Analysis of the action of useful molds and bacteria in the making of vinegar and cheese.

The making of a satisfactory tooth powder.

Canning of foods.

Oxygen-consuming experiments involving the lighted candle in a glass jar over water, or done with a mouse instead of a candle.

Testing for starch and sugar in various foods.

Experiment—Starch

Directions for the Pupil

Problem
a. How can we test for starch in foods?
b. Do milk and the other foods listed have starch in them?

Materials

cornstarch	test tubes
baking soda	iodine
milk (dry)	dropper
sugar	test tube holders (optional)
potato	test tube rack (optional)
hard-cooked egg	
knife	

What to do
a. Place about one-half teaspoon of cornstarch in a test tube. Fill the test tube one-half full of water. Add a drop of iodine. What happens? Make the same test with baking soda. Does the same thing happen?
b. Try each of the other foods suggested under "Materials." In all cases soften the food thoroughly with water as is suggested for the cornstarch. In the case of potato and other solid foods, it is best to use scrapings. Look for any change in color in the water or on the bits of food.
What did you observe?
What do you think this experiment shows?

Supplementary Aids for the Teacher's Use

The test
When a blue color is formed with iodine, starch is present. Cornstarch, which children know as a form of starch, gives the blue color as does potato. Soda, sugar, egg whites, and milk do not.
Testing additional foods
Other foods may be brought from home to test, such as bread, oatmeal, cornmeal, ripe banana, apple, meat. The test shows best on solid foods. Omit dark-colored foods since the test is a color test. Of the above foods, only bread and cereals give the test for starch.
Equipment
Cups might be used in place of test tubes. However, children like to use test tubes, and this test offers an easy experience in handling chemical equipment. Test tubes, test tube holders, and a test tube rack might be borrowed from children's chemistry sets.

Use a tincture of about 1 per cent iodine. The test does not show well with strong iodine. It may be made weaker with alcohol or water.
Related questions and activities
Plants make starch. Where do they store their starch? Read to find out.

Do we use many foods that contain starch in our daily meals? If so, why?

What happens if you eat more food than your body uses for energy? If you are fat, name some foods of which you might eat less.

Babies, at first, use only milk in their diets. How, then, do they get what starch supplies in your food?

If a microscope is available, observe starch grains under the microscope. Drop a solution of iodine on the slide and observe again through the microscope. (Each grain of starch takes on a shiny bluish-purple appearance.)

The following animal experiment illustrates better than almost anything else the powerful motivational force inherent in a properly conceived and implemented experimental method. Throughout the experiment there is demonstrated a sustained interest of high degree. This is the report of a sixth grade experiment conducted, written up, and presented to the author by Annette Marco Penan of Jacksonville, Florida.

A Rat Experiment in the Sixth Grade

We received two white, albino, laboratory raised mice, 28 days old, from the National Dairy Council. Both were males; one weighed approximately 48 grams, the other 50 grams. They were brought to us on a Thursday morning complete with instructions regarding their care, a pair of white workman's gloves, and a gram scale.

Thursday and Friday we discussed the habits of rats, types, and differences, diseases, control, etc. We used the encyclopedias, science books, nature books, read the Pied Piper of Hamlin and played games. We compared rat ages with human ages, and made charts. Some of the boys made age comparison charts on many different types of animals—dogs, horses, elephants, etc.

The first thing I did was to go up and down the aisles and let every child touch the rats while I held them. I did not insist on everyone touching. I then explained how to pick them up so as not to frighten or bruise them, made them all promise to wear at least one glove to protect both the rat and themselves, and opened the rats' mouths and showed the little sharp teeth. The entire time I caressed and petted the little things so that all the children could see how very gentle I was with them.

For fear of injury we all decided that possibly they had been handled too much already. After each and every child came by me and touched them again, we put them back in their box and they were not handled any more that day.

As soon as they settled down (both rats and children), we began to plan. I would have liked cages but the children made different arrangements—a bird cage and the case from a record player brought from home. (I still wonder what happened to the record player, but you never in your life saw such a fancy rat cage: the top with wire, the sides painted glass, fancy food dishes, little decorated boxes for them to sleep in, etc.) We kept the rats together until Monday when we began our experiment.

We discussed what we might be able to prove, and we decided to use good and poor breakfasts. We made rules for the care and feeding as well as the handling of the rats, agreed that the children would have to bring a note from home if they wanted to take one home to care for over the weekend, and that they would give the rats

only the diets we planned. We would schedule the weekend home visits after the notes arrived. I took them the first weekend to avoid confusion.

Friday, while their cage was being cleaned, the children were permitted to handle the rats themselves, and those poor little things visited on every one of 36 desks that day.

Both rats had the same diet until Monday at which time they were both weighed and measured; there was still approximately 2 grams difference in their weight. The children put the heavier one on the good diet; the other on the poor.

After being weighed, each rat was put in a separate labeled cage. The class suggested names which we voted upon, and the rats' charts read like this:

Name of rat—Mr. Kingsize
Weight of rat at beginning———————
Weight of rat at completion———————
Age of rat at beginning———————
Age of rat at completion———————
Date demonstration starts———————
Diet of rat: Whole grain bread or cereal, plus milk, plus fruit, plus bread and butter, plus egg

Name of rat—Mr. Regular
Weight of rat at beginning———————
Weight of rat at completion———————
Age of rat at beginning———————
Age of rat at completion———————
Date demonstration starts———————
Diet of rat: Sweet roll and coffee

The children brought in the food which we kept in containers. Milk and coffee were fresh every day from the lunch room.

Daily records were kept of their appearance, activity disposition, etc. Every Monday morning they were weighed and their weight charted on a large line graph. The children kept a small graph on graph paper in their note books.

During the weeks that followed we studied about the basic foods, had posters and charts on display, made posters and charts, wrote stories, kept a diary on the daily changes in the rats, made booklets, worked arithmetic problems comparing ages, plotted weights (gains and losses), studied weights and measures, graphs (line and bar), charts, printing. The children took care of the rats—committees to clean, others to feed, others to weigh and chart, etc.

Rat cartoons appeared, booklet covers were made, the mothers came to see the progress, and children started eating good breakfasts. Other children in the school came into the room to see the rats, so we issued a weekly bulletin on the changes appearing, the weights and dispositions.

The rats performed beautifully. Mr. King-size became tremendous, developed full of mischief. Poor little Mr. Regular developed a scaly, spotted tail, feet and ears became dry and rough, hair shaggy and dull, a definite contrast to the beautiful ermine coat of Mr. Kingsize. Mr. Regular became sulky and twice I was afraid we were going to lose him, but I cheated after the children went home and I gave him a little milk and dry oatmeal and he'd perk up a little. After four weeks the contrast was great and the children were beginning to worry. Since one of the purposes had been served, the children were delighted when I suggested not continuing for the full six weeks that we had originally decided upon.

We voted to see if we should reverse the diets or to just put Mr Regular on the same diet as Mr. Kingsize. It was unanimous that the diets *not* be reversed, so both rats then had the same diet. Within two weeks' time Mr. Regular started catching up to Mr. Kingsize and there was a sharp upsweep on the graphs. By the end of four weeks they weighed almost the same, and Mr. Regular's tail lost its scaly look, his eyes became larger and brighter, and his fur grew in thickness and became shiny. (As one of the little boys pointed out to me though, there was still a difference in their sex organs. I hadn't noticed, but there was.)

All these weeks the children had been making booklets about the experiments. We took pictures each week and then made a booklet to give to the Dairy Council containing selections from the children's booklets and pictures by the children together with the photographs.

The experiment over, and the children much more aware of the needs of a balanced diet, they became more conscious of their own growth and development. They were more alert in the mornings; only one or two ever fell asleep in class (TV late show—not lack of breakfast). Some mothers complained that they had to fix breakfast now, others were happy. One child fixed his own breakfast, but became a problem when selecting food; he insisted on buying certain items.

Any child who brought a note from home saying he could have a rat had his name put in a box. At the Christmas party we drew the names, and the rats went home with two little girls. The last week of school Mr. Regular came back to visit with us for the day. The children greeted him with great excitement—their little friend was hale and hearty. They were sorry that Mr. Kingsize had been sent to rat heaven by a neighborhood dog, but they were glad that it hadn't been Mr. Regular, who had been such a good sport and had taught them so much.

The number of health-related learnings that can be brought about through experimentation is great indeed. In one city classroom in Niagara Falls, New York, elementary level children experimented with the incubation of fertile chicken eggs and caring for the chicks through adulthood. They were active

students in the process exhibiting the following behaviors:[15]

Observed the daily development of the embryo by candling the eggs and viewing slides.

Used a stethescope to discover that no heartbeat was heard until after the third day of incubation

Saw eyes develop from tiny specks within a day's time

Made charts recording incubator temperature, stages and rate of growth, and later food consumption

Explored mitosis, fertilization and birth

Preserved specimens of growth stages from a three-day-old embryo to a nineteen-day-old chick, using formaldehyde

Discussed dominant strains after a Columbia Wyandotte rooster fertilized the eggs of Rhode Island Red hens one year

Tested chickens response to noises

Gave talks on hatching chicks to other classes of students

Explained to visiting primary grade pupils that the incubator takes the place of the mother hen

Described how chicks are able to peck their way out of shells

Investigated why chicks must be inoculated by a veterinarian to prevent respiratory ailments

Investigated differences between chickens bred for egg laying and for meat

[15]Adapted from the report of Isobel K. Hobba. "Hatching Chicks and Concepts," *Instructor*, April 1971, p. 42

Compared the baby chicks brief period of helplessness at birth with the longer period for the human baby

Identified gestation periods for several animals and noted how early they adapt to their environment

Shared fresh eggs laid by hens they had grown from incubator to maturity

Help in setting up a number of experiments for students to carry out may be obtained from several sources. Fodor and Glass, in their manual, set up numerous sixth grade experiments that tie in directly with preconceived concepts and behavioral objectives.[16] Experiments cover such topics as pulse rate, blood pressure, emphysema, bell jar activity, senses of taste and smell, mini-lung, goldfish and water demonstrations, and others. Somewhat along the same line, but to a far lesser degree of concentration, is the U.S. Public Health Service booklet, *Smoking and Health Experiments, Demonstrations and Exhibits* which is available through the U.S. Government Printing Office (20 cents). Experimentation with foods in the classroom is advanced in the booklet, *The Evaporated Milk Story*. It is available from the association, 910 Seventeenth Street, N.W., Washington, D.C. 20006. The National Dairy Council has done the same with foods, but in greater detail in their two booklets, *Let's Take Milk Apart.*

Demonstration. Children like to be entertained; they like to see things done before their eyes, especially if there is an element of the mysterious which they do not understand. The teacher who describes some phase of the body function through skillful demonstration encourages the class to want to do it themselves.

A sixth grade health class, in studying the principles of respiration, may observe a demonstration of artificial resuscitation and follow this by a practice period in which everyone gets an opportunity to "revive" and "be revived." In one primary grade the cleanliness of animals was discussed. In class the children watched a real cat clean itself with its paws. One of the pupils combed and brushed a long-haired dog. Another pupil demonstrated how elephants in South Africa saunter down to the nearest river toward sundown and drink and bathe. This was effective.

Actually, there are three kinds of demonstrations: teacher demonstrations, individual pupil demonstrations, and group demonstrations. All three require pre-planning in order to be effective. Individual and group demonstrations often promote more class interest than those performed by the teacher.

Examples of demonstrations that may be performed by class members for everyone to see are as follows:

A. *Air Pollution and Smog*
  1. The best way to see that the air is clean is to keep as much dirt as possible from getting into it.
  2. Controls have included "smog alerts" that have closed down factories and stopped motor traffic when serious pollution threatened.
  3. *Produce smog* by the condensation of water vapor on solid particles like smoke.
     a. Insert a lighted match in a gallon jug to make a small amount of smoke.
     b. Blow, with the mouth pressed firmly on the mouth of the jug, and release the compressed air quickly. A smog will form in the jug.
     c. Repeat the activity without the smoke from the match.
B. *Ecology and Clean Water*
  1. Most of the earth's surface is covered with water, and every type of water area supports living creatures, each interdependent in the life chain.
  2. Our limited water supply must be preserved and in some cases purified.

[16]Fodor, John T., and Glass, Lennia H. *Cigarette Smoking and Health—A Teacher's Guide.* Granada Hills, California: HRA Inc., 1971.

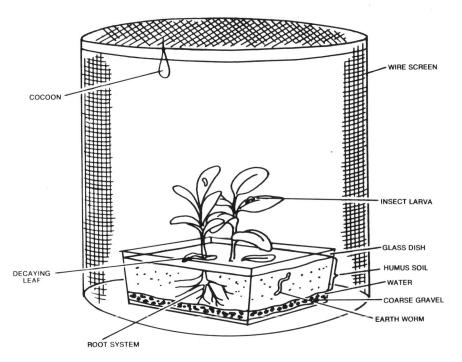

3. *Illustrate the life chain.*
   a. Put together a glass dish view of water, soil, roots, and soil animals. (Details may be obtained from *Water World Heroes Teacher's Guide*, supplied free from Nabisco, Inc., Cambridge, Massachusetts 02139.)

Glass dish allows view of water, soil, roots, and soil animals. Screen confines insect larvae and adults.
This shows the requirements for plant growth, water, nutrients (soil), support (soil), and light.

The plants are producers, insect larvae feeding on the leaves are examples of consumers. Dead leaves and insects drop to soil and decay. Soil animals, like the earthworm, help to break down this material and return it to the soil.

C. *Water Pollution*
   1. Water flows because of land elevations, from high mountains to streams, and into lakes, rivers, and swamps, and eventually to the sea.
   2. *Illustrate land erosion and water pollution.*

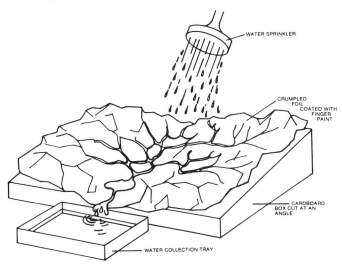

Water sprinkled on the painted foil will flow down "gullies," collect in "lakes," overflow these into larger streams or "rivers" on the way to collection tray (ocean). Paint will wash off where water flows leaving a chart of a "watershed."

 D. *Smoking Machine*
  1. The amount of tar in one or more cigarettes can be shown by a tar separating apparatus.
  2. Varying amounts of tar in different brands of cigarettes can be compared by "smoking" filtered and unfiltered cigarettes and collecting the residue.
  3. *Assemble a smoking machine.*

Equipment:
Large gallon jar with a two-hole stopper
Cigarettes
Delivery tubes (glass)
Cigarette holder
Vacuum pump
Procedure:
Assemble cigarette tar separating apparatus as shown in diagram.
Fill the gallon jar half full with water.
Place cigarette in intake and light.
Pump vacuum pump so as to draw smoke from cigarette into gallon jar and water.
Pump until cigarette is burned completely. Replace with additional cigarettes until tars can be seen in water.
Examine color of water and smell the liquid.

 E. *Breathing and Disease*
  1. Respiration depends upon lung elasticity and the power to contract.

 2. *Assemble a Bell jar* for demonstration.

Equipment:
Bell jar
Forked glass tubing
One-holed rubber stopper
Rubber sheet or membrane
Balloons similar in size and elasticity
Procedure:
Blow up one balloon and allow it to remain inflated for a day or two. When ready for demonstration deflate the balloon and note that it remains enlarged and stretched.
Insert an unused balloon into the used one and note the space or air pocket surrounding the new balloon.
Attach a new single balloon to one of the ends of the forked glass tube and the double balloon to the end of the other tube. Fasten a rubber sheet or membrane across the bottom of the bell jar to simulate the diaphragm.
Pull down on the center of the rubber membrane and observe the balloons fill with air. Note the effect of the double balloon on amount of expansion which takes place. Push the rubber membrane back up into the jar a short way to simulate exhaling. Note the difference in the deflation of the "lungs."
The action of filling and emptying the balloons may be compared to respiration; if both lungs are functioning properly they inflate and deflate properly. But if the alveoli of the lungs have been stretched too thin, as in emphysema, air pockets form in the lung tissue. The contractile power of the lungs is destroyed.

Small Group Study. Groups of children may be formed which work together to accomplish a common purpose. Small groups generally work independently on a problem in which all are

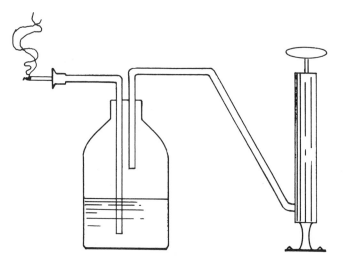

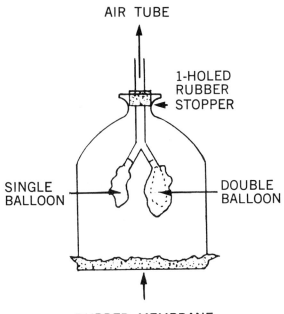

AIR TUBE

1-HOLED RUBBER STOPPER

SINGLE BALLOON

DOUBLE BALLOON

RUBBER MEMBRANE

interested. Three or four pupils may work together, or there may be as many as ten or twelve. One health topic may be initiated by the creation of four or five small groups who will consider the several aspects of the topic.

Dramatic Play and Dramatization. To the child, play is real. It is full of meaning. Through this natural expression a wealth of learning is acquired. Mimetics and action stories are common activities in the play of growing boys and girls. One sees children imitating the athlete, the mother, the physician, the nurse, and many other personalities from everyday life.

Dramatic play is unrestrained and unrehearsed. In the kindergarten and first grade the pupils generally prefer to play alone. Eight year olds will begin to play as a group. The teacher often finds that she has only to suggest a theme, and eager, creative children will start to dramatize it as they see fit. Because of the high pupil interest in dramatizations, the method is a good one to use in teaching health.

All seasons of the year lend themselves to dramatizations in the health line. At Thanksgiving time, for example, the story of the nutritious and tasty cranberry can be told. It is a colorful fruit to consider for stories.[17] So highly were cranberries prized by the Indian tribes in southeastern Massachusetts that they made a gift of them to the Pilgrims who cooked them into a sauce to serve with wild turkey and geese. It is believed that cranberries brightened the Pilgrims' first Thanksgiving feast in 1621. Moreover, the health-giving qualities of cranberries were recognized almost immediately, and in the early period of America's development, whenever vessels left New England's shores, they carried barrels of cranberries in the hold — not for trade but for the sailors to eat. Just as the English seamen prevented scurvy by eating limes, so American sailors ate cranberries, and in the Middle West, where scurvy was a scourge of the logging camps, cranberries were served regularly.

Health plays, created by the pupils from a classroom experience, are gener-

---

[17]For a useful teacher's guidebook, *Cranberries, America's Native Fruit,* write to Ocean Spray Cranberries, Inc., Hanson, Mass.

ally the most valuable. In discussing the maintenance of one's personal health through proper physical examinations, the class may decide to dramatize a visit to the school health service or the office of the family physician.

For many years puppets have been successfully used to put across certain concepts in elementary education. Puppets are fascinating to the average boy and girl; they can make statements that will be remembered longer than those made by the teacher. Interest is maintained at an even higher level when the puppets are made by the members of the class.

In using puppets for health teaching, fantasy and imagination must be separated from accurate health information.

Sometimes the dramatization takes the form of an organized play. There are a number of practical ways of making the play effective:

1. Try to get as many pupils associated with the play as possible.

2. Use a small stage or platform instead of the crowded classroom if this can be arranged. Do not worry about the absence of backdrops and props; it is part of the fun, and, after all, "the play's the thing."

3. Try an arena style performance. Here the audience surrounds the actors on all four sides, adding to the intimacy of the situation and helping even the most detached pupil to feel that he is a part of the performance.

4. Simply assign children to parts and proceed to read the play without attempting to act it out. Although less effective than the acted version, this method does promote discussion.

The Health Project. This has much in common with the problem-solving method. It calls for the study of a problem which is organized by the teacher and pupils in the form of a project or task to be accomplished. It may mean experimenting or carrying on a survey, interview, or discussion in an effort to ascertain the facts applicable to the particular health question.

The first requirement in a project is to identify and define a health problem which merits study. Goals are established as in the problem-solving method, but they appear to be broader in the project method.

Creative Activities. When children express themselves without restraint and without teacher control, they are usually being creative to some degree. Imaginative and creative children may develop and act upon a health topic in several ways — through dramatizations, mimetics, and creative play. These have already been referred to. Another way is through creative writing. Older children who enjoy writing are capable of treating a health problem rationally by writing about it. The outlet for this activity is through the school paper or possibly through the local newspaper.

Creative rhythms is another technique in teaching that is generally overlooked. Creative dance permits the child to express, communicate, and enjoy. In the process of dance-making the pupil plans, experiments, selects, and appraises a number of movements with the help of the teacher. His dance may be interpretive, such as playing the part of a "happy toothbrush," or it may be dramatic and be a part of a story danced by the whole group. Usually it is descriptive — a poem, song, or an idea is conveyed through movement — high like a cloud, low like a caterpillar, fast like a squirrel, or slow like a snowman melting in the sun.

Teachers have to be creative too. Their task is to encourage pupils to see new relationships. They need to ask the question: "Can you imagine" more often. Food, for example, can be discussed unimaginatively in terms of vitamin and mineral content, or it can be explored in terms of its color, taste, smell, and general attractiveness where it is served. Torrance and Myers stress the raising of imaginative questions that will puzzle youngsters.[18] So they ask: "Why does this?", "When was tomorrow?", and "Where is never?" After a while even slow children respond to such

---

[18]Torrance, E. Paul, and Myers, R. E. op. cit., pp. 217–219.

questions, because they start to work on them. A question is raised by the authors for which there are the usual answers and the unusual:

Where does the cold go?

usual answer: It is absorbed by objects into the air, which may later be warmed up by absorbing heat.

unusual answer: Heat expands. Cold contracts; cold contracts into a minute snowball and retreats to the top of a cumulus cloud to wait until the sun gets tired of being so gay.

Once the imagination is stimulated it is possible for creativity to emerge. Furthermore, it is fostered when each pupil is allowed to think about a health issue all by himself—with no right or wrong answer required immediately. William Glasser, who wrote *The Identity Society*, would agree; for he sees the problem of school failure in all subject matter areas very much related to pupil feelings and personal identity. This is another reason why value clarification, mentioned earlier in this chapter, is so important in health teaching.

Consider the opportunity for creative activity in a health unit where the teacher gets close enough to children to reach value indicators. This can be accomplished by choosing somewhat innovative learning activities. For example, upper elementary students studying mental health will find the coat of arms activity most rewarding.

Each student is given a mimeographed sheet with the outline of a coat of arms. It is divided into six different sections. In each of the sections the children use symbols, pictures, and numbers to correspond to: 1) Two things I do well, 2) Three things I would wish for, 3) My proudest moment, 4) A value I wouldn't budge from, 5) The saddest moment of my life, and 6) Two words I would like people to use to describe me and two words I would not like people to use to describe me. Or, there could be variations for third or fourth grade children as follows:

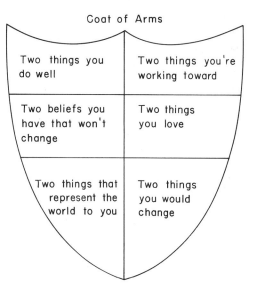

Coat of Arms

Two things you do well	Two things you're working toward
Two beliefs you have that won't change	Two things you love
Two things that represent the world to you	Two things you would change

Field Trips. The field trip, like any other experience, is planned from the earliest stage through its final evaluation and follow-up. Even before planning, the teacher attempts to find out whether the children are ready for the trip, i.e., possess the capacity and background that is needed.

In one New York school the second grade planned a trip to the zoo to observe the eating habits of animals. They asked the following questions:

"What do we want to know?"
"How shall we go?"
"How shall we prepare?"
"How shall we behave on the trip?"
"What will we need to do?"

They decided on the following:

Talk with parents, friends, neighbors, and teachers
Obtain further information from books and other aids
Trace the route on a map of the city
Use money
Estimate time and distance
Prepare a report about the trip

Although the trip was a short-term experience, it was beneficial in terms of health instruction and in relating to other subject matter fields such as art, music, mathematics, science, language arts, and social studies.

The health area is rich in opportunities for impressive field trips. Worthwhile excursions may be taken to the dentist's office, the police department, the cannery, the bakery, the dairy, the food-processing plant, and the water works. Exercise caution because it is easy to abuse rather than use this method of instruction. Trips should be made only when there is a real reason for going. The excursion is made as an integral part of the school health lesson that is in progress. Children studying the source of a water supply and how and why it is made pure may have a natural curiosity for wells, streams, types of soil, germs, purification, and the city water works. At this stage in the topic they are ready to plan a trip to the water works to see how water is purified, what filter beds look like, how chlorine and sodium fluoride are added to the water supply to protect the health of the people, and many other items that are appropriate to consider at the time. A follow-up discussion is engaged in upon returning to the classroom; this tends to anchor the experience in the minds of the pupils. Thus "going to see" can be a most enjoyable and instructive way to learn.[19]

Construction Activities. Construction activities include everything from using the hammer and saw to build a model playground, to using paste, tape, and staples to set up a novel three-sided health exhibit. There can be as much real work involved in this method of instruc-

tion as there is in the project or problem solving methods. Research, reading, discussion, and creative expression are background activities for the successful completion of an item under construction.

Pupil interests have much to do with method. In one study of Chicago schoolchildren it was discovered that about 92 per cent of the first and second graders said that they like to make or construct things. It is possible, therefore, that teachers have underestimated the value of working with the hands.[20]

Health teaching in the primary grades permits the sandbox to be used for building grocery stores, farms, irrigation ditches, and city roads and parks. Several work tables, complete with tools, encourage the construction of models of such items as teeth from clay, toothbrush holders from wood, safety patrol emblems from tin, napkin rings from leather, metal, or wood, shower room slippers from cardboard, attractive handkerchiefs from colored pieces of cloth, and many other health related items. The object, of course, is to make sure that all constructed items are directly related to the health instruction topic.

Some examples of construction activities which may be related to health teaching are:

1. Construct simple wastebaskets.

---

[19]For a practical approach to the task of arranging field trips, see Jack Zusman, "Field Trips: How to Plan and Use Them," *American Journal of Public Health*, 57:661–664, April 1967.

[20]Pupils must do things with their own hands. Because the potter works with his hands in shaping the clay, and because he is sensitive to the properties of the mix and its relationship to firing, color, and texture, he becomes changed as a person. He is as much transformed by his art as the clay is.

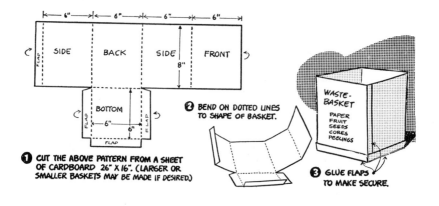

❶ CUT THE ABOVE PATTERN FROM A SHEET OF CARDBOARD 26" X 16". (LARGER OR SMALLER BASKETS MAY BE MADE IF DESIRED.)

❷ BEND ON DOTTED LINES TO SHAPE OF BASKET.

❸ GLUE FLAPS TO MAKE SECURE.

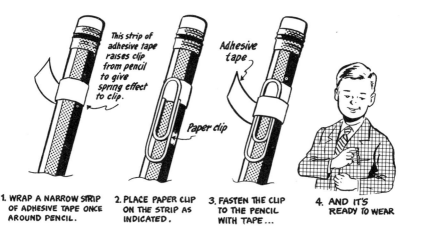

1. WRAP A NARROW STRIP OF ADHESIVE TAPE ONCE AROUND PENCIL.

2. PLACE PAPER CLIP ON THE STRIP AS INDICATED.

3. FASTEN THE CLIP TO THE PENCIL WITH TAPE...

4. AND IT'S READY TO WEAR

2. Make simple pencil clips to help impress children with the need for carrying pencils safely.

3. As a workship project, intermediate grade boys can make a baseball equipment rack.

Although cleverly constructed items encourage other children to try their skill and do likewise, their greatest value is obtained at the moment the individual or small group works on the particular project. There is genuine meaning to the child in a spot map built with colored pins to show the different types of accidents in the school and on the school grounds. There is value in mounting pictures, building charts and graphs, painting a picture of human anatomy, assembling a collection of foods, diagramming the local fire alarm system, putting together bird feeding trays, constructing a health museum, and dozens of similar purposeful activities.

Educational Games. The use of games to teach almost any topic adds ginger to the program. Play is to the child as work is to the man; it is full of meaning. Almost everyone knows that if something can be made to seem like play, it can be learned quickly. Pur-

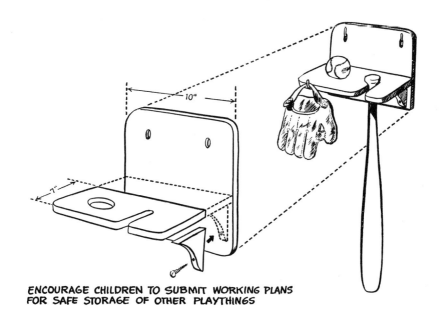

ENCOURAGE CHILDREN TO SUBMIT WORKING PLANS FOR SAFE STORAGE OF OTHER PLAYTHINGS

posely making a game of something, therefore, is sound methodology.

Slow learners, say researchers, are the chief beneficiaries of games — especially when games supplement other educational programs, making real and vivid material that sometimes seems abstract in a textbook. Carlson speaks at length about how games spur enthusiasm and how many students try harder at games than in some courses.[21]

Games should be carefully planned, and the children should know what the real goals are. Games provide many opportunities for an expression of characteristics conducive to optimum social health. Properly conceived, there are many chances for each child to demonstrate cooperation, group loyalty, leadership, and fair play.

Numerous examples can be cited showing how to use a game situation to further the learning of a particular health topic. Some illustrations follow:

1. Use a posture relay in teaching about posture. This is a regular relay race, except that the pupils running must carry a flat object such as a blackboard eraser on their heads. Point out to the class the difficulty in this feat when one does not assume a plumbline posture.

2. Make up riddles. Divide the class into two teams. For example, in discussing the teeth, one pupil says, "I am thinking of something we should do before going to school each morning." Using her watch, the teacher notes the time it takes for the other team to guess the correct answer. Riddles are alternated between teams, with the winning team being the one that has the lowest total time.

3. To teach pedestrian safety to primary graders, have pupils draw a floor map of a busy intersection. Assign children as policemen, pedestrians, automobile drivers. Cardboard discs may be fashioned as steering wheels. Simulate normal traffic conditions.

4. Use a playhouse situation and em-phasize home safety. Children play the parts of different family members.

5. A simple group game of "squat tag" may contribute to mental health, especially if the pupils realize that they are accepting the rules of the game and are having fun playing. The person being chased simply has to squat down to keep from being "It."

6. Play a game of "Health Detectives." Children report on what they have seen and heard each day that pertains to health. One child may have seen the soccer team practicing; a bicycle rider may have seen someone else riding at night without a light; one child may have noticed that children do not run up and down the stairs in the school; someone else may casually point out that Sally Jones has a runny nose — and many more.

7. Use mimetics in primary grades. When discussing pets and home safety have the class walk like cats, run like dogs, or hop like rabbits. Music may be used and rhythm developed around a theme. For example, sunflowers grow tall in the sun. As a posture activity the children may stretch high with their arms in an effort to grow high like sunflowers.

8. Identify objects by taste, odor, or sound while blindfolded. Divide the class into teams. This will help motivate the class in studying the interrelationship of the senses. Some materials to have on hand for the game might include a piece of chocolate, a spoiled orange, sour milk, or a musical record.

9. Obtain a copy of the *Game of Pretend* from Pflaum/Standard, 38 West 5th Street, Dayton, Ohio, 45402. It is part of the Dimensions of Personality series for grade three. It is a board game in which children take turns spinning a pointer and then acting out how they would respond to a situation. Example activities: "Make the face you make when eating ice cream"; "Walk like a boy who is taking home a very poor report card"; "Jump up and down like a three-year old having a temper tantrum."

10. Distribute copies of the smoking crossword puzzle available from the National Tuberculosis and Respiratory Disease Association.

---

[21]Carlson, Elliot. "Games in the Classroom," *Saturday Review*, April 15, 1967.

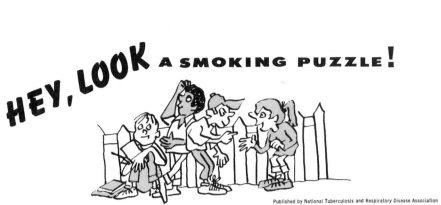

HEY, LOOK A SMOKING PUZZLE!

Published by National Tuberculosis and Respiratory Disease Association   12/70

CHRISTMAS SEALS FIGHT
Emphysema...TB...Air Pollution...Smoking
IT'S A MATTER OF LIFE AND BREATH

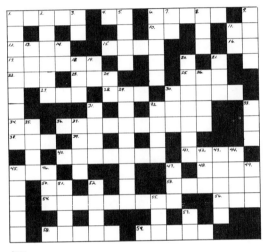

*41. Many emphysema sufferers actually have to _____ for breath.
45. Contemporary clothing style.
48. Solar system twinkler.
*50. From, as a cause or motive. (To die _____ lung cancer.)
*53. Every time you _____ a cigarette you let in a complex mixture of smoke particles and gases, many of which are poisonous.
*54. Leaves a bad taste in your mouth and smells up your clothes.
56. Bright color.
*58. The _____ rate of smokers is about 70% higher than that of nonsmokers.
*59. Cilia act like little brooms to _____ the dirt from the lungs.

Down

*1. A respiratory disease. The lungs lose their elasticity and hold in too much air.
*2. Smoking can cause shortness of _____. (One of the reasons athletes don't smoke!)
3. Abbreviation for "William".
*5. Smoking stains and yellows the _____ on one's fingers.
*6. Efficient little brooms which clean our lungs, but can be paralyzed by cigarette smoke.
7. Opposite of "off".
8. Automobile fuel.
*9. If a cigarette smoker will _____ smoking, his life expectancy will increase.
11. See #10 across.
13. Name of boy or girl.
14. Short for Albert.
*18. Mixture in cigarettes that coats the lungs and slows down their normal action.
19. Short for "hello".
*20. Cigarette manufacturers are required by law to print a _____ on all packages.
21. Small insect which makes honey.
24. Syllable on the musical scale between "do" and "mi".
26. Farm animals from which we get ham.
*29. A poison in cigarettes that makes the heart beat faster and quickens breathing.
*30. If a person is unable to quit smoking, he should at least _____ down.
*31. The preferred entrance for outside air into the respiratory system.
*32. A cigarette smoker can take as many as 8 years off his _____.
*33. A great many fires are caused by people who smoke in _____, and fall asleep.
35. A repetition of sound, a resounding.
*37. Lung cancer was a _____ disease until smoking became widespread.
*42. Smoking is messy, and often leaves _____ on clothing and furniture.
*43. It is smart not to even _____ smoking.
44. People who are ill often have little color and are _____.
*45. Cigarettes are costly and a waste of _____.
46. Nickname for doctor.
*47. Many more smokers than nonsmokers _____ from heart disease and lung cancer.
49. #56 across.
*51. One-fourth of all accidental _____ is caused by careless smokers.
*52. Heavy smokers often puff and _____ as they climb stairs.
55. A type of truck which pulls cars.
57. #34 across.

* Terms which apply to smoking and health.

Across

1. Arm Joint.
4. We.
*6. Smokers often suffer from annoying, chronic _____.
10. Opposite of "out".
11. In a game of tag, the person who must catch the others is _____.
*12. An appeal. (Begging someone to stop smoking for their own good health.)
*15. To cause death (Cigarettes _____ many smokers.)
16. Opposite of "yes".
*17. Freedom from physical disease or pain. (Everyone wants to have good _____.)
22. Rhymes with "bet".
*23. Cigarette smoke pollutes the _____ we breathe.
25. A large monkey.
27. He and she, or him and _____.
*28. If one must smoke, it is best not to smoke the cigarette to the _____ because the tar and nicotine become more concentrated.
30. Past tense of cry.
*32. A cigarette smoker runs ten times as great a risk of death from _____ cancer as a nonsmoker.
34. Myself.
*36. A serious lung disease characterized by an inflammation in the lining of the bronchial tubes.
38. In playing cards it is higher than a King and lower than a Two.
39. To the same extent. (She swam _____ well as he did.)
*40. Emphysema patients find it hard to _____.

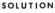

(May be torn off)

SOLUTION

11. Play the game where a pupil spins a wheel made out of oaktag or heavy cardboard. The wheel is divided into triangle sections. Each section contains a group of unassociated words. The pupil writes sentences using one of the words in each section.

Sample sentences:

> The dentist filled my tooth.
> I brush my teeth after eating.
> Milk is good for my teeth.
> I will eat candy only at the end of meals.

12. Ask children to bring colorful pictures of food clipped from magazines. Mount these illustrations on lightweight cardboard and cut to make a jig-saw puzzle.

13. Write "mixed-up" words on the chalkboard or duplicate lists and distribute them to children. Let pupils unscramble the letters to make words which are names of foods. Here are examples:

iklm	milk
draeb	bread
gge	egg
epalp	apple

14. Food charades. Pupils may take turns acting out something to do with food, such as making a cake, peeling an apple, and so on. Whoever guesses the answer has the next turn of being "It."

Programmed Instruction. Programmed health instruction has been employed in a number of communities because it provides the individual pupil with organized health information which can be learned with an immediate knowledge of results.

The Behavioral Research Laboratories programmed a *First Aid* manual which Johnson & Johnson took over for distribution. It has been used with thousands of students throughout the country and is designed for sixth grade use. There is a procedure for using the manual and the first aid film strip which accompanies it. A teacher's instruction manual and a test manual are also available on a complimentary basis. Students work with their own manual, and, since it is different from most workbooks, the novelty seems to appeal to children.

Other health programs which are a part of the American Health and Safety Series and are distributed by Behavioral Research Laboratories include programmed instruction titles: *Body Structure and Function, Personal Health, Nutrition, Safety,* and *Prevention of Communicable Disease.* These programmed learning experiences provide continuity between the easier and the more difficult health concepts by acquainting the pupil with the organized nature of knowledge. Because the learner can proceed at his own speed, he

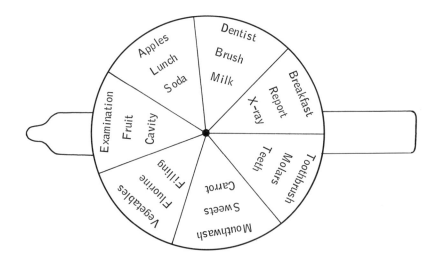

is not threatened by the task; he knows he is learning, and anxiety should be somewhat reduced.

Youth to Youth. As already indicated in Chapter 8, under smoking education, the use of older children to instruct younger children can be a very effective kind of education for healthful living. In this case the relationship between the "teacher" and the "pupil" is often an exciting experience for both, with the enthusiasm of the one affecting the other. Such a person-to-person contact frequently stimulates student actions that no other teaching ingredient can match.

Miscellaneous Techniques. *Storytelling,* an age-old device, has always been a powerful way of impressing youngsters with health facts, especially if the information is accurate and the storyteller skilled in the art. Numerous good health stories are available in textbooks and supplementary readers.

The *guest speaker*, for example, the physician, dentist, policeman, or dogcatcher, is often a welcome relief in the average classroom. He brings life to the class. He is from the world of reality outside the school and is sometimes able to put across a particular health recommendation where the regular classroom teacher has difficulty.

Oral presentations have their place in health teaching. Good reports resulting from research, problem-solving, experimentation, library, and readings need to be skillfully presented to the class. Individual pupil presentations of this nature, followed by class discussion, represent a useful instruction technique.

The *anecdote* represents an interesting tale, narrative, or description of some person or event in health. It is used, for example, to give an account of the life of a man like Lister or Pasteur, or to depict the conditions present in a disease-ridden land such as Egypt.

Counseling with groups or with individuals has become one of the most successful ways of changing health behavior. In dealing less with health facts and more with individual personalities, it tends to "hit home" and bring about real changes in health practices and attitudes. It is not a classroom technique, but is one especially suited to the school setting where the teacher has a few moments here and there to talk with and guide the members of her class.

The use of *student leaders* is a first-rate method of teaching. Leaders may assist in the classroom and on the playground. They may help the teacher inspect for cleanliness or form patrols for safety. New leaders should be chosen as often as possible.

Examinations may be related to educational method as well as to the topic of evaluation. Primary and intermediate graders sometimes like the challenge of a test or short quiz, and use it very well as a pure and simple learning situation. Self-testing activities, where pupils measure their progress against their previous records and against the records of their classmates, are useful in health education. This is particularly true when there is no pressure to excel purely for the purpose of receiving grades.

Independent study may be employed when certain individuals show a keen interest in a health topic. It may be a short-term topic, but some phase of it is of such concern to some pupil or pupils that permission is granted to pursue the topic further to satisfy personal curiosity. This may be done with or without infringing on class time, and it permits the teacher to provide challenging work and study for the especially gifted child.

Research, even in the grades, is an effective learning technique. Almost every kind of child can find some satisfaction in "looking something up." They may learn to be thorough and carefully appraise their findings. Problem-solving and experimental methods employ various forms of research. School surveys, interviews, and questionnaires are useful in elementary health research.

A *Health Education Fair* has been carried on with much general interest in a number of schools. Its purpose is not only to motivate students in health education, but to enlist the support of community groups in assisting the schools. Students prepare health projects which are exhibited and judged by representatives of the community health agencies. In Norfolk, Virginia, the fair has gone on for several years and health projects have been judged on the basis of their originality, scientific accuracy, and overall quality.

The *analysis of current events*, both in the community and the world at large, is one method that has been used for years to make geography and science stimulating. Not a day goes by that there is not some occurrence, phenomenon, or discovery taking place which has either direct or indirect health consequences. Radio, television, and local newspapers invariably refer to such news items as an improved sewer system for a nearby town, a child rushed to the hospital because he swallowed poison, a search for a rabid dog, an automobile and bicycle accident, news of a new method of aiding some disease, or another city setting up plans to fluoridate the water supply. Using current events so that they tie in with the health topic of the moment requires little extra planning and represents an easy technique to employ. From news articles may come group discussions relative to misbehavior in social situations, such as stealing, lying, fighting, or drunkenness. This is an opportunity for intermediate graders to better understand human relationships, thus leading to a better comprehension of mental health.

School-Community Activities. The day has long since passed when the school was considered a self-sufficient agency occupying a building in the center of town. Today, community life is the life of the school, and much of school life is the life of the community. Education is a two-way street. Community personnel and their accompanying ideas come into the school, and classroom health facts and figures arrive in the home to indirectly educate the parents.

There is direct learning through community experiences because they involve immediate sensory contacts with reality. It is difficult to question a properly planned and executed field trip, interview, camping excursion, work project, or survey. One raises a question only when this educational method is employed too often, or when the attending classes are not properly orientated.

The services of the community resources will vary in the degree to which they make a health contribution. Finding and using these resources is the teacher's job. A good place to begin is *people*; this is followed by *places* and *materials*.

People in the community who are usually willing to give assistance to health teachers include:

Health officer	Sewage disposal
School physician	plant operator
School nurse	Statistician
Public health	Laboratory
nurse	technician
Dentist	Health educator
Sanitary engi-	Safety director
neer	Welfare director
Practicing physi-	Hospital super-
cian	intendent
Water plant	Social worker
operator	Farmer
Home demon-	Dairy plant
stration agent	operator

Places in the community that are especially helpful in health instruction include:[22]

Health depart-	Recreation
ment	facility
Dairy	Water purifica-
Milk pasteuriza-	tion plant
tion plant	Sewage disposal
Industrial plant	plant
Food Freezer	Housing project
plant	Fire department
Experimental	Police depart-
station	ment
Dental clinic	Restaurant
Laundry	City playground
Bakery	Home water
Home garden	supply
Utility company	Meat packing
Farm	plant

Parents, perhaps more than any other group in the community, are equipped to

---

[22] For a useful list of voluntary, professional, and commercial organizations see Chapter 10.

work closely with the schools in the program of health teaching. If there is any one modern method of teaching health, it is to get pupils to carry out at home what they have learned in the classroom. Teachers, therefore, assign homework in health that involves real action about the home, and encourages classroom-home cooperation.

In every community there are groups of people who are in some way interested in child welfare and school health. Sometimes an organization will actually be searching for a "project of the year." They may decide to do something like financing an eyeglasses program or purchasing prophylactic tablets for a rheumatic fever campaign.

CORRELATION AND INTEGRATION OF HEALTH INSTRUCTION

There is an interrelationship between direct teaching, correlation, and integration. It is difficult to say that one is better than the other, for all three methods of instruction may be used in health instruction.

There is a distinct difference between correlation and integration. *Correlation involves the use of other areas within the curriculum by which health material is taught.* Health, therefore, is correlated with physical education, science, and social studies. It may also be correlated with additional areas such as art, arithmetic, and English. In the elementary classroom, in which there is less formality and the teacher has her own pupils most of the day, it is not difficult to relate the materials in one subject matter discussion to that of another. True correlation means that the teacher, when thinking of English, must plan for some health teaching in the English lesson. The same is true for other lessons. In discussing ventilation and heating in the sixth grade science period, some definite reference to the personal and community health aspects of the topic would be provided. In social studies the teacher purposely

plans to talk about health conditions and the practice of bloodletting during the colonization days at Plymouth and Jamestown. Likewise, health is correlated with physical education games, stunts, and dances by definitely organizing the time available so that specific reference may be made to such items as playground safety, exercise, food, rest, and personal cleanliness. There are many opportunities for correlating health teaching with art through the preparation of posters and charts relating to health problems under study and in the making of puppets to dramatize an idea.

It may be seen that almost any school activity can be correlated with health.

Social Studies
  History of foods
  Eating habits over the world
  Food preparation for the party
Art
  Discussing and arranging flowers for table
  Making place mats
  Poster drawing
  Foods modeled from clay
Arithmetic
  Counting: "How many will eat with me?"
  Building number vocabulary: quart of milk, one-half slice of toast, pound of butter
  Concept of time: time needed to eat breakfast
Science
  How foods grow
  The effect of climate and weather on foods
  Animal experiments with foods
Physical Education
  Food and energy for play
  Rest and recreation
  Overeating and undereating
Reading
  Health textbooks
  Charts and posters about good foods
  Captions under food ads in magazines and newspapers

Good health instruction helps make correlation a two-way process. Not only is health taught through English, but proper speech, writing, and spelling are taught through health activities. An example of this kind of cooperation is illustrated by the story of what happened in one elementary school. The teacher of a third grade class felt that the parents were not always aware of what meals were served in the school cafeteria. So the class copied the cafeteria menu for the next day as part of their writing lesson. This was taken home to the family.

The children were encouraged to use their best handwriting so that their parents would really know what they were going to have to eat. Another example from the English area involves the use of the school library. Health assignments require familiarity with books, card catalogs, encyclopedias, and guides. The pupil not only discovers information about a health topic, but he also improves his concept of the use of basic library tools.

Integration involves an organization of learning experiences around a central objective. It differs from correlation by relating parts to the whole. The "whole" can be anything. A well-integrated bicycle, for instance, is one in which all parts—wheels, chain, nuts, bolts, seat, handlebars, fenders—fit perfectly together to afford the rider a safe and pleasant journey. By the same token, a well-integrated child is one who has been exposed to the hundreds of educational stimuli and has emerged to take his place in society as a "whole" person. He is like a giant mosaic—all the unique parts make a complete being. This may be accomplished by the well-integrated curriculum, one which is balanced and refined, and embraces many areas of instruction.

Instruction in the lower grades is very often based on centering the attention of pupils on broad topics rather than dividing the school time into periods for different subject matter areas. Here, arithmetic, art, spelling, social studies, science, and health are interrelated as part of a broad learning experience. As an example, third grade children in Baltimore studied housing problems. A dilapidated old house being rejuvenated according to the Baltimore Plan was dramatized by the children. They acted the parts of germs, trash, garbage, and mice, and declared that this was no longer a home for them. In the same school there were other examples of integration. One second grade study was built around the quality of Baltimore's water supply. Health aspects were considered with social study aspects. Moreover, the choice of words and ease in speaking gave proof to the observer that these lower grade children understood the importance of good water.

No subject in the elementary curriculum can long remain divorced from the total program. An overlapping of topics is necessary in order to give appropriate meaning to the various pieces of information. As it is, too many children know a great many health facts but fail to see their usefulness in the world they live in. This may be due to the fact that we live in an integrated or whole society, but we often continue to formally study the parts without in any way relating them to the whole. This is somewhat true at all educational levels. It has only been in recent years that physiology, sociology, and psychology have been examined together with the resulting emphasis today on human ecology.

MATERIAL AIDS IN HEALTH TEACHING

Thinking directly in terms of color, tones, images, is a different operation technically from thinking in words. . . . If all meanings could be adequately expressed by words, the arts of painting and music would not exist. There are values and meanings that can be expressed only by immediately visible and audible qualities and to ask what they mean in the sense of something that can be put into words is to deny their distinctive existence.

—John Dewey
Art as Expression

Education is more than just exposing a learner to information. Somehow he must be involved in the process by taking part in it. He has to *do* something *with* something. And because it is purposeful activity, he feels, listens, smells, and acquires health concepts *through the use of material things.* Homer once said, "Greater glory hath no man than that which he wins with his own feet and hands." Therefore, we may say that children learn some from what they hear, more from what they see and hear, and most from what they do. If something appeals to a child because he has heard or read about it, he usually wants to "try it out," "feel it," and "work it"—himself. He seeks a rich, full-bodied experience that is the bedrock of all education. It is the unabridged version of life itself—commonly referred to as "something you can sink your teeth into." This alone is reason enough for the existence of good instructional materials and the continuous search for better ones.

THE NATURE OF INSTRUCTIONAL MATERIALS

Instructional materials, by definition, exist to aid in the instructional program. They are not a substitute for good teaching—they are only a supplementary item. They are *aids*, and as such are a bona fide part of educational method.

As a whole, instructional materials are well supported by research. When properly used in the teaching situation they accomplish the following:

They supply a concrete basis for conceptual thinking and hence reduce meaningless word-responses of students.

They have a high degree of interest for students.

They make learning more permanent.

They offer a reality of experience which stimulates self-activity on the part of pupils.

They develop a continuity of thought; this is especially true of motion pictures.

They contribute to growth of meaning and hence to vocabulary development.

They provide experiences not easily obtained through other materials and contribute to the efficiency, depth, and variety of learning.

THE PROPER USE OF HEALTH TEACHING MATERIALS

The numerous audio-visual materials and other teaching aids cannot take the place of the teacher. It is the teacher who determines the opportune time for each type of instructional material. It is the teacher who selects the health materials because they are needed by the child in a particular learning situation. Materials used in this way become an integral part of instruction and perform a special function in achieving health goals.

Whether teaching aids are successful or not depends upon preplanning and effective usage. In one grade five class, for example, a filmstrip was shown to start pupils thinking about drug use and drug abuse. Following this a display of pertinent materials was set up:

Empty containers of various drugs (medicines)

aspirin
BC or Stanback (powder and tablet containers)
cough syrup
cough drops
Milk of Magnesia (liquid and tablet)
rubbing alcohol
Merthiolate or Mercurochrome
Ex-lax
Bufferin
prescription drugs
Anacin
Contac
Spec-T
Zestabs
Sominex
Stanback
Ionized Yeast
Blistex

Empty containers of household substances

lighter fluid	flea powder and
airplane glue	tick spray
spot remover	garden spray
nail polish	hair spray

After examining the materials the students became involved in making a working definition of the word "drug," and a discussion of the differences between prescription and non-prescription drugs.

It is interesting to note when considering the proper use of instructional materials that Comenius, in his *Orbis Pictus* (a book of "sense objects" numbered to tie in with English and Latin words), warned his students about making pictures and other materials the main part of education. Materials were to be used chiefly to avoid verbalistic teaching. They were not to be an end in themselves.

Edgar Dale stresses eight ways of evaluating these materials.[23] They may be readily applied to the general use of all health teaching materials:

"Do the materials give a true picture of the ideas they present?" Is there some distortion of truth in order to make a point? Is there a built-in bias of some kind? Several existing films on alcohol present this weakness.

"Do they contribute meaningful content to the topic under study?" The only way to really answer this question in a health class is to evaluate the results of teaching. Do the pupils know any more about the topic? Are practices improved and attitudes changed because of the materials used? We say that "a picture is worth ten thousand words," but is just any picture that effective? One may have an elaborate and highly authentic display of alcohol and tobacco pictures, pamphlets, and other supplementary materials, but it may not alter behavior any more than a movie or a talk by the school nurse. Probably the chief reason more television is not used in schools is not because sets and programs are difficult to obtain; it is because, in the minds of some people, there is a question whether television is a highly effective educational aid.

"Is the material appropriate for the age, intelligence, and experience of the learners?" One of the common mistakes of inexperienced teachers is to use materials with the wrong age group. A cancer film that appears interesting to the teacher may leave her primary grade class "cold." A lesson on the making of

tooth powder may insult the intelligence of an upper grader, yet be most appropriate for the second grade boy and girl. Certain health textbooks are difficult when used alone, but supplemented with other materials, they become usable.

The appropriateness of materials is best determined by ascertaining the common custom and practice in their use. Many school systems today employ personnel to manage a materials center and to be of service to teachers. These people have the evidence and the educational listings; they make it their business to know which teaching aids are satisfactory for a certain grade level. Beyond this, some experimentation by the teacher is necessary.

"Is the physical condition of the materials satisfactory?" Few things can detract more from a teaching aid than untidiness and uncleanliness. A broken working model of the eye, a dirty graph, a grimy poster, or a film with a noisy sound track can hurt the teaching lesson measurably. Health teaching exhibits, drawings, and models should be fresh and almost sparkling in appearance.

"Is there a teacher's guide available to provide help in effective use of the materials?" Ideally, every teacher should preview materials before she ever uses them. A good guide can provide a detailed understanding of the items being used and offer numerous practical suggestions. Time is at a premium today; there may be little time to experiment with a certain model or film — only time to read what others have previously done with it.

One of the finest sources of teaching aids may be found in the teacher's guides distributed with the health reading books of several of the larger book publishers.[24] These guides are often as well prepared as the texts they are made to accompany.

"Do they make students better thinkers, critical-minded?" Because children usually enjoy moving pictures, it is

---

[23]Dale, Edgar. *Audio-Visual Methods in Teaching.* New York: Dryden Press, revised 1964.

[24]Notably Scott, Foresman, & Co., Lyons & Carnahan, Laidlaw Brothers, Bobbs-Merrill Co., 3M Co., Ginn & Company, and J. B. Lippincott Co.

not difficult for them to be lulled into accepting and believing something that they might otherwise challenge if they had examined it critically. On the other hand experience demonstrates that children become quite critical of smoking when they experiment with a simple smoking machine such as the Mini-lung. (See Fig. 9–8.)

"Do they tend to improve human relations?" Children learn to live together harmoniously not only by studying about it but also by practicing it as they live together in the school. Human relations is a continuous process. It is a kind of health education that is most desirable and often comes about as a concomitant learning in the everyday activities of the pupils. The use of a wide variety of materials in teaching health tends to pave the way for cooperative effort, sharing of ideas and objects, and understanding the skills and feelings of the other fellow.

"Is the material worth the time, expense, and effort involved?" This, of course, is the culminating question. In every educational endeavor it becomes necessary sooner or later to appraise fully the expended efforts of teachers. It is at such a time as this that the criteria of economy is applied. Just how costly, in terms of time and money, is the project? In a third grade class studying cleanliness, is it better to draw posters for a poster contest than to view a ten-minute film on some phase of community sanitation? In a fifth grade class studying the relationship of food to personal vigor, is a rat-feeding experiment worth all the time it takes to feed the animals, clean the cages, keep the records, and secure the food?

Other things being equal, it is possible to show that some aids are far superior to others. In the Pittsburgh public schools, for instance, the use of a film was found to be the most successful way of teaching the pertinent facts of diet early in childhood.[25] This conclusion was reached after many aids had been tried.

VARIETIES OF TEACHING AIDS IN HEALTH EDUCATION

There are few fields of educational endeavor that are as fertile for the use of teaching aids as health education. Health has a biological, sociological, psychological, and philosophical basis that cuts across all areas of effort. It is concerned with total human welfare: mind, body, and spirit. Because of this, practically every known teaching aid can in some way be used in the health instruction program. But school time is at a premium; one must be scientific in the use of methods and supplementary aids.

Variety in the use of material aids is as

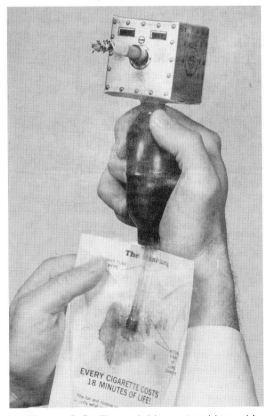

Figure 9–8 The mini-lung teaching aid fosters critical thinking. (Courtesy Spenco Corporation, Waco, Texas.)

[25]The film used: *Bill's Better Breakfast Puppet Show* (25 min., 16 mm., color), the Cereal Institute. Recommended for kindergarten through fourth grade.

important as varying the method of teaching from time to time. Children welcome a change, and since some pupils prefer one aid to another, it is only fair to everyone to be flexible in the use of the various materials. By the same token, some material aids are better than others at a particular grade level. To children who cannot read, a typical poster may be less effective than a flat photograph. A colored slide, for instance, may do a better job of depicting the relationship of food colors to one's appetite than almost any other available means.

Numerous errors are committed in the name of variety. Care must be taken not to forget eye and ear appeal nor lose sight of the fact that materials should be pertinent to the health lesson. Also, materials should be free from objectionable commercial advertisements.

MATERIALS AVAILABLE TO THE CLASSROOM TEACHER

The following materials are not easily made in class and should be available to the teacher:

Essential in Health Teaching

Catalogs of films
Catalogs of equipment
Card file of films
Model boards
Bulletin boards
Chalkboard
Picture file
Filmstrip projector and filmstrips
Motion picture projector
Portable screen
Overhead projector
Record player

Desirable in Health Teaching

Daylight projection screen
Camera (bl. & wh. and 35 mm. color)
Movie camera
Opaque projector
Tape recorder
Public address system
Slide projector and 35 mm. slides

In the larger elementary schools in which there are satisfactory materials centers the average classroom teacher

will have little trouble securing the necessary aids. In fact, by selecting from the "Desirable" list, it will be possible to experiment somewhat with other items. She may try out a tape recorder in class or borrow a 35 mm. camera and take her own pictures of the pupils in action to be shown on the slide projector at a later date.

SOURCES OF INSTRUCTIONAL MATERIALS

The classroom teacher, possibly more than any other teacher, needs a working knowledge in instructional materials. Selecting, preparing, and utilizing these materials has become almost a science. The teacher in most areas will have to become proficient by virtue of her own efforts and experimentation. And in the special area of health teaching, a trial and error approach will prove helpful in weeding out ineffective teaching aids that do not appeal to the pupils. This last point is worth dwelling on, for there are several ways to "skin a cat" and each teacher has a favorite way. Where photographs may appeal to one teacher, another may dislike bothering with them and find success in the use of stick drawings.

It is no small task to find new techniques and clever materials for putting across a particular health lesson. Magazines such as *Instructor* and *The Grade Teacher* are rich in ideas for new teaching materials every month. (Creative ways of developing inexpensive materials appear in the November, 1972 *Instructor* in full detail.)

The teacher with an open mind, who is searching for new ideas and sources of information on the selection, preparation, and use of audio-visual materials, will find most of the following sources helpful:

Printed Materials

Aids to Learning, grades one to eight, a project of Creative Playthings, Inc., Princeton, N.J.

*Educator's Grade Guide to Free Cur-

riculum Materials, edited by Patricia H. Suttles, and published annually by Educator's Progress Service, Randolph, Wisconsin.

Educational Media Index, a project of the Educational Media Council, New York, McGraw-Hill Book Co. Contains a vast range of materials; volumes 1 and 2 refer to health and safety materials for kindergarten through sixth grade.

Free and Inexpensive Learning Materials, published annually by George Peabody College for Teachers, Nashville, Tenn.

Guide Book Describing Pamphlets, Posters, and Films on Health and Disease, published periodically by the Maryland State Department of Health, Baltimore, Md.

1001 Valuable Things You Can Get Free, by Thelma Weisinger, published periodically by Bantam Books, Inc., New York, N.Y. Contains an extensive list of materials that are bona fide giveaways.

Lacey, Richard A. *Seeing With Feeling: Film in the Classroom*, Philadelphia: W. B. Saunders Co., 1972.

Lowndes, Douglas. *Film Making in Schools*, New York: Watson-Guptill Publications, 1968.

Mallery, David. *The School and the Art of Motion Pictures*. Revised ed. Boston: National Association of Independent Schools, 1965.

Sources of Free Pictures, edited by Merton B. Osborn and Bruce Miller, published periodically by Bruce Miller Publications, Riverside, California.

Sources of Information on Educational Media, edited by John R. Molstad of Education Media Council in cooperation with U.S. Office of Health, Education, and Welfare, Washington, D.C. (available from U.S. Government Printing Office).

Vertical File Index, published monthly with an annual cumulative volume by R. R. Bowker Co., New York, N.Y. Lists free and inexpensive materials from private and public sources.

Periodicals

Audio-Visual Instruction. Washington, D.C.: National Education Association Department of Audio-Visual Instruction, 1201 Sixteenth Street, N.W. Nine issues.

Educational Screen and Audio-Visual Guide. Chicago: 2000 Lincoln Park West. Ten issues.

EFLA Film Review Digest. New York: Educational Film Library Association, 345 E. 46th Street. Eight issues.

Journal of Health, Physical Education, and Recreation. Washington, D.C.: American Association for Health, Physical Education, and Recreation, 1201 Sixteenth Street, N.W. Nine issues. Each issue contains an audio-visual section.

Journal of School Health. Kent, Ohio: The American School Health Association, 515 E. Main Street. Ten issues. Most issues contain specific references to new teaching aids.

Junior Scholastic. New York: Scholastic Magazines, 33 West 42nd Street. A weekly for grades six to eight. Features material on plays, short stories, science, health, radio, TV, records, personal guidance, and hobbies.

School Health Review. Washington, D.C.: American Association for Health, Physical Education and Recreation, 1201 Sixteenth Street, N.W. Nine issues. Each issue contains a section on resources for school health programs.

Audio-Visual Materials in Health Instruction

Of the dozens of techniques and aids being used in the elementary schools, some are more common than others. A brief discussion of each follows this paragraph. It begins with the more spectacular projected materials involving motion, sound, electricity, and electronics, and moves to the older and more elemental forms of non-projected materials. One cannot accurately say that a certain material aid is superior to another without qualifying the statement in terms of the objectives. To say that one material aid is better than the other depends upon a number of variables — variables such as the teacher's ability and the make-up of the class. Each classroom teacher will have to determine to what extent the following material aids can be successfully used in classes of health instruction.

1. Motion Pictures. In one breath we can say that the use of motion pictures to convey health messages is almost as badly abused as the use of pamphlets; they cannot stand alone in putting messages across. In the next breath, however, we can state with certainty that motion pictures may well be one of the finest mediums for presenting health ideas in readily acceptable terms. Why the extreme difference in these two statements? One answer lies in the meaning of the film. Lacey asks, "Meaning for whom?"[26] Aren't children different? Don't they find a variety of meanings in a film? They should react with feelings ("Fantastic movie") as well as thoughts, and they shouldn't be *compelled* to intellectualize the movie, says Lacey, or they will miss the experience.

Another answer lies in planning. *When good planning takes place, health interest and health understanding increase.* Specifically, health education instructional films are planned to reach certain goals. They may be used:

As an introduction to a unit to stimulate interest or give an overview.

In the direct teaching of a health lesson, i.e., to help develop an idea or attitude, to convey certain facts, or to help solve or correct certain problems.

As a review or summary of previous learnings.

  a. The *preliminary steps* are:

    Familiarize yourself with the film before showing it.

    Make a list of the important points in the film that you want the audience to understand and remember.

    Prepare some thought-provoking questions which will stimulate discussions.

    Introduce the film to the class, bringing out the points you want them to look for.

  b. The *presentation* is a challenge:

    The viewing distance of the farthest

seat from the screen is approximately six times the width of the picture for pupils in the front row.

The room should be effectively darkened.

Acoustics are better when the room is filled with people or has many drapes to muffle reverberations.

Room ventilation should not be overlooked.

The projectionist must know how to maintain and care for the machine.

Before the showing, check cords, lamps, reels, position of speaker, amplifier, and film gates.

Test run and focus picture.

In starting the picture dim the room lights, turn on the motor, then the lamp, check focus, increase volume, and adjust the tone respectively.

During the showing check the loops, volume, and frames, and stay with the operation until the film is over.

In ending the picture turn off the lamp, fade the volume, turn on room lights, turn off motor respectively.

Following the showing rewind the film, clean film channels, put all parts in their proper places, get film ready for return to film library, and make out required records.

  c. The *follow-up* "sets" the experience:

Review with the class the main points of the film.

Clear up any existing questions concerning the film.

Ask the class questions (oral or written) for the purpose of evaluating the film and its effectiveness.

Repeat film showing if time permits and some points appear to need re-emphasis.

Engage in follow-up activities, i.e., tests, papers, drawings, demonstrations, experiments, as neces-

---

[26]Lacey, Richard A. *Seeing With Feeling: Film in the Classroom*, Philadelphia: W. B. Saunders Company, 1972. p. 18.

sary to insure a practical understanding of the topic.

d. The *evaluation* is as important as
any of the above points. Standard
evaluation forms may be obtained
from the Educational Film Library
Association, Inc. Teacher-made
forms for elementary classroom appraisal should include answers to a
number of questions.

It takes time to become familiar with
the large number and variety of health
films appropriate for the primary and intermediate grade levels. Such a list
would more than fill this book. A good
start may be made by reviewing Chapter
10 which deals with the sources of materials. Also the lists of producers and distributors are continually being revised.
For a wide coverage of current sources
consult the following:

The Blue Book of Audio-Visual Materials, Chi-
cago: Educational Screen, 64 East Lake Street.
Included here are films, filmstrips, slides, and
recordings.
*Educator's Guide to Free Films, Educator's
Guide to Free Film Strips, Educator's Guide to
Free Transcriptions, Tapes and Scripts*, Ran-
dolph, Wisconsin: Educator's Progress Service.

An annually revised guide with title index, subject classification, brief descriptions, and cross
references.
Public Health Service Film Catalog, Washington, D.C.: U.S. Public Health Service, U.S. Government Printing Office, annual.
Visual Materials in Safety Education, Supplement II. Washington, D.C.: National Commission
on Safety Education, 1201 16th Street, N.W. A
bibliography. (Revised periodically.)
*U.S. Government Films for Public Educational
Use*, compiled for the U.S. Dept. of Health, Education, and Welfare and published by the Government Printing Office, Washington, D.C., annual.

It sometimes makes a good project to
produce a health film at school. The
teacher who can operate a movie camera
and knows something about the composition of pictures can often make an 8
mm. or 16 mm. colored film that may be
used from year to year. A good homemade film does not outgrow its usefulness very soon. Future classes enjoy
seeing their older friends in the moving
picture, and the class that makes the
film has a wonderful opportunity to
integrate the health message with other
subject matter areas. In writing the

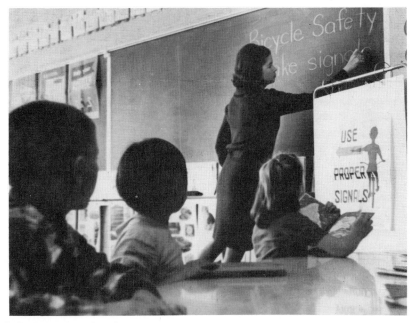

Figure 9–9 Following the showing of a safety film the teacher reviews key points. (Courtesy
National Safety Council.)

script, the various scenes are tied in closely with the narration. This, like everything else in the aids line, takes conscientious planning, but it can be quite worthwhile for there is a tremendous range of health problems which can be approached by this teaching technique. Some examples of films produced by classes include first aid to the injured child, boating safety, swimming safety, garbage disposal, shopping for safe vegetables and fruits. Even a simple on-the-spot movie of a field trip to the dairy or of a group of happy youngsters surrounding an animal feeding demonstration can be a motivating device for children that follow. Also, a good amount of fun may be had in filming the bicycle skills of several children riding about the school playground. Ideas for a local film could come from reviewing the excellent Eastman Kodak Company booklet, *Movies With a Purpose* (Free), which is a teacher's guide to planning and producing 8 mm. movies for classroom use. Also available from Kodak at a small charge is the filmstrip and record for teachers, *Putting New Excitement into School Pictures*.

A very fine teaching aid is the silent cartridge *loop film*. This is a short (several minutes) presentation to drive home a point. Shown on the single-concept film projector, it can be used with other media. A number of health related films are now available from Popular Science, Hank Newenhouse, Guidance Associates, Ealing Corporation, and Encyclopaedia Britannica Educational Corporation.

2. Filmstrips. Much that has already been said about the selection, presentation, and evaluation of movie films can be applied to the utilization of filmstrips.

Filmstrips are a very convenient technique of showing a series of still pictures. They are mounted on a continuous strip of 35 mm. film and vary in length from 18 frames to several times that number. The film is threaded through the filmstrip projector and engaged with the teeth of a sprocket wheel. A knob connected with the sprocket wheel makes it possible to advance the filmstrip, frame by frame, as needed.

The advantages of filmstrips for elementary health teaching are:

They are lightweight and easy to handle in the classroom. The projector is simple enough for a primary grade pupil to operate.

They are relatively inexpensive—one of the cheapest projected visual aids.

They are available in vivid colors.

They may be obtained for use with a sound recording.

There is a wide variety to choose from in health.

Body functions and specific health implications can be effectively broken down and presented through a sequence of filmstrip projections.

The teacher can pause as long as she likes on any one picture.

Many filmstrips are designed to accompany textbooks.

3. Slides. Slides, like filmstrips, are easy to use and relatively inexpensive. One can make a slide or filmstrip from anything that is drawn, written, typewritten, printed, or photographed—and it can be done in full color. Drawings may be made with pencil on etched glass or with special slide ink. It would not be difficult in an intermediate grade class, for example, to sketch the skeleton of the body on glass and project it life-size on a screen. So many slides are readily available today that it often proves more economical in terms of teacher time to purchase ready-made slides.

Most slides are 2 inches × 2 inches; however, the 3½ inch × 4 inch variety are sometimes employed. The latter are more readily used in adapting charts, pictures, tables, and the like from magazines and books since more detail can be shown. Also they can be made by hand more easily. Most slides of a health and biological nature are photographically produced. They may be shown on any one of a number of easy-to-operate projectors. One type of tape recorder is available which will automatically change the slides in a slide projector. This can be a very effective means of putting over a health topic at an exhibit or as part of a display in the main corridor of the school.

4. Opaque Projector. The light from any flat picture may be reflected directly on the screen by means of mirrors and lenses. The opaque projector is flexible enough to handle anything up to six inches square; anything larger can be inserted into it and moved around until the desired part of the picture is on the screen. Its use in the lower grades for showing almost any flat object is great. Although it is heavy to move about, it is inexpensive to use. Small clippings from a newspaper or magazine can be greatly enlarged on a screen. The same is true for poison labels and medical prescription instructions. It is a good health motivating device, for children love to see their own health pictures, drawings, charts, and graphs projected on a big screen before the whole class.

5. Overhead Projector. For the teacher of health it is a simple matter to sketch, write, or draw on a strip of cellophane with a ceramic or wax pencil, and in color if desired. The chief advantage of this projector is that the teacher can readily project all the details of a lecture while facing the class.

6. Transparencies. With the use of the overhead projector has come an increasing amount of good transparencies.

Some of the finest prepared health education transparencies, ready to use and in sharp colors, are distributed by such companies as the Minnesota Mining and Manufacturing Company (3M), National Dairy Council, American Dental Association, Popular Science, Milton Bradley in Springfield, Massachusetts, American Cancer Society, Western Publishing Company, Hubbard Scientific Company and Dennoyer-Geppert Company. Other full-color transparencies especially good in depicting physiological functions are distributed by Medi Visuals, Inc., 342 Madison Avenue, New York, N.Y., 10017.

Overlay transparencies are useful in showing the structure of such items as body organs, cells, muscle tissue, human skin as it would appear under the microscope, sense organs, and major areas of the brain. The American Dental Association, in its booklet, *How Teeth Grow*, uses overlay transparencies to clearly illustrate the changing pattern of dental development from infancy to the early teens. The booklet is especially practical when children are permitted to look it over and finger the transparencies.

7. Radio. One teacher has said, "Our boys and girls like to listen to others their own age. It seems to me they learn more from them."

The radio in the classroom is an inexpensive device that is realistic, is authentic, and has emotional impact. It may be used directly by scheduling classes to coincide with some radio programs in order to hear health lectures, interviews, or panel discussions. It may also be used within the classroom as a simulated broadcast with class members taking part in the production.

From the point of view of health actions, pupils need to be taught how to use the radio and be selective and critical of radio programs. Just as children are taught not to accept everything that appears in print, so they must learn to appraise that which is presented over the radio and television channels.

8. Portable Conference Telephone. A whole class can talk on the telephone with the help of one set. While all listen a public health official can explain the need for precautions against the flu germ, or a senator can be engaged in conversation a thousand miles away. This device weighs less than 20 pounds and can plug into any standard telephone jack. There are dozens of ways it can enliven health teaching.

9. Television. A number of schools have access to educational television. Health programs are staged for school audiences. Both professional personnel and schoolchildren may be employed as performers. This can be a fine medium for motivation providing, as, in the case of moving picture films, there is some pertinent discussion prior to and following television presentation. Here sight and sound are combined to teach an entire community. Several intermediate grade school classes, for example, could watch the actual pulling of a bad tooth in a dentist's chair, this to be followed by a special message from the dentist.

Each material aid has its own unique advantages and limitations. Television is a powerful medium, but it is expensive and is often only a one-way communication. Attempting to regiment health classes by means of television would be to violate certain principles regarding pupil interests, needs, and differences. If programs are carefully related to classroom activity, especially following the presentation, it seems logical to expect television to become an effective tool in the promotion of health. However, it must always be evaluated against alternate tools that are available.

Cassettes are now available from several educational film makers for classroom use. Columbia Broadcasting System has a selection (EVR cassettes) at 51 W. 52nd Street, New York, N.Y., 10019. Videotaping is also becoming popular in the schools. All kinds of student activities, trips, and experiments are recorded on videotape and replayed later.

Home television may be used for pupil assignments somewhat the same way as radio has been used for years, i.e., to appraise "health" commercials and advertising, and to listen to special health talks, demonstrations, news, and plays.

10. Records. Records are easy to play, are relatively inexpensive, and are available in many schools today. Disc recordings are owned by children who often enjoy sharing their records with the rest of the group. They give meaning to numerous events, bring authentic sounds into the classroom, and improve the listening habits of boys and girls. They constitute two-way communication and can be stopped and discussed with the class.

In the teaching of health, commercial records may be used for health songs and action stories. The Stanley Bowmar Company, Valhalla, N.Y. 10595, has a wide selection of these. Other health records may be obtained from the American Medical Association, Encyclopaedia Britannica Films, American Cancer Society, National Interagency Council on Smoking and Health, The National Safety Council, Maryknoll Lending Library, and the United States Rubber Company.

11. Tape Recordings. The tape recorder opens a great many areas to the teacher of health. Tape recorders are not difficult to operate, and the tape is easy to edit and repair. In many respects the tape recorder has more uses in the classroom than the radio or television set. Tape recordings may be purchased. (The periodical, *Tape Recording*, lists most of the tapes available from commercial companies. See also, *Educator's Guide to Free Transcriptions, Tapes, and Scripts*, Educator's Progress Service, Randolph, Wis.)

From a health instruction viewpoint tape recordings make learning more complete by:

a. Bringing health authorities into the classroom. A committee of two or three pupils can visit a busy physician, bakery manager, or water department superintendent and record the answers to prearranged classroom questions. Distance is no problem. The world is brought to the classroom.

b. Recording home radio and television commercials, plays, and talks to be used for class discussion and appraisal.

c. Providing a variety of approaches to the same subject. A recording of a health lesson may be reviewed two weeks later with profit. Gives both pupils and teacher an opportunity for self-evaluation.

d. Bringing to the classroom some of the health problems of the community. The teacher's ability to verbalize about a health problem—alcoholism and drug abuse, for example—is at best limited. The tape recorder brings to the students the actual voices of community members who know the problem at first hand. The teacher can use this information, emphasize it, and elaborate upon it; but the raw material of life is here, not lost in abstract verbiage. Moreover, it can be identified in a social peer group setting where it is especially revealing.

One of the most valuable uses of a

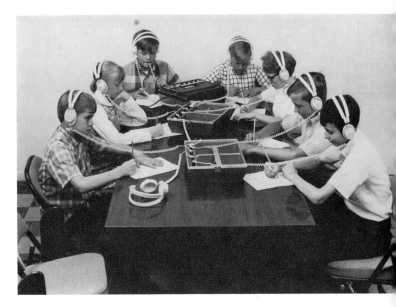

Figure 9–10 Headset listening assures student attention. (Courtesy Anedex, Incorporated.)

tape recorder is to play it back to the pupils so that they hear how their own voices sound. Several statements pertaining to a health lesson may actually be read into the machine and played back the next day for class consumption. A "traveling recorder team" may survey the pupils and teachers for their opinions relative to some current health idea, or they may venture into the business area of town to interview the "passing citizen." A sixth grade class in one New York State community questioned quite a number of leading citizens on their opinions relative to fluoridating the city water supply. Another idea often used is to put together a simple story and have it taped exactly as desired for future presentation. A single topic combining humor with good advice is "How to Burn Down Your House."

12. Textbooks. Earlier, textbooks were reviewed as a method of teaching. If they are up-to-date and are more than just another reading book, they have value. If not, then they are very much the way historian Oscar Handlin described them—"dogmatic and dull, an obstacle rather than an aid to learning." When the book is accurate in the presentation of facts and illustrations and orderly in the arrangement of materials, it

can be used as an effective guide to the health program at a certain grade level. This is particularly true if the pupil is asked to discover things for himself, answer questions, engage in learning activities, and respond to diagrams and situations. Listed below are the publishers of textbooks primarily concerned with health in the elementary school:

Benefic Press, Chicago, Ill., *The Health Action Series*, grades 1–8 (1962).

Benziger, Inc., *Becoming a Person Grades 1–8.* (1972) 866 Third Ave., New York, N.Y. 10022.

The Bobbs-Merrill Co., Inc., Indianapolis, Ind., *Health for Young America Series*, grades 1–8 (1965).

D. C. Heath Co., Boston, Mass., *Health Science Series K–8.* (1965).

Ginn and Company, Boston, Mass., *New Ginn Elementary Health Series*, grades kindergarten–8 (1969).

Houghton Mifflin, Boston, Mass. *Investigating Your Health.* (Grade 6) (1971).

Laidlaw Brothers, River Forest, Ill., *Laidlaw Health Series*, grades 1–8 (1970).

J. B. Lippincott Co., Philadelphia, Pennsylvania *Basic Health Science Series*, (Grades 1–6) (1972).

Lyons & Carnahan, Chicago, Ill., *Dimensions in Health Series*, grades 1–8 (1965).

Scott, Foresman & Company, Glenview, Illinois, *Health and Growth K–8* (1971).

Prentice-Hall, Inc. *Systems of the Body Series* — Ages 8–12 Englewood Cliffs, New Jersey 07632 (1972).

13. Pamphlets. Probably no other health medium is more wisely used — or mis-used — than the leaflet or pamphlet. Thousands are distributed in school each year, only to end up in wastebaskets. Pamphlets need to be simple and have a definite message. They should be in bold print with lots of color and illustrations and contain some white space so that what is written will stand out. These criteria should also be followed when health leaflets or "handouts" are made in class for home distribution. The accompanying illustration is included in a leaflet which has been widely distributed in Florida. Although limited to black and white, note how attractive it is and the message it has for the parents.

Pamphlets for school use may be obtained from numerous official and nonofficial health agencies. (See Chapter 10.) Most of the large insurance companies, the American Medical Association, the Florida Citrus Commission, The Cereal Institute, National Society for Prevention of Blindness, and the National Dairy Council represent organizations which distribute particularly well-fashioned leaflets suitable for elementary school classroom use. In recent years there has been a reduction in the number of free materials available for teachers. However, the quality of the inexpensive materials has improved measurably. For years the National Dairy Council has made its wide variety of health leaflets available to teachers, and in sufficient quantity so that each pupil may have his own. *The Story of the Cow* has been written for 12 different grade levels. Third graders are able to use the little 3 inch × 4 inch colored leaflet on the four basic food areas, both in the classroom and at home. Attractive "handouts" such as these may be used in a number of effective ways; however, a pamphlet cannot be expected to influence attitudes and behavior without being used in conjunction with other methods of health education. They must be informative and motivating, and they must be adapted to each age level.

To meet the health and safety needs of pupils, it is recommended that careful consideration be given to the selection of pamphlets, textbooks, and other printed materials. How each applies in a given instance depends upon the specific teaching objectives which have been set up to meet particular needs.

Finally, a word about the use of magazines. The Research Division of the National Education Association has discovered that some of the most imaginative classroom projects are sparked by materials appearing in magazines. Their most common usage is to develop bulletin board displays. They are also employed for useful reference information, for free reading, and for stimulation of student

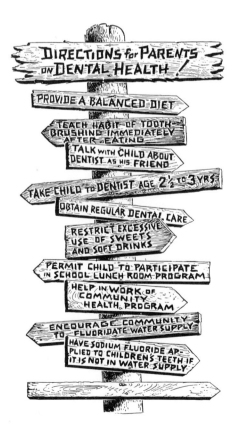

Leave hitch-hiking to the kangaroos. They are built for it, and you and your bike are not. Only one person belongs on your bike . . . and that's YOU. Never hitch rides on cars, trucks or buses. Never follow bikes or cars too closely; allow plenty of room for a safe stop.

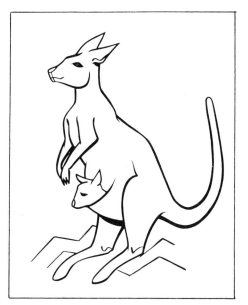

Figure 9-11 A page from the attractive pamphlet, *Good Biker Today . . . Good Driver Tomorrow.* (Courtesy Employers Mutual of Wausau.)

writing. Health articles may be read in class or summarized in understandable language.

14. Encyclopedias. Sets of encyclopedias form a wealth of background materials for the classroom. By following the library method of teaching real use may be made of this two-way reference material. Many a statement in an encyclopedia has triggered ideas for pupil activities. Even more important, perhaps, encyclopedias can be used directly by pupils in their search for facts and comments relative to the health unit being studied. It covers all related fields of health, contains bibliographies for the teacher, and provides excellent background material to look over before viewing films, filmstrips, or TV programs. And it often contains a quantity of illustrative diagrams, charts, and maps.

15. Clippings. One of the finest uses of the health clipping is to tack it to a designated space on a bulletin board where everyone can see it. Clippings from magazines and newspapers include pictures, stories, reports, research, and advertising. Every health topic, particu-

larly in grades four to six, can be bolstered with appropriate clippings. Hardly a week passes by without some of the magazines having an item suited for a health lesson. Pictures of foods, drawings of body parts, and facial expressions may all be posted on a bulletin board or projected on a large screen.

16. Study Guides and Workbooks. There is some use in health teaching for these aids providing they encourage students to be active—to try something out, to experiment, to listen, to observe, or to discuss.

A good elementary school workbook is attractive. It has directions for study, self-instructive techniques, and self-corrective exercises. It contains pictures, practice exercises, and testing material. Provision is made for individual differences and for developing initiative and independence.

17. Pictures and Photographs. Pictures crystallize ideas and form much of the basis for thinking. Industry and business spend a fortune each year on pictures to put their story across. Pictures are everywhere today in magazines, folders, and booklets. Good pho-

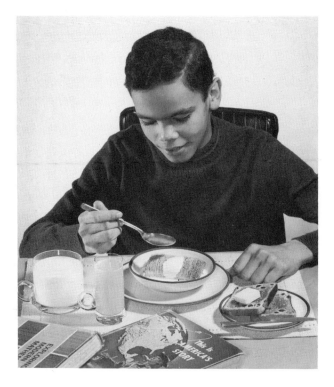

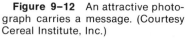

Figure 9–12 An attractive photograph carries a message. (Courtesy Cereal Institute, Inc.)

tographs are also available or may be made through a school project. Once used, the outstanding pictures and photographs should be filed in an accessible folder for future use.

Suitable health instruction pictures should include such items as groups of healthy children with smiling faces; pictures of pets and other animals eating the same foods as children (pigs drinking milk, rabbits eating green vegetables, chickens picking up grain in the barnyard); the fire engine en route to a fire, the policeman directing traffic, and the like.

A multitude of heterogeneous pictures will only confuse a student. To obtain the best results with pictures use only a few well chosen ones for a pertinent illustration. Pictorial materials may be mounted and passed around for individual inspection or exhibited on a board. They may also be projected by the opaque projector.

18. Posters. The thousands of billboards spread across the land have only one purpose: to put over an idea in one fleeting glance. Posters accomplish the same purpose.

Posters have become an expressive form of American art. Their chief purpose is stimulation. Thus they may be used to introduce a unit or call attention to some facts in a phase of instruction. A good poster should be simple, large (28 inches × 22 inches), have bold and colored lettering that is easily read and understood. If it can be interesting enough to cause a chuckle, adroit enough to promote discussion, and clever enough to haunt the memory, it has just about everything that is needed to make it a useful teaching aid. If, however, it functions only as another implement, requiring the support of more basic teaching aids, then it is of limited value. Too often posters have been used solely as a wall decoration, having been left on display far beyond the point of attracting notice. They are effective only when they are *frequently changed.*

Numerous manufacturers of foods, toothpastes, school furniture, and dairy products are excellent sources of poster

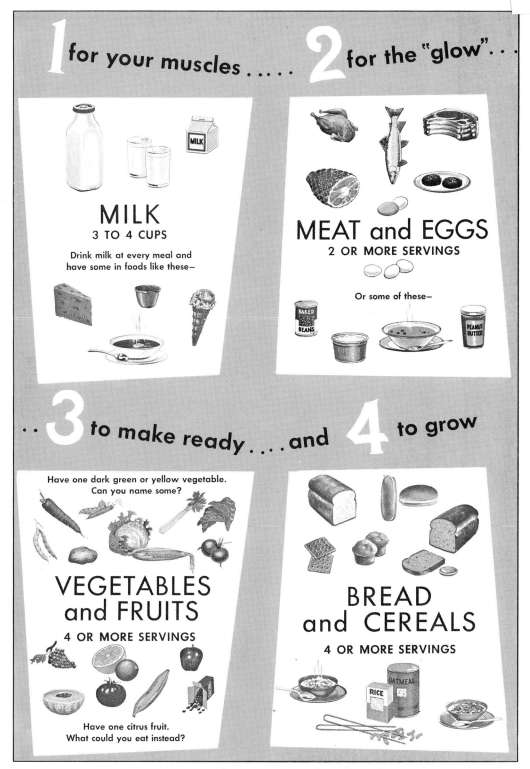

Figure 9–13 (Courtesy National Dairy Council.)

materials. Practically all of the large insurance companies distribute, free of charge, colorful wall posters relating to health and safety practices. Some examples of the more effective free posters for primary and intermediate grade use may be obtained from:*

American Cancer Society
American Dental Association
American Heart Association
American Medical Association
Bicycle Institute of America
Educators Mutual Life Insurance Co.
Employers Mutual of Wausau
Equitable Life Assurance Society
Florida Citrus Commission
Instructor (Every month in this magazine)
The National Dairy Council
National Institute of Mental Health
National Livestock and Meat Board
Personal Products Corporation
National Commission on Safety Education
Sunkist Growers
The National Safety Council
Travelers Insurance Co.

In working with posters the best learning probably takes place when children make their own. This is especially true when the poster making is directly re-

*Addresses may be found in Chapter 10.

lated to the particular health topic, is clear and forceful, is well designed, is colorful, and has easily understood titles with brief captions. An example of a poster that meets these qualifications and would be attractive on a fourth grade bulletin board is Figure 9–13.

Artistic posters may be fashioned from wrapping paper, scrap tin, tinfoil, box tops, magazine pictures, wallpaper, and the usual art supplies. Even comic book clippings and newspaper cartoons may be used in making the poster. These sometimes serve to make the poster more attractive and humorous.

Once health posters are discussed in class they may be hung about the room for a short period. The better ones may be selected for a main corridor bulletin board, the lunchroom, or the physical education locker room.

More and more posters are employing cut-out figures and superimposed materials over the foundation surface. Items are readily tacked, stapled, or glued to the surface and provide another dimension for observation. Simple line expressions can tell more sometimes than fancy drawings. Mental health is well depicted this way:

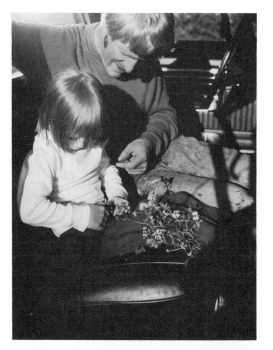

Figure 9–14 Poster. (Photograph by John R. Crane, reprinted from *Instructor,* Copyright © 1972 by the Instructor Publications, Inc., used by permission.)

SIMPLE LINE EXPRESSIONS

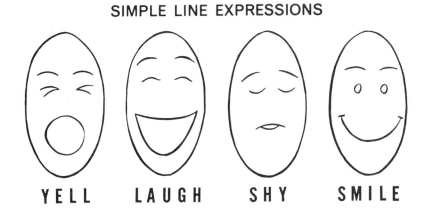

YELL   LAUGH   SHY   SMILE

19. The Health Mobile. Under the direction of the clever teacher a rather stimulating health "mobile" may be constructed. This may consist of wooden signs, printed on both sides, a wire frame, and string. To learn about food values a fourth grade class might build and hang a mobile such as the following: This mobile is different enough from the usual display that the pupils can learn the four basic food groups more easily. Here they also see the values inherent in each group. The wooden signs may be made in class or in the elementary industrial arts laboratory. These are superior to cardboard signs. Also, as an alternative to using signs for vitamin and mineral values, the class might cut out and hang pictures of the various human organs affected. Example, the eyeball for vitamin A, or the skeleton for calcium.

20. Cartoons. The perfect cartoon needs no caption. The symbolism conveys the message, for the best cartoons make their point immediately.

If the teacher will watch carefully for cartoons having to do with health, she will find a number of excellent ones appearing each week in popular magazines and newspapers.

In some respects cartoons work better with intermediate grade children, probably because a first-rate cartoon has emotional impact. This is arranged by the clever cartoonist who is able to play with humor, mockery, satire—qualities that are generally appreciated more by older children.

In using such a medium in health teaching, one must be careful that pupils do not accept the message of the cartoon uncritically. Cartoons are very often all

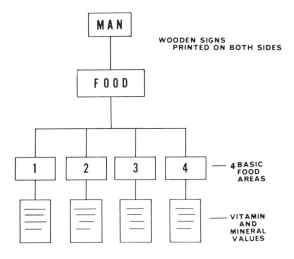

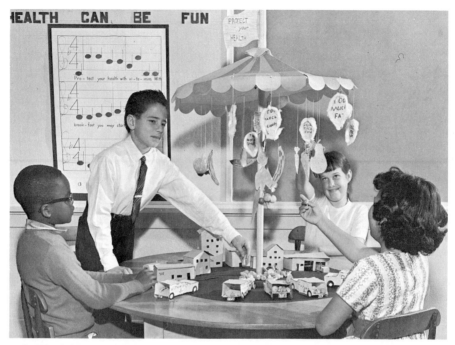

Figure 9–15 A variety of mobile. (Courtesy *Health Education Journal*, Los Angeles City Schools.)

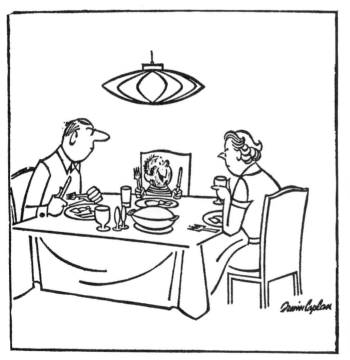

"Why should I wash—I'm inoculated against everything, ain't I?"[27]

[27]Reproduced through courtesy of Irwin Caplan, McNaught Syndicate, Inc., and the *American Legion Magazine*.

"black" or "white," or they oversimplify without qualification. Moreover, they cannot be used repeatedly as can pictures and photographs. They become outdated rapidly. They must be considered because surveys indicate that they are among the most popular aids used by teachers. And where they are not obtained from initial sources they may be made in the classroom. In fact, original health cartoons frequently help students think for themselves and apply what they know about health to the cartoon.

21. Sketches and Drawings. A pencil sketch or drawing made with a pen, pencil, or special crayon may make health facts more vivid. A class studying posture, for example, may see what is involved in a straight line type of posture when a simple sketch is drawn of building blocks.

Drawings and diagrams are valuable at all age levels. Primary grade children seem to appreciate the line drawing that outlines a process. In a study of foods, an outline of how the grain passes from the farmer's field to the bakery and ultimately to the bread on the table is of real interest. The diagram of a water supply from the original source to the clean glass or the story of milk from the cow to the table are other examples that may be nicely diagrammed. Some of these items

may be put on transparencies by pupils themselves.

Drawings, sketches, and diagrams may also be put together by the teacher or the class using magazine prints, newsprint, wrapping paper, window shades, or anything else that can be brought to class to work with. These materials may be large sheets of paper, chart cloth, old bedsheets, large paper panels, or classroom chalkboards.

22. Strip Drawings ("Comics"). Here a story is told through a series of drawings, frequently called "comics."

A number of free health comic books are available from the Food and Drug Administration, U.S. Public Health Service. The comic *Dennis the Menace Takes a Poke at Poison* is especially well written. So are the several "Sparky" fire stories distributed by the National Fire Protection Association: *Early Man and Fire, Man Learns More about Fire, Hello, I Am Fire, Is This Your Home?*

23. Writing Pads. These pads of paper may be as big as or bigger than 2 feet × 3 feet. They are usually supported on an easel and used very much the same as a chalkboard. They have a distinct advantage over the chalkboard in that sketches, diagrams, and notes may be prepared well in advance of the class period. This is especially helpful in the

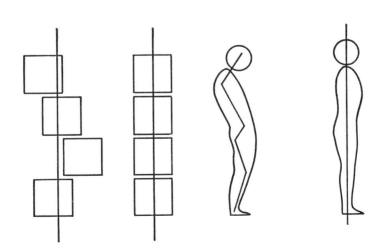

crowded school with inadequate blackboard space. To many children it is simply a different medium—a fact to keep in mind when new sources of motivation are sought.

24. Charts and Tables. Information is arranged in lists. Facts, figures, and even pictures are organized in some way so that the visible parts are related to the whole. The ramifications of a whole concept or idea are presented at once. The danger here is that the table or chart may include too much detail or too many words.

A proper chart should have a title large enough to be seen across an ordinary classroom. Lettering should be clear with strong colors on a neutral or light background. It may be several square feet in size and hung from the ceiling, or small enough to be duplicated and distributed to each pupil. It may be mounted on heavy paper, a bulletin board, or ordinary flannel. In any case it should not remain on display beyond its period of usefulness.

It is not difficult to make an elaborate table or chart when it comes to depicting health and disease statistics, the nutritional breakdown of food into calories, or something similar. Care must be taken, however, to limit the detail to the primary and intermediate grade level of comprehension.

Health charts with the most instructional value are those which the pupils make themselves, and are based on data which they have assembled. In one Southern school the primary grade boys and girls put together a chart which they called *A Trip Through Healthland*.[28] It was constructed with felt mounted on heavy paper. The medium of light colors was also applied to make it attractive.

At each "stop" on the "trip through healthland" the importance of that area was discussed and personal problems were raised and talked about.

Every elementary teacher should have a chance to look over the *Good Health Record* charts distributed by the Kellogg Company, Battle Creek, Michigan. The students keep these current on a day-to-day basis, recording habits of cleanliness, eating, sleeping, and helping at home and at school. Most children enjoy charting their progress and keeping their own records. This becomes a kind of self-testing activity—a means of comparing oneself today with what one did yesterday or with someone else in the class.

Another attractive chart used especially in health teaching is one for measuring pupil height in the ordinary classroom. The *How Tall Chart* of the

---

[28]Originated and reported by Mary Charles Garrett of Gainesville, Fla.

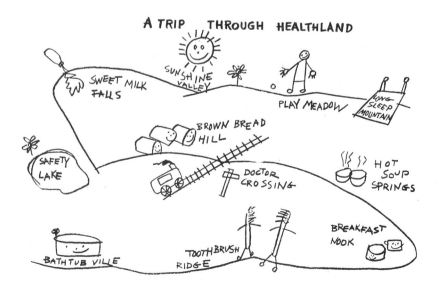

A TRIP THROUGH HEALTHLAND

Travelers Insurance Company, Hartford, Connecticut, fits inconspicuously on a closet door or wall. It hangs so that the bottom of the chart is 2½ feet above the floor. Height may be measured to the nearest quarter inch.

25. Graphs and Maps. A graph diagrams quantity, development, function, or relationship of factors. There are graphs that are horizontal or bar, line, pictorial, and circular or pie. All may be effectively used in health teaching. Excellent multi-colored bar graphs for health teaching may be obtained from the Evaporated Milk Association and the National Dairy Council.

The graph on page 332 has a message for upper grade children. It clearly illustrates how well cereal and milk "go together" to furnish a breakfast meal.[29] It may be seen that cereal contributes most of the nutrients supplied less generously by milk and vice versa.

A map is something more than a diagram or line drawing. It generally starts somewhere and goes somewhere. A map may be made on any health subject. It is different from the physical, economic, and political maps made available by a supplier and used in geography and social studies; it is generally made by the students. Primary graders, for example, may derive considerable benefit from mapping the route from home to school. In one school, as a part of a lesson on safety, all pupils drew a picture map showing the route from home to school. They were encouraged to make them complete, even to including such hazards as water holes, angry dogs, inviting junkyards, houses under construction, a pile of dirt, and the like. When the maps were completed they were studied by the class so that the hazardous places could be discussed. Some new routes were created to avoid the hazards. The routes were further appraised from the point of view of the bicycle rider. The maps were so revealing that the pupils carried the discussion beyond walking and bicycling to automobile and bus safety.

Another map particularly suited to health teaching in the elementary school is the spot map. It may be a map of the community or an ordinary road map. It could be stuck with a small colored-head pin to show the exact spot where an automobile accident occurred during the preceding month. In one school the pupils marked the spots on the map of the school grounds where accidents occurred. They counted everything from cut elbows, scraped knees, and blisters, to serious falls and minor emergencies. Once the map was well covered with pins, the class stopped to analyze the situation in an attempt to do something about it.

26. Flash Cards and Flip Charts. Flash cards have titles printed on each side for use in flashing certain information before the pupils. An idea is brought home on a small card. These cards may be in the form of charts, such as the food value charts of the National Dairy Council, and they may be mounted on hinged display panels and flipped one at a time by the teacher.

Flash cards and flip charts may be used to develop quick reaction and correct responses. To many pupils they are a novelty, and, as such, command attention. A series of questions and answers on school safety may be displayed before the class on 13 inch × 22 inch panels, or the logical progress of a certain food may be followed through the processes of assimilation, digestion, and elimination.

A series of 36 large flip charts, expressly created for kindergarten or grade one pupils, are the *How About You?* health charts published by Ginn and Company. These 17 inch × 20 inch full color charts were described on page 130, Chapter 7.

Teaching with flash cards permits the teacher to put over a concept that is brief and to the point. The word *Stop* or *Go* or *Caution* has a message all by itself. A series of words arranged to cover health instruction in one class period might read (1) Health, (2) Food, (3) Music, (4) Rest, and (5) Happiness. As the es-

---

[29]Adapted from the graph in the booklet, *The "Cream of Wheat" Story*, distributed free by the Cream of Wheat Corp., Box M, Minneapolis, Minn., 55413. (Used by permission.)

Cereal and Milk—Nutritional "Go-Togethers"

Enriched Quick "Cream of Wheat" with fresh whole milk and sugar is a perfect breakfast combination. This chart shows you how these nutritious foods complement each other. For example, when you eat 1 ounce (dry weight) of Enriched Quick "Cream of Wheat", along with 4 ounces of fresh whole milk and a teaspoon of sugar, about 99% of the Iron comes from the cereal and the remaining 1% from the milk. But then, from this same combination you will get about 71% of the Riboflavin from the milk. The cereal contributes most of the nutrients supplied less generously by the milk and vice versa.

Nutritionists recommend a "Basic Breakfast Pattern" which supplies about 600 calories and makes a good contribution of almost every essential nutrient. Enriched Quick "Cream of Wheat" with milk plus a serving of citrus fruit fills the bill!

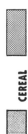

Chart — horizontal bar chart with x-axis: 0 10 20 30 40 50 60 70 80 90 100%

Rows: IRON, NIACIN, THIAMINE, CARBOHYDRATE, PHOSPHORUS, CALORIES, CALCIUM, PROTEIN, RIBOFLAVIN, FAT

  (SUGAR)

Legend: CEREAL   MILK

sential ingredients of a healthy person are mentioned, the particular key word on the chart or card is flipped for the class to see. Finally, if the flip chart is helpful in keeping the pupils' minds on the speaker's track, it is equally helpful in keeping the speaker's mind on it.

27. The Bulletin Board. Practically every classroom has some kind of bulletin board which is used from time to time to display health materials. The materials displayed should have a unifying theme. They should be authentic and easy to read. Simplicity should be the rule in organizing material for elementary schoolchildren. One should ask these questions:

Is there a center of interest?

Is there beauty of line and form?

Do the materials go well together?

Is the total arrangement well-balanced?

Is there repetition of color?

Is a feeling of unity created?

Does the arrangement tell a story?

Captions for bulletin boards have great value. A challenging question or statement accompanying the material may have much to do with the value derived from the display. Captions which tell little, such as *Foods for Health*, or *This Is Posture Week*, can be improved by making them read *Eat Your Way to Good Health* and *How Do You Look to Your Friends?* Other captions which relate to health clippings or the

health topic being studied might read: *Have You Seen These? Do You Know? Stop — Look — Read.*

Notice that in arranging the pictures or other materials the teacher places the largest number of pictures in the bottom row to give strength to the arrangement. The same procedure is followed when color is used — the darkest colors are concentrated near the bottom of the display.

The bulletin board, when used in health teaching, can arouse interest in many things such as special health week (safety, heart), seasonal wearing apparel, current discussion topics, or local health events. If bulletin boards are especially colorful and make a good first impression early in September, there is a fairly good chance they will be purposely seen by pupils whenever they pass by them. Needless to say, the materials must be changed frequently.

Three-dimensional display can enhance the appearance of the bulletin board. Real objects brought from home may be hung or tacked to the board with particular attention given to space, color, and shape. In fact, when children help plan and organize the bulletin board display, it is more apt to be read than otherwise. The pupils may print their own captions, mount their materials, and take care to label each item with the name of the child who made it or brought it to school. An odorless and stainless bulletin

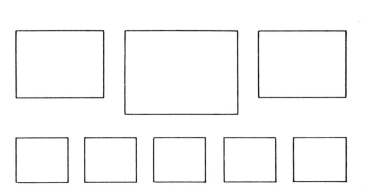

board wax may be used in place of thumbtacks to hold three-dimensional as well as flat objects.

At Chautauqua Central School, Chautauqua, N.Y., what started as a health project of one class became the interest of the entire school. The project was a *Health Bulletin Board* that was extremely colorful and was changed weekly. Students gathered regularly to review it, and parents even visited the school each week to see what was new. Here short interesting items were posted. Here is an example of a notice to all sixth grade athletes:

— NOTICE —

100 words —

Best advice for amateur and professional athlete alike, say Dr. Jean Mayer and Beverly Bullen: Eat a variety of foods daily — Enriched or whole grain bread and cereal, milk or cheese, meat or an alternate, fruits and vegetables.

Special Pre-Event Meal Instructions for Strenuous Contests:
- Avoid a heavy meal within three to four hours before the game.
- For endurance events, concentrate on foods high in carbohydrate, low in fat. Include generous amounts of cereal, bread, jam, honey.
- To prevent disabling discomfort during the game, avoid high protein and bulky foods.
- Omit coffee, tea, alcohol to avoid a depressing effect later.

---

28. Flannel Boards and Felt Boards. Flannel or felt is unique in that once the background is constructed it may be developed into any type of diagram, graph, chart, or bulletin board. Moreover, this may be done while the class watches, and, like a blackboard or chalk talk, the teacher can add portions of the chart or diagram as the lesson unfolds until the story is complete.

The flannel or felt it stretched over a 2 foot × 3 foot stiff board, usually on an easel. Velvet, velveteen, suede cloth, or flocking may also be used. Material which will cling to this includes coarse sandpaper, flannel, felt, terry cloth, or Floktite. All titles, captions, letters, and models are pasted to one of these adhering substances. It is a simple matter after this to arrange and rearrange the board materials. In one school a pie graph of the four basic food groups was put together piece by piece in four operations while the teacher told the class about each category of food. By the time she added piece Number 4 the class was well on the way to visualizing how the parts make up the whole — the balanced diet. Here, the pie graph and the felt board techniques were effectively employed to give meaning to a health lesson which would be difficult to duplicate through some other medium.

In a second grade class in Garden City, New York, the children made up a large number of food items which were attached to the board. They were then asked to select from the board those foods that would make a good breakfast, lunch, and dinner. With practice the pupils were able to do a reasonably good job in planning a full day's diet. Such a technique in learning is another worthy way to help boys and girls of varying abilities engage in a stimulating learning experience.

29. Magnetic Boards. Closely associated with the flannel board is the magnetic board. This is essentially a metal sheet upon which magnets may be attached for a number of purposes of representation. The board may be covered with a thin layer of cardboard or oilcloth or some other material which will not hinder the action of the magnet. One form of this board is truly flexible in all situations. Not only is it permanently magnetized, but it has a chalk writing surface and is available with brightly colored plastic symbols and indicators enabling the teacher to plan and illustrate al-

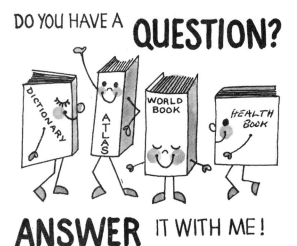

DO YOU HAVE A **QUESTION?**

ANSWER IT WITH ME!

most anything. In terms of health instruction, this aid may be used to teach such things as fire routes for fire drills or air raids, moving foods from one plate to another, showing the spread of cold germs, illustrating the hands of the clock at bedtime, placing children and equipment on the school playground, and as many others as the teacher's imagination will permit.

30. Collections and Specimens. Newspaper clippings, magazine articles, and cartoons may be collected for bulletin board display. Other items such as eight or ten animal teeth for a dental health lesson present a challenge to the average nine or ten year old if he is asked to locate them. In one fourth grade class the boys and girls made a collection of empty cereal boxes. Every known cooked and dry cereal was represented and displayed. This was done to initiate a unit on breakfasts. It promoted much interest, especially after the boxes were examined to see what food values the cereals contained. In a fourth grade class that was talking about food spoilage, several persons were asked to bring a good item and a spoiled one to class, for example, a good grapefruit and a bad one, a sound potato and an unsound one, a fresh stalk of celery and a withered one. There was as much interest created by the bad specimen as by almost anything else brought to class that school year.

Other ideas for collections of health-centered articles include:

Canned food labels	Candy bar wrappers
Foods that clean teeth (apples, celery)	Samples of good and poor sneakers
Household cleaning agents	Varieties of apples
Animals and human teeth (also bones and hair)	Drinking utensils used over the years
Potentially dangerous implements (knives, axes, sharp pencils, chisels)	Pressed leaves and stalks of eatable plants (wild)

31. Models. The true value of a model lies in its degree of accuracy. It helps also if it has several characteristics to attract the eye.

A number of biological supply houses sell excellent models of the various body parts. Merely demonstrating or exhibiting these, however, does not necessarily promote understandings and appreciations. Associating a model of the digestive system with a machine that processes foods, or a model of the heart with a mechanical instrument is not enough. The teacher must project the idea that the digestive tract or heart or anything else is merely a part of the whole man, that man is not a machine—for no ma-

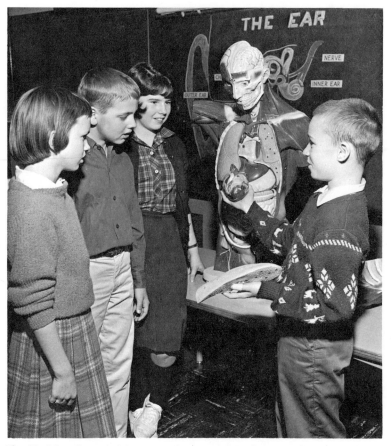

Figure 9–16   Studying the special senses via the model. (Courtesy Cincinnati Public Schools.)

chine repairs itself or reproduces itself. In other words, a model is, at best, only a poor copy of the real thing, but it may be quite helpful in creating favorable concepts. A model of the human ear, for instance, may help teach the fact that careless blowing of the nose can be dangerous. This is more important to understand than learning all of the names of the parts of the inner ear. An exploratory examination of the mechanics of the inner ear, however, may be the item that impresses the children the most. The way the model is used is probably more important than the model itself. If somehow the student can get the idea that the human body is the greatest of wonders, a real appreciation will be born. Man wonders over many things, said St. Augustine, but "man himself is the most wonderful."

32. Mirrors.   A large share of health teaching is concerned with personal appearance. The use of a single full length mirror can do much to impress growing boys and girls. Children may look at themselves in terms of cleanliness and neatness. They may view their own eyes, teeth and tongue at close range. Many children have never seen themselves in a full length mirror. Also, when it comes to posture improvement, there is no finer medium than the mirror. Full length mirrors hinged together are the most desirable for they allow several viewing angles.

33. Exhibits and Museums.   The educational exhibit, whether a simple affair in the corner of a classroom or an elaborate museum layout, has considerable value in the health instruction area. It tends to have its greatest value when it is a product of the pupils who help to design and develop it.

A good health exhibit takes careful

planning and time to prepare. Here are some useful standards to follow for making school exhibits:

Use only one central idea in the exhibit.

Place the exhibit where it is certain to be seen.

The exhibit is something to look at, not to read.

Make all labels short and simple, uniform and legible.

Motion attracts attention.

See that the exhibit is well lighted.

Use color to add interest and attractiveness.

Employ sound and various mechanisms to add charm to the exhibit.

The construction method of teaching is applicable to the building of displays for exhibits and museums. Children have excellent ideas when it comes to presenting these materials. The exhibits that stand out in almost any room are those which employ color and motion. Colored posters, colored paper, paint, or cloth add spice to the display. A simple battery-driven device or a turntable from a discarded phonograph puts motion into the exhibit. Music and other sounds may be supplied by automatic record players. Questions may be asked and answers given over a simple telephone circuit. Most local telephone companies are happy to cooperate in such a project by lending the necessary equipment to the teacher. In fact, there are many people in every community who willingly go out of their way to help the classroom teacher. An orthodontist, for example, will lend plaster casts of teeth, which may be

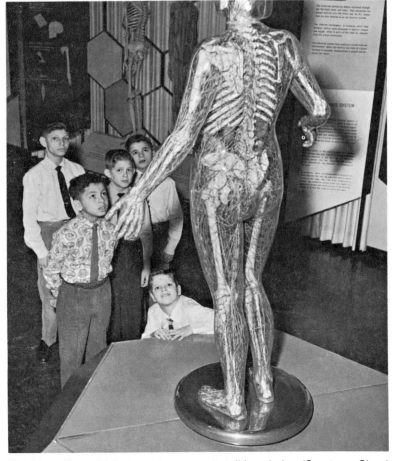

Figure 9–17 "Juno," world-famous transparent talking lady. (Courtesy Cleveland Health Museum.)

displayed along with the teeth of horses and cows and the jawbones of other animals. A taxidermist in Florida will lend alligator teeth, while his contemporary in Wyoming will lend one of the elk.

At almost any time of the year displays may be obtained for exhibit purposes from official and non-official health agencies. Many state health departments have such displays. In New York State two of the most popular have dealt with tuberculosis and fluoridation. Other displays may be obtained from the local heart or mental health association, the county health association, the National Foundation, the American Red Cross, the American Dental Association, the National Safety Council, and many other health organizations. Safety displays are often prepared by traffic safety personnel in industry and business. And, of course, one should not overlook the local police department and its safety efforts.

The way an exhibit is used is the key to whether or not pupil behavior is changed in any appreciable way. Generally, there is an intrinsic interest in pupil-built exhibits—an interest that may accompany a particular display *if the teacher requires the pupils to use the materials.* Children should be permitted to touch, feel, and otherwise examine much of the exhibit. There should be answers to their questions. Even a formal listing of questions on a sheet of paper may help to guide some students in securing answers from the exhibit. More than one teacher has employed a simple version of the true-false questionnaire for the pupil to complete as he studies the exhibit.

Additional activity may be involved when electric buttons are pressed or little doors are opened. In the Cleveland Health Museum there is a food facts and fallacies exhibit which employs the "lift-up door" technique.[30] Here, a question is

asked, such as "Are celery and fish special brain foods?" After the pupil ponders the answer for a few seconds he simply lifts the hinged door and finds the answer. "No. There are no such things as brain foods." Other examples from this excellent display which support this method of teaching include the following:

Q. "Are raw eggs more digestible than cooked eggs?"
A. "No. Soft or hard cooked eggs are more digestible."
Q. "Is Vitamin A margarine as good as butter?"
A. "Yes. Vitamin A margarine contains the same amount of vitamin A as butter."
Q. "Is it safe to leave food standing in open tin cans?"
A. "Yes, if food is properly refrigerated."

True-false questions may also be used with this "lift-up door" technique. Following are two examples used for sixth graders in the Cleveland Health Museum:

Q. "Potatoes have more minerals and vitamins than a head of lettuce. True or false."
A. "True. Lettuce has few minerals and vitamins while potatoes contain iron, vitamins B and C."
Q. "Calcium pills are a good substitute for milk. True or False."
A. "False. Milk contains valuable minerals, vitamins, and proteins in addition to calcium."

The elementary school health museum may be built in a spare room or in the corner of a large classroom, but this is not easy to accomplish. A museum differs from the usual exhibit in that it is permanent. For this reason very few schools have a museum. Space is at a premium in most buildings, and unless the whole school has easy access to the museum, it will soon lose its usefulness. The short-term exhibit, therefore, will be more practical for elementary school use, and the museum will be more prac-

---

[30] The Cleveland Health Museum, Cleveland, Ohio, has a long history of experimenting with the more effective ways of visualizing health concepts. Among its most successful attempts has been the production of a series of suitcase exhibits created for classroom use.

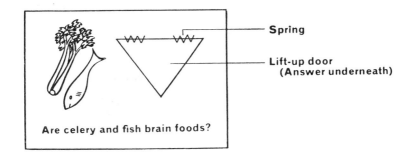

Spring

Lift-up door
(Answer underneath)

Are celery and fish brain foods?

tical if set up as a resource area in the community.

Permanent museums have been gaining in popularity since the Century of Progress World's Fair in Chicago (1933–1934). One of the first to be established was the Mayo Foundation Museum of Hygiene and Medicine in Rochester, Minnesota, opened in 1935. A year later the Cleveland Health Museum was incorporated. The Dallas (Texas) Health Museum was organized in 1946, and in 1952 the now famous Lankenau Hospital Health Museum opened in a suburb of Philadelphia. This was followed by the establishment of the Hinsdale Health Museum in a Chicago suburb in 1959, and by 1963 the Reading (Pennsylvania) Hospital had its health museum in operation. In 1972 the Hall of Health at the California Museum of Science and Industry opened in Los Angeles. It features the "Circulatory Man," the "Neuroman," and the "Transparent Woman." People of all ages are discovering that the value of a permanent health museum is great indeed; it is an educational institution, alive and vital—not a static, smelly mausoleum.

There is little doubt that the community health museum is a real force in the area of public health and school health education. The constantly replaced and modernized exhibits of the Dallas Health and Science Museum make it one of the outstanding educational forces in that section of the United States. The Cleveland Health Museum is without doubt the finest example of a museum set up to educate in matters of health. For almost three decades thousands of schoolchildren and adults have visited this institution to see such superb exhib-

its as: Human Genetics; the Hall of Health, which shows how the body is put together and how it works; the plastic engravings, "From Egg to Embryo"; the transparent talking woman; the transparent tooth; the famous Dickinson sculptured models showing human birth and growth; the sound of the beating heart; truths and misconceptions relative to food and nutrition; and many more. The educational department of this one museum supplies hundreds of schools annually with materials for use in various phases of health and human biology.

One of the most successful projects originated by the Cleveland Health Museum is that of the portable exhibits for health teaching in the classroom. These suitcase exhibits have traveled widely, and teachers and nurses have been instructed in teaching from the materials presented. To facilitate this, a seven-minute magnetic tape recording was made for each exhibit, describing in detail and giving teachers pointers on what to stress at different grade levels as well as suggestions for class projects. A mimeographed teacher's manual was also developed.

Finally, and perhaps more important than anything else, the modern health museum is a place where one goes to look at something that is available without obvious propaganda, and where one is saved from any kind of commercialism.

THE MEDIA CENTER

One of the problems confronting teachers is the storage of materials and equipment. For the teacher of several

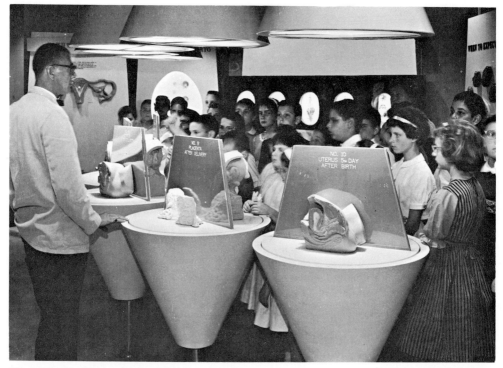

Figure 9-18 Class of schoolchildren hear a museum staff instructor talk on "Wonder of Life" display. (Courtesy Cleveland Health Museum.)

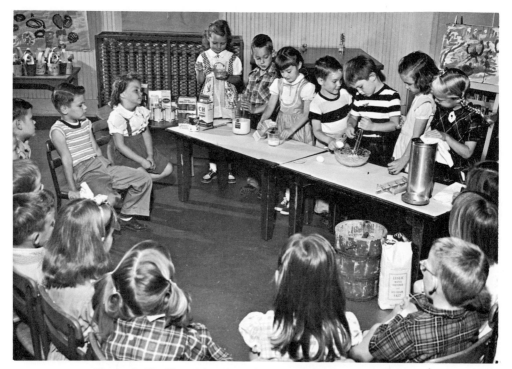

Figure 9-19 Materials galore. Making ice cream in Grade One.

decades ago who was concerned primarily with one textbook for each subject, the problem of selection, handling, and storage of these materials was relatively simple. However, with the increase in variety and quantity of instructional aids came the problem of their management. This has been resolved in some of the larger elementary schools by the organization of a resource or materials center — more recently called a media center.

Such a center is a vital force in the health instruction program, especially if one person is given the responsibility for its direction. Regardless of size, a few of the services which the center can offer classroom teachers and pupils are:

Make available a central source for all types of teaching materials.

Assist in locating and obtaining needed teaching aids.

Assist with the production of classroom materials.

Organize and keep current a file of all health instructional materials and equipment in the school building and a file of community resources.

Maintain equipment and materials in a good state of repair.

Inform teachers of new materials.

Organize in-service training in the use of equipment for pupils and teachers.

In an open plan school, whose hub is the media center, teaching is quite different. Each pupil chooses the medium which helps him learn best. Such flexibility in a center encourages real exploration, problem-solving projects and independent study.

QUESTIONS FOR DISCUSSION

1. Prepare a checklist of teaching aids, and survey one or two elementary schools to see how many of these aids are in use. Are they being employed in any unique way for health instruction?

2. Does there appear to be any one teaching method that works more effectively than others in the teaching of health at the elementary school level? Explain.

3. To what extent does the personality of the teacher influence the choice of educational method employed in health instruction?

4. In your opinion, what is the difference between seeing a good film dealing with the work of the heart or some other organ, and hearing an interesting broadcast on this function?

5. Do you see the health museum as influential in helping students form concepts of healthful living? Does it have more or less to offer than a well-run classroom program in school?

6. As a classroom teacher interested in health instruction, what value would there seem to be in coordinating the activities and materials of the community health agencies with those of the school?

SUGGESTED ACTIVITIES

1. Visit a curriculum library and look over several brands of health textbooks suitable for primary or intermediate grade pupils. Generally, the level of word difficulty and the pictures will approximate the age level of the pupils for which the text is intended. However, the content may vary considerably between brand books for a particular grade level. What are some of your specific observations?

2. Review an article or two about innovation in teaching. Are there ways of teaching that literally "turn kids on"? List the essential points set forth in the article you review; follow this up with your comments.

3. Seek out and read research data having to do with the effective use of health materials. Do you find evidence to suggest that media such as instructional television or tape recordings are more effective than the more traditional media?

4. Visit a media center that has been established to serve the many and varied needs of teachers in a school system. Find out how it functions and how regularly it is used by the elementary classroom teachers.

5. Observe the teaching method being practiced in an elementary school classroom. After the class is dismissed ask the teacher

why the particular method was chosen. Ask also if the method has replaced another method or has been changed at any time during the last year or two. In short, are teachers flexible in the use of methods?

6. Design an experiment to appraise the effects of three different methods of teaching on health behavior. The health topic and methods selected may be of your own choosing.

7. Plan and produce a short 8 mm film with children interested in a health topic. The short reference will be helpful.

SELECTED REFERENCES

Benningsohn, Lorraine. "A Kindergarten Resource Center." *School Health Review, 3:*26, December 1972.

Cox, Helen M. "Sex Education via Instructional Television." *Journal of Health, Physical Education, and Recreation, 37:*71–72, April 1966.

Cox, Mary Jane. "Environmental Awareness Projects for Children." *School Health Review, 3:*19–23, July-August 1972.

Erickson, Carlton W., and Curl, D. C. *Fundamentals of Teaching Audio-Visual Technology.* New York: Macmillan Co., 1972.

Fox, Willard. "Care and Feeding of Bulletin Boards." *Education, 83:*362–363, February 1963.

Funk, Hal D., and Olberg, Robert T. *Learning to Teach in the Elementary School.* New York: Dodd, Mead and Co., 1971.

Glasser, William. "Roles, Goals, and Failure." *Today's Education,* October 1971, p. 21.

Hainfield, Harold. "Home-made Mannequin for First Aid Classes." *Journal of Health, Physical Education, and Recreation, 37:*65–67, February 1966.

Healy, Mildred. "Thinking-Cap Creations." *Instructor, 82:*45–50, November 1972.

Hubbard, Nancy E. "Motivation for Health Learning: Taped 'Live Experience'." *Journal of School Health, 42:*548–550, November 1972.

Kinder, James S. *Using Audio-Visual Materials in Education.* New York: American Book Co., 1965.

Kohlberg, Lawrence. "Understanding the Hidden Curriculum." *Learning, 1:*10–12, December 1972.

Lacey, Richard A. *Seeing With Feeling: Film in the Classroom.* Philadelphia: W. B. Saunders Company, 1972.

Leigh, Terrance M. "Nationwide Profile of Health Instruction." *School Health Review, 4:*35–39, May-June 1973.

Mallan, John T., and Hersh, Richard. *No G.O.D.s in the Classroom.* Philadelphia: W. B. Saunders Company, 1972.

Mayshark, Cyrus, and Foster, Roy A. *Methods in Health Instruction: a Workbook Using the Critical Incident Technique.* St. Louis: C. V. Mosby Co., 1966.

McTaggart, Aubrey C. "The Readability of Health Textbooks." *Synthesis of Research in Selected Areas of Health Instruction.* The School Health Study, National Education Association, 1963, pp. 129–140.

Raths, Louis E. "Values in the Classroom." *National Education Association Journal, 56:*12–15, October 1967.

Raths, Louis E., Harmon, Merrill, and Simon, Sidney B. *Values and Teaching.* Columbus, Ohio: Charles E. Merrill Co., 1966.

Reichert, R. *Self Awareness Through Group Dynamics.* Dayton, Ohio: George A. Pflaum Co., 1970.

Schneider, Robert E. *Methods and Materials of Health Education,* 2nd Ed. Philadelphia: W. B. Saunders Company, 1964.

Shart, Philip A. "Sixth-Grade Filmmaking." *Instructor, 81:*43, June-July 1972.

Teaching Toward Inquiry. Washington: National Education Association, 1972.

Torrance, E. P., and Myers, R. E. *Creative Learning and Teaching.* New York: Dodd, Mead and Co., 1971.

Tuck, Miriam L. "Experimental Demonstration as a Method of Stimulating Learning." *Journal of School Health, 35:*172–175, April 1965.

VanTil, William. *Curriculum: Quest for Relevance.* Boston: Houghton Mifflin Co., 1971.

Ylvisaker, Paul N. "Beyond '72: Strategies for Schools." *Saturday Review,* November 11, 1972, p. 33.

10 SOURCES OF FREE AND INEXPENSIVE TEACHING AIDS

Today boys and girls acquire the practice at an early age of keeping up with what is happening in the world by seeing and hearing contemporary material—pamphlets, films, filmstrips, tape recordings and much more. And in the field of health a vast amount of good material is available. One of the reasons for this is that many organizations are interested in child health.

The health curriculum, having lost its old-fashioned rigidity, now employs a variety of health materials to supplement books and teacher lectures; this is a more practical means of recording and reporting the current scene. But it requires considerable work on the part of the teacher to locate and select these materials for classroom use. Even when there is a media center in the school, it is still helpful to have some knowledge of what is available and from what official, voluntary or commercial agency it may be obtained.

A number of organizations and agencies have educational consultants who are of real help to teachers, providing they have sufficient information to work with. When ordering materials, it is well to mention the age group to be served, the number of children in the class, the type of materials desired, and the special area of interest. Some companies or agencies will then go out of their way to

supply useful aids to learning. In fact, in several instances they will develop new materials if the teacher can show that there is a need for them.

The Reliability of Health Information

Teachers are becoming more and more aware of health materials and sources of health information. They are being exposed from all sides to a variety of pamphlets, booklets, and products designed to overcome health problems or, at least, to bear on mental and physical well-being. How reliable is this material? Is it loaded with advertising in order to sell a product?

Health information must be evaluated before it is used in the classroom. Ordinarily there is little reason to question the materials and aids of a well-known organization such as the American Red Cross or the American Medical Association. And there are numerous commercial organizations that conscientiously promote health as their primary purpose, followed by the promotion of their own product. This is well demonstrated by the fact that it is sometimes difficult to find the name of the commercial organization or its product on the school health literature.

The evaluation of health information, whether it is read, heard, or seen, may be determined in part by appraising the publisher, association, or agency. One might ask the following questions:

Is the agency recognized as having a good reputation in the field of health?

Why has the health information been presented?

Is the purpose of the communication to give facts on which to base personal opinion and beliefs? To improve living?

Is the purpose to sell specific products or ideas without reference to the scientific value of the product?

Is the purpose simply to entertain?

What are the qualifications of the specific author?

Is the material up to date?

What is the opinion of others, such as medical experts, public or private agencies, and reliable friends familiar with the topic?

OFFICIAL HEALTH AGENCIES

Organizations that have been established by law to accomplish specific health maintenance, promotion, and control are generally designated as official health agencies. These include city, county, state, and Federal government organizations. Very often a wealth of free teaching aids is available from these groups:

City and County Health Departments—Child health material in the form of pamphlets for teacher use. Films and certain poster material may also be on hand.

State Health Departments—In almost every state there is much in the way of child and teacher health pamphlets, monthly magazines or bulletins, films, special health exhibits, and speakers available for school use. In addition to this, several states publish catalogs dealing specifically with health education sources of materials and selected audiovisual aids.

State Universities—In many states the unit of the state university having to do with public health or school health provides pamphlets, bulletins, and special charts for school use within the state. Other institutions, such

as Indiana University, Syracuse University, or Boston University, have an extensive division which supplies a wide variety of audiovisual aids. Sample materials are generally available for out-of-state use.

Federal Government—

Department of Health, Education, and Welfare Office of Education Washington, D.C. 20025	Special booklets, primarily for teacher use, on food, alcohol, drugs, environmental pollution, consumer health, prevention and control of illness. Lists of materials are available with no charge for single copies.

General Services Administration—

National Archives and Records Service National Audiovisual Center Washington, D.C. 20409	Extensive list of films on all major health problems. For rent or sale. Extensive material on smoking research and smoking education programs.
National Interagency on Smoking and Health P.O. Box 3650 Arlington, Virginia 22203	Program materials relative to drug abuse; for school and community use.
National Coordinating Council on Drug Abuse P.O. Box 19400, Washington, D.C. 20036	
Superintendent of Documents U.S. Government Printing Office Washington, D.C. 20025	Considerable health information for teacher use which may be adapted to healthful school living and health teaching. A

	catalog should be secured before materials are ordered.
U.S. Public Health Service Washington, D C. 20201	This organization has many health interests including the National Institutes of Health, health research, statistics, and promotion.
U.S Children's Bureau Division of Reports Washington D C. 20025	Numerous catalogs, child health pamphlets, and lists.
The United Nations World Health Organization Geneva, Switzerland (or New York, N.Y. 20006)	A large number of picture booklets dealing with world health conditions. Useful in studying community health and social studies.

NON-OFFICIAL HEALTH AGENCIES

In almost every American community there are groups of citizens banded together for the express purpose of promoting health. Generally their interest is centered on some special disease or abnormality such as malnutrition, tuberculosis, mental illness, heart disease, or crippled children. These groups are, without a doubt, in a position to be of immense service to the schoolteacher if the teacher will call upon them.

Non-official agencies generally include *voluntary health agencies, commercial organizations,* and *professional associations.* Their scope of influence is great and includes health education services for the entire community, its industries, and its schools. If the agency is a state or national one, its sphere of influence is almost unlimited.

With the tremendous growth in the number of charitable institutions and foundations in this country over the last quarter century, it is becoming increasingly difficult to differentiate between a purely voluntary health organization and a professional association. Many voluntary health organizations began at the local level with a handful of volunteers and blossomed through the years into full-fledged national groups with considerable professional zeal. In any case, both categories of organization exist to help in any way they can.

The staff and members of these citizen and professional worker groups help the schools enrich curricula, add resources, carry on research, and improve the school health programs. The schools in turn offer to these agencies an excellent channel for working towards personal and community health. Certainly there are common goals; "child health is everybody's business." Moreover, there are common activities involving the home and the school. Some of the agency activities include:

Making available to school personnel the latest health information.

Providing teaching aids.

Helping in the preparation of resource units.

Helping with special short-term projects.

Helping with in-service education of teachers.

Providing the means for demonstrations and studies.

Enriching the curriculum.

Interpreting the school health program and needs of the community.

Helping in interpretation to the parents.

Voluntary and Professional Health Agencies

A selected number of the more productive voluntary and professional health agencies that have proven to be of immeasurable service to elementary teachers are as follows:

Alcoholics Anonymous, 305 E. 45th Street, New York, N.Y. 10017.

American Academy of Pediatrics, 1801 Hinmon Avenue, Box 1034, Evanston, Ill. 60204.

American Association for Health, Physical Education, and Recreation, Department of the National Education Association, 1201 16th Street, N.W., Washington, D.C. 20036.

American Association of Poison Control Center, c/o Academy of Medicine of Cleveland, 10525 Carnegie Ave., Cleveland, Ohio 44106.

American Cancer Society, 219 E. 42nd Street, New York, N.Y. 10017.

American Dental Association, 211 E. Chicago Avenue, Chicago, Ill. 60611.

American Foundation for the Blind, 15 W. 16th Street, New York, N.Y. 10011.

American Hearing Society, 919 18th Street, N.W., Washington, D.C. 20006.

American Heart Association, 44 E. 23rd Street, New York, N.Y. 10010.

American Hospital Association, 840 N. Lake Shore Drive, Chicago, Ill. 60611.

American Institute of Family Relations, 5287 Sunset Boulevard, Los Angeles, Calif. 90027.

American Medical Association, 535 N. Dearborn Street, Chicago, Ill. 60610.

American Optometric Association, Department of Public Affairs, 700 Chippewa Street, St. Louis, Mo. 63119.

American Public Health Association, 1790 Broadway, New York, N.Y. 10019.

American National Red Cross, 17th and D Streets, N.W., Washington, D.C. 20006. (Contact local chapters for materials.)

American School Health Association, 515 E. Main Street, Kent, Ohio 44241.

American Social Health Association, 1740 Broadway, New York, N.Y. 10019.

Arthritis Foundation, 10 Columbus Circle, New York, N.Y. 10019.

Better Vision Institute, 630 Fifth Avenue, New York, N.Y. 10020.

Child Study Association of America, 132 E. 74th Street, New York, N.Y. 10021.

Cleveland Health Museum, 8911 Euclid Avenue, Cleveland, Ohio 44106.

Hogg Foundation for Mental Health, University of Texas, Austin, Tex. 78712.

Muscular Dystrophy Associations of America, 1790 Broadway, New York, N.Y. 10019.

National Association of Hearing and Speech Agencies, 919 18th Street, N.W., Washington, D.C. 20006.

National Association for Mental Health, Inc., 1800 North Kent St., Rosslyn, Virginia 22209.

National Congress of Parents and Teachers, 700 N. Rush Street, Chicago, Ill. 60637.

National Education Association, Division of Elementary Education, 1201 16th Street, N.W., Washington, D.C. 20036.

National Foundation, 800 Second Avenue, New York, N.Y. 10017.

National Multiple Sclerosis Society, 257 Park Avenue South, New York, N.Y. 10010.

National Nutrition Education Clearing House, P.O. Box 931, Berkeley, Calif. 94701.

National Recreation Association, 8 W. 8th Street, New York, N.Y. 10011.

National Safety Council, 425 N. Michigan Avenue, Chicago, Ill. 60611.

National Society for Crippled Children and Adults, Inc., 2023 W. Ogden Avenue, Chicago, Ill. 60603.

National Society for the Prevention of Blindness, Inc., 79 Madison Avenue, New York, N.Y. 10016.

National Tuberculosis and Respiratory Disease Association, P.O. Box 500, Boston, Mass. 02117.

Nutrition Foundation, Inc., 99 Park Avenue, New York, N.Y. 10016.

Planned Parenthood Federation of America, Inc., 515 Madison Avenue, New York, N.Y. 10022.

Public Affairs Committee, 381 Park Avenue South, New York, N.Y. 10016.

Rutgers Center for Alcohol Studies, The State University, Rutgers, New Brunswick, N.J.

Sex Education and Information Council of U.S. (SEICUS), 1855 Broadway, New York, N.Y. 10023.

United Cerebral Palsy Associations, Inc., 321 W. 44th Street, New York, N.Y. 10017.

Commercial Organizations and Associations of Industry

There are many business and commercial agencies which publish materials especially fitted for elementary school use. The list of individual industries that offer printed matter is a long one. It is customary today for practically every commercial organization to promote its product through bulletins, brochures, posters, and other advertising media. Many of these companies have suitable products that are legitimate in terms of health promotion. In the area of foods there are a number of firms that sell a healthful product and employ sound health teaching techniques to promote it. There are also a large number of companies which promote a valid health concept as a public service item. For instance, a company promoting dental health through charts, leaflets, and films puts over a basic idea. This in turn is good business for it sells more dental products. When people buy more dental products, this is an indication that their health behavior has been favorably changed. In view of this, a number of commercial firms in several areas have formed their own associations. These associations of industry make available, often in unlimited quantity, a number of health items for the classroom teacher to use with her pupils.

There follows a partial list of national sources of especially reliable and generous companies and associations of industry. No attempt is made here to list specific materials offered by these sources, but in many cases catalogs are available, and in most cases the name of the agency will indicate to some extent the subject matter and scope of its material.

Aetna Life Affiliated Companies, Education Department, 151 Farmington Avenue, Hartford, Conn. 06115. Leaflets and motion pictures on safety for teachers and pupils, special tests.

American Automobile Association, Traffic Safety Department, 1712 G. Street, N.W., Washington, D.C. 20036. Pamphlets and films on traffic safety; also safety project materials.

American Bakers Association, Public Relations Department, 1700 Pennsylvania Avenue, N.W., Washington, D.C. 20036. Booklets on bread for intermediate grades. Contact state bakers associations for additional materials.

American Institute of Baking, Consumer Service Department, 400 E. Ontario Street, Chicago, Ill. 60611. Pamphlets, posters, self-testing charts, colorful guides to eating, record forms.

American Insurance Association, Safety Department, 85 John Street, New York, N.Y. 10038.

Armour and Company, Public Relations Department, 401 N. Wabash Street, Chicago, Ill. 60690. Maps, charts on foods.

Association of American Soap and Glycerine Products, Inc., Cleanliness Bureau, 295 Madison Avenue, New York, N. Y. Pamphlets, posters, radio and TV scripts.

Athletic Institute, 805 Merchandise Mart, Chicago, Ill. 60650.

Behavioral Research Laboratories, Box 577, Palo Alto, Calif. 94300.

Bicycle Institute of America, 122 E. 42nd Street, New York, N.Y. 10017.

The Borden Company, The Borden Building, 350 Madison Avenue, New York, N.Y. 10017. Pamphlets on milk values and uses.

Cereal Institute, Inc., Educational Director, 135 S. LaSalle Street, Chicago, Ill. 60603. Classroom teaching units, food charts, and graphs.

Colgate Palmolive Company, 740 North Rush St., Chicago, Illinois 60611. Toothbrushing kits and dental health teaching materials.

Colorado Wheat Administrative Commission, Mr. Dwayne E. Williams, Administrator, 1636 Welton Street, Denver, Colorado 80202.

Connecticut Bakers Association, Mrs. Lee Silva, Secretary, 85 Belcher Road, Wethersfield, Connecticut 06109. (Honors requests from Connecticut only.)

Cream of Wheat Corporation, Box M, Minneapolis, Minn. 55413. Educational Activities Inc., Box 392, Freeport, N.Y. 11520. Action records for physical fitness and rhythmics.

David C. Cook, Elgin, Illinois 60120. Charts and posters covering major health topics.

Educational Activities, Freeport, New York 11520. Variety of health records and filmstrips.

Eli Lilly and Company, Indianapolis, Indiana 46206. Materials on safety and control of infectious diseases.

Employers Mutuals of Wausau, 407 Grant Street, Wausau, Wisc. 55402.

Encyclopaedia Britannica Educational Corporation, Britannica Building, 425 N. Michigan Avenue, Wilmette, Ill. 60611. Filmstrips, slide films, movies, cartoons, and records. (Rentals only.)

Evaporated Milk Association, 910 17th Street, N.W., Washington, D.C. 20036. Flash cards, graphs, and leaflets on milk equivalent values.

Films Incorporated, Public Relations Department, 1150 Wilmette Avenue, Wilmette, Ill. Cartoons and catalogs for all age levels.

Florida Citrus Commission, P.O. Box 148, Lakeland, Fla. 33802. Posters, pamphlets, movies on citrus fruits.

Ford Motor Company, Information Department, Dearborn, Mich. 48127. Traffic safety materials.

General Mills, Inc., Education Section, 9200 Wayzata Boulevard, Minneapolis, Minn. 55426. Nutrition education teaching aids.

Gillette Company, Toiletries Division, 100 Charles River Plaza, Boston, Mass. 02114.

H. J. Heinz Company, P.O. Box 28, D-32, Pittsburgh, Pa. 15230. Food charts and stories of origin of various foods.

Indiana Bakers Association, Mr. Ferd A. Doll, Secretary, 1941 E. 30th Street, Indianapolis, Indiana 46218. (Honors requests from Indiana only.)

International Education and Training, Inc., Box GT-10, 1776 New Highway, Farmington, N. Y. 11735.

Johnson & Johnson, Educational Division, New Brunswick, N.J. 08903. Charts, pamphlets, films on first aid and safety, and programmed instruction first aid for grade six.

Kansas Wheat Commission, Mr. G. C. Fowler, Administrator, 1021 N. Main Street, Hutchinson, Kansas 67501.

Kellogg Company, Department of Home Economics Services, Battle Creek, Mich. 49016. Breakfast food pamphlets and charts.

Kimberly-Clark Corporation, Educational Department, Neenah, Wis. 54947. Menstrual physiology chart and films; pamphlets, guides on common cold.

Kraft Cheese Company, 500 Peshtigo Court, Chicago, Ill. 60690. Nutrition items.

Lederle Laboratories Division, American Cyanamid Co., Pearl River, N.Y. 10965. Child health and nutrition.

Licenced Beverage Industries, Inc., 155 E. 44th Street, New York, N.Y. 10017.

Metropolitan Life Insurance Company, Health and Welfare Division, 1 Madison Avenue, New York, N.Y. 10010. Catalogs, exhibits, films, filmstrips, booklets for teachers on all diseases and the school health instruction program; health bulletin for teachers.

Missouri Bakers Association, Mr. Louis F. O'Konski, Jr., Secretary, 1016 Central Street, Kansas City, Missouri 64105. (Honors requests from Missouri only.)

Money Management Institute, Prudential Plaza, Chicago, Ill. 60601. Consumer health materials.

National Board of Fire Underwriters, 85 John Street, New York, N.Y. 10038.

National Dairy Council, Program Service Department, 111 N. Canal Street, Chicago, Ill. 60606. Health education materials, exhibits, films, filmstrips, displays, animals for feeding experiments. Local chapters are rich in materials especially suited for primary and intermediate grades; health bulletins for teachers.

National Fire Protection Association, Public Relations Department, 60 Batterymarch Street, Boston, Mass. 02110. Posters, pamphlets, safety lists, comics, fire inspection blanks, charts, quizzes.

National Livestock and Meat Board, 36 S. Wabash Avenue, Chicago, Ill. 60603. Self-testing charts, food graphs, colored posters of the various cuts of meat, pamphlets on food values of meat.

National Social Welfare Assembly, Inc., 345 E. 46th Street, New York, N.Y. 10017. Health comic books.

North Dakota State Wheat Commission, Mr. Paul E. R. Abrahamson, Administrator, 316 N. Fifth Street, Bismarck, North Dakota 58501.

Ocean Spray Cranberries, Inc., Executive Offices, Hanson, Mass. 02341. Pamphlets, films, food recipes, and food record charts.

Pennsylvania Bakers Association, Mr. Robert H. Maurer, Secretary, 407 N. Front Street, Harrisburg, Pa. 17101. (Honors requests from Pennsylvania only.)

Personal Products Company, Milltown, N. J. 08850. Charts, posters, leaflets regarding menstruation.

Pet Milk Co., 1406 Arcade Building, St. Louis, Mo. 63101. Nutrition pamphlets and charts.

Pharmaceutical Manufacturers Association, 1155 15th Street, N.W., Washington, D.C. 20005. Films and booklets on general health topics.

The Procter and Gamble Company, P.O. Box 171, Cincinnati, Ohio 45201. Booklets and materials for dental health. Several excellent posters in color.

Scott Paper Company, Home Service Center, Philadelphia, Pa. 19113. Menstrual health pamphlets.

Sealtest Foods Consumer Service, 605 3rd Avenue, New York, N.Y. 10016. Food charts and graphs.

South Dakota Wheat Commission, Mr. August Snyder, Executive Director, P.O. Box 549, Pierre, South Dakota 57501.

Stanley Bowmar Company, Inc., Valhalla, N. Y. 10595. Records for creative activities and rhythmics.

Sunkist Growers, Box 2706, Sunkist Building, Los Angeles, Calif. 90054. Teaching units on nutrition, posters, pamphlets.

Swift and Co., Union Stockyards, Chicago, Ill. 60609.

Tampax, Incorporated, Educational Director, 5 Dakota Drive, Lake Success, New York 11045. Anatomical charts, student pamphlets, and special instruction materials for teachers on the subject of menstruation.

Texas Gulf Bakers Council, Mr. Robert H. Ruhe, Exec. Dir., P. O. Box 11125, Houston, Texas 77016. (Honors requests from Texas only.)

The Travelers Insurance Company, Hartford, Conn. 06115. Charts on growth, height-weight, and posture, and several colorful posters.

United Fresh Fruit and Vegetable Association, 777 14th Street, N.W., Washington, D.C. 20005. Leaflets on foods for elementary level.

United States Beet Sugar Association, Tower Building, Washington, D.C. Teaching kits and charts.

J. Weston Walch Publisher, Portland, Maine 04104.

Washington Wheat Commission, Mr. Wayne B. Gentry, Administrator, 409 Great Western Building, Spokane, Washington 99201.

Wheat Flour Institute, Supervisor of Distribution, 14 E. Jackson Boulevard, Chicago, Ill. 60604. Posters, filmstrips, pamphlets, and catalogs pertaining to nutritious breakfast foods.

SOURCES OF AIDS FOR HEALTH TEACHING UNITS

A list of sources of health teaching materials for a major area of study cannot contain every known aid, nor would one want it to, because some sources are better than others for teaching a certain health topic. The teacher's time is at a premium, and following up several leads to sources takes time. It is the purpose of the author, therefore, to limit the following list to those sources of *teaching aids which have proved to be especially valuable in the health instruction program in the elementary schools.*[1] All sources listed are for the students to read or see themselves. They have been carefully selected with this in mind.

---

[1] For additional sources see *Educator's Guide to Free Films, Filmstrips, Transcriptions, Tapes and Scripts*, Educators Progress Services, Randolph, Wis. (annual).

The sources are set up by health topics which are in keeping with the major activity areas referred to in Chapter 8. The type of teaching aid (i.e., film, pamphlet, poster), the specific name of the aid, and the name of the agency supplying it are listed.

1. Personal Cleanliness and Appearance*

a. Pamphlets or Leaflets

Everybody Smile, American Dental Association.
Facts about Vision, American Optometric Association.
Hearing Is Priceless — Protect It, American Hearing Society.
It's Smart to Protect your Sight, U.S. Public Health Service.
Only One Pair of Ears for Life, American Hearing Society.
Professor Ludwig Von Drake's IQ, National Society for the Prevention of Blindness.
Signs of Eye Trouble in Children, National Society for the Prevention of Blindness.
Sunglasses, National Society for the Prevention of Blindness.
Take Care of Your Eyes, National Society for the Prevention of Blindness.
The Eye in Sight, American Optometric Association.
The Language of Light, National Society for the Prevention of Blindness.
The Little Seeing Book, Pharmaceutical Manufacturers Association.
The Story of Soap, Procter and Gamble Company.

b. Films**

Alexander Has A Good Day, Coronet Instructional Films.
A More Attractive You, Modern Talking Picture Service.
Body Care and Grooming, McGraw-Hill Book Company.
Care of the Hair and Nails, Encyclopaedia Britannica.
Care of the Skin, Encyclopaedia Britannica.
Choosing Clothes for Health, Coronet Instructional Films.
Cleanliness and Health, Coronet Instructional Films.
Eyes and Their Care, Encyclopaedia Britannica.
Hear Better: Healthy Ears, Coronet Instructional Films.
Health: The Dirt Witch Cleans Up, Encyclopedia Britannica.
How Billy Keeps Clean, Coronet Instructional Films.

How the Ear Functions, Knowledge Builders.
Joan Avoids a Cold, Coronet Instructional Films.
Johnny's New World, National Society for the Prevention of Blindness.
Kitty Keeps Clean, Young America Films.
Let's be Clean and Neat, Coronet Instructional Films.
Platform Posture, Young America Films.
Running for Sheriff, Charles Cahill and Associates.
See Better: Healthy Eyes, Coronet Instructional Films.
The Doctor Is Your Friend, National Tuberculosis Association.
Ways to Good Habits, Coronet Instructional Films.
Your Cleanliness, Young America Films.
Your Ears, Young America Films.
Your Eyes, Young America Films.
Your Friend the Doctor, Coronet Instructional Films.
Your Health at School, Coronet Instructional Films.
Your Teeth, Young America Films.

c. Filmstrips

Care of the Hair and Nails (Health story), Encyclopaedia Britannica.
Care of the Skin (Health story), Encyclopaedia Britannica.
Health Habits (Health story), Encyclopaedia Britannica.
Healthy, Happy, and Wise, Popular Science.
How Your Ears Work, Popular Science.
Keeping Clean, McGraw-Hill Book Company.
Keeping Well, McGraw-Hill Book Company.
Keeping Well and Happy, National Tuberculosis Association.
Let's Stand Tall, Society for Visual Education.
Neat Is a Girl's World, Gillette Company.
Neat Is Not a Dirty Word, Gillette Company.
Protecting Our Eyes and Ears, McGraw-Hill Book Company.
Special Senses, Keystone View Co.
The Ears, Young America Films.
The Eyes, Young America Films.
The Science of Personal Appearance, McGraw-Hill Book Company.
This Is You, Encyclopaedia Britannica.
You and Your Clothes, Young America Films.
You and Your Ears, Encyclopaedia Britannica.
Your Eyes at Work, Popular Science.
Your Skin and Its Care, Popular Science.

d. Posters

Be Fair — Cover Your Coughs and Sneezes, National Tuberculosis Association.
How to Catch a Cold, Kimberly-Clark Corporation.
Only One Pair of Ears for Life, American Hearing Society.
Physical Fitness Posters, National Dairy Council.
Reading Takes Seeing, American Optometric Association.
School Time, Vision Exam Time, American Optometric Association.

---

*Includes the care of the special senses.
**The addresses of film and filmstrip sources may be found on page 370.

Seeing and Hearing, American Medical Association.

To Fight Germs—Wash Your Hands, National Tuberculosis Association.

Wash Thoroughly, National Safety Council.

e. Charts

Cross Section of the Eye, National Society for the Prevention of Blindness.

One Out of Four Children Needs Eye Care, National Society for the Prevention of Blindness.

Singer Picture Story Study Prints, Society of Visual Education.

Snellen, Symbol E Charts, National Society for the Prevention of Blindness.

The Ivory Inspection Patrol, Procter and Gamble.

f. Radio Scripts

(From University of Texas, Bureau of Research in Education by Radio)
Care of the Skin
Cleanliness
Importance of Good Vision
We Wash Our Hands Before We Eat

g. Tape Recordings

Health Is Wealth (HC15), New York State University College of Agriculture, Cornell University, Ithaca, N.Y.

Are We Responsible for Our Own Good Health? Audio-Visual Aids Service, University of Illinois.

h. Selected Stories for Children

(P) Primary Level, (I) Intermediate Level

About Glasses for Gladys (I), Mary K. Erickson (Melmont).

All Ready for Winter (P), Leone Adelson (McKay).

Health Can Be Fun (P), Munro Leaf (Lippincott).

Lesson in Loveliness (I), J. W. Scott (Macrae, Smith).

Look at Your Eyes (I), Paul Showers (Crowell).

Manners Can Be Fun (P), Munro Leaf (Lippincott).

Nothing to Wear but Clothes (I), F. K. Jupo (Aladdin).

Our Insect Friends and Foes (I), W. A. Dupuy (Winston).

Our Senses and How They Work (I), H. Zimm (Morrow).

Our Wonderful Eyes (P), J. Perry (McGraw-Hill).

Somebody Called Boo (P), L. Gardner (Watts).

Story of Your Coat (P,I), Clara Hollos (International Publishing Co.)

The Clean Pig (P), Leonard Weisgard (Scribner).

Tim and His Hearing Aid (I), E. C. Ronnei and Joan and Max Porter (Dodd).

Time Out for Living (P), D. E. Patridge and C. Mooney (American Book).

True Book of Health (P), O. U. Haynes (Children's Press).

World of Invisible Life (I), Mary Stephenson (Wilcox and Follet).

You and Your Senses (I), L. Schneider (Harcourt).

Your Ears (I), Irving and Ruth Adler (John Day).

Your Eyes, (I), Irving and Ruth Adler (John Day).

Your Manners Are Showing (I), D. Betz (Grossett).

2. Activity, Sleep, Rest, and Relaxation

a. Pamphlets or Leaflets

A Boy and His Physique, National Dairy Council.

A Girl and Her Figure, National Dairy Council.

A Girl and Her Figure and You, National Dairy Council.

Eat and Grow, Evaporated Milk Association.

Fit for Fun, American Medical Association.

Exercise and Fitness, American Medical Association.

How to Get in Shape—and Stay There, Florida Citrus Commission.

Johnny Makes the Team, American Medical Association.

Letters to Tony, Evaporated Milk Association.

Physical Fitness, U.S. Government Printing Office.

Relax! You're a Bundle of Nerves, The Borden Company.

Seven Paths to Fitness, American Medical Association.

What the Classroom Teacher Should Know and Do about Children with Heart Disease, American Heart Association.

Working and Playing, Evaporated Milk Association.

b. Films

America Goes Camping, Bicycle Institute of America.

American Square Dance, Coronet Instructional Films.

Day at the Fair, Coronet Instructional Films.

Dress for Health, Encyclopaedia Britannica.

Exercise and Health, Coronet Instructional Films.

Fun That Builds Good Health, Coronet Instructional Films.

How the Body Uses Energy, McGraw-Hill Book Company.

Improving Your Posture, Coronet Instructional Films.

Physical Fitness and Good Health, Walt Disney Productions.

Play in the Snow, Encyclopaedia Britannica.

Playtown U.S.A., The Athletic Institute.

Safety: Playground Spirits, Encyclopaedia Britannica.

Ski the Outer Limits, Bicycle Institute of America.

Sleep for Health, Encyclopaedia Britannica.

Water Safety, Young America Films.

You and Your Helpers, Coronet Instructional Films.

Your Child's Health and Fitness, AAHPER, Washington, D.C. 20036.

Your Exercise and Posture, Coronet Instructional Films.

c. Filmstrips

At Home in the Evening, Popular Science.

Checking Your Health, Encyclopaedia Britannica.

Exercise for Happy Living, Encyclopaedia Britannica.

Getting Ready for Bed, Popular Science.

Learning About Growth and Exercise, Encyclopaedia Britannica.

Learning About Sleep and Rest, Encyclopaedia Britannica.

Rest and Sleep, McGraw-Hill Book Company.

Rest and Sleep, Young America Films.

Sleep and Rest, Popular Science.

Sleep for Health, Encyclopaedia Britannica.

The Muscular System, Encyclopaedia Britannica.

The Skeletal System, Encyclopaedia Britannica.

Working and Playing Together, McGraw-Hill Book Company.

d. Posters

A Day with the Wide Awakes, General Mills, Inc.

Health Is Not Just Luck, General Mills, Inc.

Keep Physically Fit, Florida Citrus Commission.

Lift with Your Legs, Not Your Back, American Medical Association.

Physical Fitness, American Medical Association.

Physical Fitness (4), Educational Activities, Inc.

Physical Fitness (9 posters), National Dairy Council.

Physical Fitness Posters (4), Stanley Bowmar Co.

Sleep Tonight for Pep Tomorrow, National Tuberculosis Association.

We Help You Keep Fit, Florida Citrus Commission.

e. Charts

Ball Handling Skills, Athletic Institute, Chicago, Ill. 60654.

Day to Day Good Health Records, Kellogg Company.

Your Heart and How It Works, American Heart Association.

f. Radio Scripts

Batter Up, National Safety Council.

Fresh Air and Sunshine, Bureau of Research in Education by Radio, University of Texas.

Sleep and Rest, Bureau of Research in Education by Radio, University of Texas.

Swimming Is Fun, National Safety Council.

Vacation Daze, National Safety Council.

g. Comics

The Adventures of Eva, Pora, and Ted, Evaporated Milk Association.

h. Records

Another Rainy Day Record, Educational Activities.

Around the World in Dance, Educational Activities.

Classroom Rhythms, Stanley Bowmar Co.

Exercise Every Day, Educational Activities.

Honor Your Partner Records, Educational Activities, Inc.

Let's Do Some Posture Exercises, Educational Activities.

Lullabies for Sleepy Heads, Dorothy Olsen, RCA Victor.

Modern Square Dancing, Stanley Bowmar Co.

Music for Relaxation, Melochrino Strings, RCA Victor.

Play Party-Singing Games, Stanley Bowmar Co.

Physical Fitness Activities, Album 14, Primary Grades (Durlacher), Stanley Bowmar Co.

Rhythms and Game Songs, Stanley Bowmar Co.

Rhythmic Play Series (K-3), Educational Record Sales.

The Sleepy Family (A35), Children's Record Center, 2858 W. Pico Boulevard, Los Angeles, Calif.

Toy Shop Album (A4—Grades 1–6), Activity Records.

Why Do I Have to Go to Sleep? (P156), Children's Record Center.

i. Selected Stories for Children

(P) Primary Level, (I) Intermediate Level

Bedtime for Frances (P), H. Hoban (Harper and Bros.).

Boo, Who Used to Be Scared of the Dark (P), Munro Leaf (Random House).

Child's Good Night Book (P), Margaret Wise Brown (W. R. Scott).

Child's Treasury of Things to Do (P), Caroline Horowitz (Hart).

Do You Move As I Do? (P), Helen Borten (Abelard).

Forty Rainy Day Games and Plan Alone Fun (P), Caroline Horowitz (Hart).

Going to Camp (P,I), Helen Beck (Daye).

Health Can Be Fun (P), Munro Leaf (Lippincott).

Hustle and Bustle (P), Louis Slobodkin (Macmillan).

Jimmy's Own Basketball (I), M. B. Renick (Scribner).

Joey Gets the Golf Bug (I), J. Sherman (Little, Brown).

Lifeline (I), L. Schneider (Harcourt).

Mr. Tall and Mr. Small (I), Barbara Brenner (W. R. Scott).

Not Bad for a Girl (I), Isabella Taues (M. Evans).

Shotput Challenge (I), Berman Lord (Walck).

Sleepy ABC (P), Margaret Wise Brown (Lothrop).

Switch on the Night (P), R. Bradbury (Pantheon).

The Dream Book (P), Margaret Wise Brown (Random House).

Time for Sleep (I), Millicent Selsam (W. R. Scott).

Touchdown for Tommy (I), M. Christopher (Little, Brown).

While Susie Sleeps (P), Nina Scheider (W. R. Scott).

Who's Afraid of Thunder? (I), H. E. Sandman (Sterling).

3. Nutrition and Growth

a. Pamphlets or Leaflets

A Guide to Better Nutrition, H. J. Heinz Company.

A Nutrition Guide, General Mills, Inc.

Animals That Give People Milk, National Dairy Council.

Better Breakfast Activities, Cereal Institute, Inc.

Breakfast Your Way to a Better Day, Kellogg Company.

Breakfast Cereals Part of Modern Life, Cereal Institute.

Build a Better You With Fresh Citrus, Sunkist Growers.

Cereals a Food for Today, Cereal Institute.

Citrus as Aid to Health and Beauty, Florida Citrus Commission.

Citrus Fruit And Nutrition, Florida Citrus Commission.

Can Food Make the Difference?, American Medical Association.

Citrus Industry Story, Sunkist Growers.

Cooking Is Fun, National Dairy Council.

Cranberries, Ocean Spray Cranberries, Inc.

Eat a Good Breakfast, Kellogg Company.

Eat a Good Breakfast to Start a Good Day, Cereal Institute, Inc.

Eat and Grow, General Mills, Inc.

Eat to Live, Wheat Flour Institute.

Elementary School Nutrition, National Livestock and Meat Board.

Enriched Bread, American Institute of Baking.

Facts About Cereals and Good Nutrition, Cereal Institute.

Facts about Evaporated Milk, Evaporated Milk Association.

Facts About Foods, H. J. Heinz Co.

Facts about Nutrition (PHSP-917), U.S. Public Health Service.

Foods for Growing Boys and Girls, Kellogg Company.

Foods to Grow On, National Livestock and Meat Board.

Foodway to Follow, American Institute of Baking.

Fresh Citrus for Vitamin C, Sunkist Growers.

From Flour to Bread, Kansas Wheat Commission.

Fruit and Vegetable Facts and Pointers on Nutrition, United Fresh Fruit and Vegetable Association.

Functions of Food in Nutrition, National Livestock and Meat Board.

Hello U.S.A., National Dairy Council.

How to Conduct a Rat Feeding Experiment, Wheat Flour Institute.

How Much Do You Know About Bread?, American Bakers Association.

How Your Body Uses Food, National Dairy Council.

Ice Cream Is Good, National Dairy Council.

If You Think Breakfast Is for the Birds — Think Again, Cereal Institute.

It's Smart to Eat Breakfast, Kellogg Company.

Jane and Jimmy Learn about Fresh Fruits and Vegetables, United Fresh Fruit and Vegetable Association.

Light and Lively — Low-Fat Milk, Sealtest Foods.

Maybe I'll Be a Milkman, National Dairy Council.

Meal Planning Guide, Pet, Inc.

Meat Builds Better Breakfasts, National Livestock and Meat Board.

Meat Snacks for Better Health, National Livestock and Meat Board.

My Friend the Cow, National Dairy Council.

Nutrition Aids Grade One Through Eight, Kellogg Company.

Nutrition Information Test (Grade 3), General Mills, Inc.

Nutrition Information Test (Grades 4, 5, 6), General Mills, Inc.

Our Bread and Butter, in Pioneer Days and Today, National Dairy Council.

Our Food — Where It Comes From, National Dairy Council.

Pick a Breakfast Pattern, Cereal Institute.

School Lunch, National Dairy Council.

—Some Foods Just Go Together, Sealtest Foods.

Teaching About Meat, National Livestock and Meat Board.

The Grains Are Great Foods, Kellogg Company.

The Nutrition Ladder, Florida Citrus Commission.

The School That Learned to Eat, General Mills, Inc.

The Story of the Cereal Grains, General Mills, Inc.

The Story of Food Preservation, H. J. Heinz Company.

Toast Talk, American Institute of Baking.

Tots at the Table, National Livestock and Meat Board.

Uncle Jim's Dairy Farm, National Dairy Council.

Vitamin Supplements and Their Correct Use, American Medical Association.

What Did You Have for Breakfast This Morning?, National Dairy Council.

What's on Your Table?, Aetna Life Affiliated Companies.

What Is a Balanced Diet?, Sealtest Foods.

Wild Bill Hickock Breakfast Games, Kellogg Company.

You and Your Engine, National Livestock and Meat Board.

Your Daily Bread, American Bakers Association.

b. Films

Better Breakfasts, U.S.A., Cereal Institutes, Inc.

Big Dinner Table, National Dairy Council.

Dairy — Farm to Door, Charles Cahill and Associates.

Digestion of Foods, Encyclopaedia Britannica.

Eat for Health, Encyclopaedia Britannica.

Food, Energy and You, National Dairy Council.

Food and Growth, Encyclopaedia Britannica.

Food Stores, Encyclopaedia Britannica.

Food, the Color of Life, National Dairy Council.

Foods That Build Good Health, Coronet Instructional Films.

Foundation Foods, Avis Films, Inc.

Fundamentals of Diet, Encyclopaedia Britannica.

Good Eating Habits, Coronet Instructional Films.

Good Table Manners, Coronet Instructional Films.

Growing Up Day by Day, Encyclopaedia Britannica.

Journey Into Nutrition, Indiana University Audio-Visual Center.

Judy Learns About Milk, Young America Films.

Health — You and Your Helpers, Charles Cahill and Associates.

Learning About Foods We Eat, Coronet Films.

Milk, Encyclopaedia Britannica.
Save Those Teeth, Encyclopaedia Britannica.
Something You Didn't Eat, Association Films.
Something You Didn't Eat, U.S. Department of Agriculture.
The Best Way to Eat, Florida Citrus Commission.
The King Who Came to Breakfast, Association Films.
The Wheat Farmer, Encyclopaedia Britannica.
Two Little Rats, National Dairy Council.
Uncle Jim's Dairy Farm, National Dairy Council.
Understanding Vitamins, Encyclopaedia Britannica.
Vegetables for All Seasons, Arthur Barr Productions, Inc.
Visit to Dairyland U.S.A., National Dairy Council.
Vitamins from Food, National Dairy Council.
Water We Drink, Coronet Instructional Films.
Whenever You Eat, Association Films.
You and Your Food, National Dairy Council.
Your Food, McGraw-Hill Book Company.
Your Food, Young America Films.

c. Filmstrips

A Right Breakfast, Society for Visual Education.
Alexander's Breakfast Secret, Cereal Institute.
Beef—From Store to Table, National Livestock and Meat Board.
Bill's Better Breakfast Puppet Show, Cereal Institute, Inc.
Digestive System, Young America Films.
Eat Well: Live Well, McGraw-Hill Book Company.
Food Around the World, National Dairy Council.
Foods for Health, Young America Films.
Food We Eat, American Bakers Association.
Grain from Farm to Table, Cereal Institute, Inc.
Guide to Breakfast, Kraft Foods.
How Food Becomes You, National Dairy Council.
How Food Is Digested, McGraw-Hill Book Company.
How We Get Our Foods, Society for Visual Education.
How Your Body Uses Food, National Dairy Council.
Learning About Food, Encyclopaedia Britannica.
Mix and Match for Good Meals, Evaporated Milk Association.
Nutrition for You, Educational Activities.
Project AM, Cereal Institute.
Proper Food, Encyclopaedia Britannica.
Skimpy and a Good Breakfast, Cereal Institute, Inc.
Story of Wheat, Wheat Flour Institute.
The Digestive System, Encyclopedia Britannica.
The Essentials of Diet, McGraw-Hill Book Company.
The Foods We Eat, Singer Society for Visual Education.
The Power of Food, National Livestock and Meat Board.
The Wonderful World of Freshness, United Fresh Fruit and Vegetable Association.
Vitamin C Makes the Difference, Sunkist Growers.
We Grow, National Dairy Council.

What's in Our Food, American Bakers Association.
Why Does Food Spoil?, McGraw-Hill Book Company.
Why Eat a Good Breakfast?, Cereal Institute, Inc.
You and Your Food, Young America Films.

d. Posters

A Basic Breakfast Pattern, Cereal Institute.
A Day with the Wide Awakes, General Mills, Inc.
A Guide to Good Eating, National Dairy Council.
Child Feeding Posters (3 posters), National Dairy Council.
Citrus Guards Your Health, Florida Citrus Commission.
Food Nutrient Posters (6), National Livestock and Meat Board.
Foods, United Fresh Fruit and Vegetable Association.
Foods You Need Every Day, National Livestock and Meat Board.
Foodway to Follow, American Institute of Baking.
Good Breakfast Is Fun, Florida Citrus Commission.
Good Foods Help You Grow, National Tuberculosis Association.
Grains—Origin of Breakfast Cereals, Cereal Institute.
Let's Make Butter, National Dairy Council.
Make Lunch Count, National Dairy Council.
Milk from Farm to Family (6 posters), National Dairy Council.
More Milk Please, National Dairy Council.
My Growth Record, National Dairy Council.
Nutrition Ladder to Better Health, Florida Citrus Commission.
Ready for Breakfast, National Dairy Council.
School Lunch, National Dairy Council.
Series of Posters about Citrus Fruits (8), Florida Citrus Commission.
Start a Better Day with a Better Breakfast, National Livestock and Meat Board.
Surprise for Mother Pictures, National Dairy Council.
The Four Food Groups, Florida Citrus Commission.
The Wheel of Good Eating, American Institute of Baking.
What Did You Eat for Breakfast This Morning?, National Dairy Council.
Which Are You?, General Mills, Inc.

e. Charts

A Basic Breakfast Pattern, Cereal Institute, Inc.
A Guide to Good Eating, National Dairy Council.
Availability Guide for Fruits and Vegetables, United Fresh Fruit and Vegetable Association.
Be Aware of Good Nutrition, Kansas Wheat Commission.
Better Breakfast for Primary Children, Florida Citrus Commission.
Colored Food Value Charts, National Livestock and Meat Board.
Conserving Minerals and Vitamins, General Mills, Inc.

Day to Day Good Health Record, Kellogg Company.

Facts About Foods, H. J. Heinz Company.

Follow the Foodway, Kansas Wheat Commission.

Food Chart, General Foods Corporation.

Food Mobile, American Institute of Baking.

Foods for Growing Boys and Girls, Kellogg Company.

For the Calcium You Need, Evaporated Milk Association.

Grains — Origin of Cereal Breakfasts, Cereal Institute, Inc.

Its Always Breakfast Time Somewhere, National Dairy Council.

Kernel of Wheat, Kansas Wheat Commission.

Milk from Farm to Family, National Dairy Council.

Mother Hubbard's Cupboard, General Mills, Inc.

My Daily Food Record, National Livestock and Meat Board.

My Growth Record, National Dairy Council.

Nutritive Values of Fruits and Vegetables, United Fresh Fruit and Vegetable Association.

Potato Calorie Bar Charts, United Fresh Fruit and Vegetable Association.

Safari Breakfast Game, Kellogg Company.

School Lunch Evaluation Charts, General Mills, Inc.

School Lunch Record, National Dairy Council.

School Teaching Charts on Beet Sugar, United States Beet Sugar Association.

Shield of Good Health, Wheat Flour Institute.

Teaching About Meat, National Livestock and Meat Board.

Vitamin Food Chart, The "Cream of Wheat" Corporation.

Wall Meat Charts, National Livestock and Meat Board.

We Work Together, Wheat Flour Institute.

f. Maps

Armour Food Source Map, Armour and Company.

g. Models

Better Breakfast Cut-outs, Florida Citrus Commission.

Dairy Farm, National Dairy Council.

Food Mobile, Pennsylvania Bakers Association.

Food Model, National Dairy Council.

It's Always Breakfast Time Somewhere, National Dairy Council.

Model Cow, National Dairy Council.

Story Display Banners, United Fresh Fruit and Vegetable Association.

Urban Panorama, National Dairy Council.

h. Comics

How Meat Moves to Market, Swift and Company.

i. Selected Stories for Children

(P) Primary Level, (I) Intermediate Level

About Food and Where It Comes From, (I), T. Shannon (Melmont).

Around the World in Eighty Dishes, (I), L. Blanche (Harper).

At the Bakery (P), L. Colonius and G. Schroeder (Melmont).

Baker Bill (P), Jean Barr (Whitman).

Basketful, the Story of Our Foods, (I), J. Eberle (Crowell).

Brazil, Giant to the South (I), Alice Hagar (Macmillan).

Chickens and How to Raise Them (I), L. Darling (Morrow).

Chocolate Touch (P,I), P. S. Cathing (Morrow).

Cook-A-Meal Cookbook (I), G. Clark (W. R. Scott).

Diet and Dental Health (I), (American Dental Association).

Everybody Eats (P), M. M. Green (W. R. Scott).

Farmer and His Cows (P), L. Floethe (Scribner).

Fish (I), R. Fawcett (Gawthorne).

Fun with Cooking (I), Mae Freeman (Random House).

Great Nutrition Puzzles (I), D. Callahan (Scribner).

It's Always Breakfast Time Somewhere (I), M. C. Letton (National Dairy Council).

Jimmy, the Groceryman (P), Jane Miller (Houghton).

Krista and the Frosty Foods (P,I), H. Olds (Messner).

Let's Take a Trip to a Fishery (P), S. Riedman (Abelard).

Little Pig in the Cupboard (P), Helen Buckley (Lothrop).

Milk for You (P), W. G. Schloat (Scribner).

Milkman Freddy (I), Elizabeth Hoffman (Messner).

Miss B's First Cook Book (I), Percy Hoffman (Bobbs).

Nothing to Eat but Food (I), Frank Jupo (Aladdin).

Plants That Feed Us (I), C. Fenton (Day).

Story Book of Foods (P,I), M. Petersham (Winston).

Story Book of Wheat (P), M. Petersham (Winston).

Stories from the Americas (I), F. Henuis (Scribner).

Sugar (I), R. Fawcett (Gawthorne).

The Apple That Jack Ate (P), William R. Scott (W. R. Scott).

The Lunchbox Story (P), M. Goldberg (Holiday House).

The Milk That Jack Drank (P), W. R. Scott (Cadmus).

The Wonderful Egg (I), W. G. Schloat (Scribner).

This Is the Bread That Betsy Ate (P), Irma Black (W. R. Scott).

To Market We Go (P), Jane Miller (Houghton).

Walkabout Down Under (I), K. S. Foote (Scribner).

What the World Eats (I), H. H. Webster (Houghton).

Where's the Bunny? (P), Ruth Carroll (Oxford University Press).

Who Dreams of Cheese? (P), Leonard Weisgard (Scribner).

Wonderful Baker (I), M. L. Hunt (Lippincott).

Your Food and You (I), H. S. Zim (Morrow).

4. Dental Health

a. Pamphlets or Leaflets

A Bright Smile Is to Keep, Florida Citrus Commission.

A Drop in the Bucket, U.S. Public Health Service.

A Visit to the Dentist, American Dental Association.

Better Teeth For Life: Fluoridation, U.S. Public Health Service (Pub. 636).

Cleaning Your Teeth and Gums, American Dental Association.

Dental Health Education, American Dental Association.

Dental Health Today, Procter and Gamble Company.

Dental X-Rays and Your Health, American Dental Association.

Even Dragons Have Teeth, American Dental Association.

Fluoride Helps Prevent Tooth Decay, American Dental Association.

Food and Care for Dental Health, National Dairy Council.

Food and Care for Good Dental Health, National Dairy Council.

Frank Visits the Dentist, American Dental Association.

Fresh Oranges, Important for Sound Teeth, Sunkist Growers.

Good Teeth, Government Printing Office.

How Bright the Smile, Florida Citrus Commission.

How to Take Care of Your Teeth, Procter and Gamble Company.

How Teeth Grow, National Dairy Council.

I'm Going to the Dentist, American Dental Association.

Kit Goes to the Dentist, Health Education Service.

Orthodontics, American Dental Association.

Smoking and Your Oral Health, American Dental Association.

Teeth Talk, Travelers Insurance Company.

The Way to a Smile, Procter and Gamble Company.

They Are Your Teeth, National Dairy Council.

Tom Visits the Dentist, Procter and Gamble Company.

Tommy's First Visit to the Dentist, American Dental Association.

Toothbrushing, American Dental Association.

What is a Healthy Tooth?, Procter and Gamble.

When I Grow Up, National Dairy Council.

Why You Should Use Dental Floss, Johnson and Johnson.

You Can Prevent Tooth Decay, American Dental Association.

b. Films

Billy Meets Tommy Tooth, American Dental Association.

Case of the Missing Tooth, American Dental Association.

Gateway to Health, National Apple Institute.

Healthy Teeth: Happy Smile, American Dental Association.

How Teeth Grow, Encyclopaedia Britannica.

It Doesn't Hurt, Coronet Instructional Films.

Learning to Brush, American Dental Association.

Merlin's Magical Message, American Dental Association.

Our Teeth, Knowledge Builders.

Project Teeth, American Dental Association.

Save Those Teeth, Encyclopaedia Britannica.

Set the Stage for Dental Health, American Dental Association.

Sights and Sounds Around the Dental Chair, American Dental Association.

Take Time for Your Teeth, Johnson and Johnson.

Teeth, American Dental Association.

Teeth, Films Incorporated.

Teeth Are to Keep, Encyclopaedia Britannica.

The Beaver's Tale, American Dental Association.

The Teeth, Encyclopaedia Britannica.

Tommy's Day, Young America Films.

Tommy's Healthy Teeth, Coronet Instructional Films.

What Do You Know about Teeth?, American Dental Association.

Your Teeth, Young America Films.

c. Filmstrips

Billy Meets Tommy Tooth, American Dental Association.

Brush Up on Your Teeth, Canadian National Film Board.

Dental Health Stories, Educational Activities.

Enjoy Your Teeth for Life, American Dental Association.

Johnny's Magic Toothbrush, American Dental Association.

Learning About Our Teeth, Encyclopaedia Britannica.

Let's Visit the Dentist, National Dairy Council.

Primary Grade Health Series, National Dairy Council.

Save Those Teeth, Encyclopaedia Britannica.

Strong Teeth, McGraw-Hill Book Company.

Tale of a Toothache, Society for Visual Education.

Ten Little People and Their Teeth, Canadian National Film Board.

The Mouth I Live In, Colgate-Palmolive.

The Teeth, Encyclopaedia Britannica.

The Teeth, Young America Films.

Tips on Tooth Care, American Dental Association.

You and Your Dentist, American Dental Association.

Your Teeth and Their Care, Popular Science.

You're on Parade, Society for Visual Education.

d. Posters

Armed to the Teeth, Florida Citrus Commission.

Begin Early, National Dairy Council.

Big Pains, Travelers Insurance Company.

Brush Your Teeth, Eat Good Foods, Visit Your Dentist, National Dairy Council.

Do You?, National Dairy Council.

Do's for Dental Health, Florida Citrus Commission.

Elementary School Posters (set of 4), American Dental Association.

How Teeth Grow, Procter and Gamble.

Healthy Tooth, Procter and Gamble.
How We Take Care of the Teeth, National Dairy Council.
Make Your Teeth the Best, National Dairy Council.
Swish and Swallow, American Dental Association.
Teeth, American Dental Association.
They're Your Teeth, National Dairy Council.

e. Charts

Class Toothbrushing Record, Procter and Gamble.
Development of Human Dentition, American Dental Association.
Decay in Six-Year Molar, American Dental Association.
Four Food Groups, National Dairy Council.
Honor Roll—Clean Teeth Club, Pepsodent.
How to Brush the Teeth (21″ × 25½″), American Dental Association.
Ivory Inspection Patrol Chart, Procter and Gamble Company.
Toothbrushing Chart, American Dental Association.

f. Records

Friendly Doctor Drillum Fillum, J-209 Columbia Records.
Recorded Radio Presentations, American Dental Association.
Willie and a Little Tooth, J-184 Columbia Records.

g. Toothbrushing Kits

American Dental Association (M10 kit), Procter and Gamble Company. (Third grade)
Colgate-Palmolive Company.

h. Models

Look at Your Teeth—Everyone Else Does, American Dental Association.
Toothbrushing Model (M13 new), American Dental Association.

i. Exhibits

Behind the Smile of Health (6½′ × 7½′), American Dental Association.
Break the Chain of Tooth Decay (7½′ × 5½′), American Dental Association.
Fluoridation (6½′ × 7½′), American Dental Association.

j. Comics

The Friendly Ghost, Casper, And The Friendly Dentist, American Dental Association.

k. Loop Films

Cleaning Your Teeth, Encyclopaedia Britannica.
The Nature of Decay, Encyclopaedia Britannica.
What is a Tooth, Encyclopaedia Britannica.

l. Selected Stories for Children
(P) Primary Level, (I) Intermediate Level

Child's Book of Teeth (I), H. W. Ferguson (World Book).

Diet and Dental Health (I), (American Dental Association).
Let's Be Healthy (P), W. W. Charters (Macmillan).
Let's Go to a Dentist (P), N. Buckheimer (Putnam).
Milk for You (P), W. G. Schloat (Scribner).
Milkman Freddy (I), Elizabeth Hoffman (Messner).
One Morning in Maine (P), R. McClusky (Viking).
The Serpent's Teeth (I), Penelope Farmer (Harcourt).
Your Wonderful Teeth (P,I), W. G. Schloat (Scribner).

5. Body Structure and Operation

a. Pamphlets or Leaflets

Blood as Medicine, American National Red Cross.
Clara Barton, Heroic Woman, American National Red Cross.
Contact Lenses, American Medical Association.
Good Posture in the Little Child, U.S. Children's Bureau.
Growing Up and Liking It, Personal Products Company.
Heart Disease, U.S. Public Health Service.
The Breath of Life, Aetna Life Insurance Company.
The Heart and Circulation, American Heart Association.
The Miracle of Life, American Medical Association.
The Story of Blood, American National Red Cross.
The Wonder of You, American Institute of Baking.
When I Grow Up, National Dairy Council.
Wonder Stories of the Human Machine (7 stories), American Medical Association.
Your Heart, Metropolitan Life Insurance Company.

b. Films

Back on the Job, American Heart Association.
Breath of Life, American Heart Association.
Breathing, Encyclopaedia Britannica.
Circulation, United World Films.
Cells of Plants and Animals, Coronet Films.
Digestion in Our Bodies, Coronet Instructional Films.
Digestive System, Films Incorporated.
Endocrine Glands, Encyclopaedia Britannica.
Functions of the Nervous System, Knowledge Builders.
Health: Eye-Care Fantasy, Encyclopaedia Britannica.
Healthy Lungs, Coronet Instructional Films.
Heart and Circulatory System, Films Incorporated.
Heart, Lungs, and Circulation, Coronet Instructional Films.
I Never Catch a Cold, Coronet Instructional Films.
Mechanisms of Breathing, Encyclopaedia Britannica.

Muscles and Bones of the Body, Coronet Instructional Films.
Nature of Life: Respiration in Animals, Coronet Films.
Obesity, National Dairy Council.
Our Wonderful Body: How It Grows, Coronet Instructional Materials.
Rescue Breathing, American Heart Association.
Rest That Builds Good Health, Coronet Instructional Films.
Sitting Right, Association Films.
Sleep for Health, Encyclopaedia Britannica.
The Huffless, Puffless Dragon, American Cancer Society.
The Human Body, National Dairy Council.
To Live and Breath, Aetna Life and Casualty Company.
Wonder Engine of the Body, American Heart Association.
Wonder of Our Body, Moody Institute of Science.
Work of the Kidneys, Encyclopaedia Britannica.
You and Your Five Senses, Walt Disney Productions.
Your Nervous System, Coronet Instructional Films.
You — The Human Animal, Walt Disney Productions.

c. Filmstrips

Every Body's Skin Makes Everybody Kin, American Association for Health, Physical Education and Recreation.
Harvey and Blood Circulation, International Film Bureau.
How the Heart Works, Popular Science.
How to Grow Well and Strong, McGraw-Hill Book Company.
How to Grow Well and Strong, Popular Science.
Human Respiration, Popular Science.
Learning About Our Ears, Encyclopaedia Britannica.
Learning About Our Eyes, Encyclopaedia Britannica.
Learning About Our Skin, Encyclopaedia Britannica.
Nervous System, Young America Films.
Respiratory System, Young America Films.
Skin, Hair, and Nails, McGraw-Hill Book Company.
Straight and Tall, Young America Films.
Systems of the Body, Educational Activities, Inc.
Taste, Smell and Touch, Encyclopaedia Britannica.
The Circulatory System, Encyclopaedia Britannica.
The Digestive System, Enclopaedia Britannica.
The Heart — How It Works, McGraw-Hill Book Company.
The Human Cell, American Cancer Society.
The Story of Human Life, Educational Activities, Inc.
Use of Artificial Respiration, McGraw-Hill Book Company.
We Grow, National Dairy Council.
You and the Living Machine, Encyclopaedia Britannica.
Your Blood System, Curriculum Films.

Your Bones and Muscles, Popular Science.
Your Heart and Lungs, Popular Science.
Your Posture — Good or Bad, Young America Films.

d. Posters

ACS Bulletin Board Posters (7 each), American Cancer Society.
Blood As a Medicine, American National Red Cross.
Give Blood to Give Life, American Medical Association.
Posture on Parade (for girls), National Dairy Council.
Protect Your Eyes, National Safety Council.
The Breath of Life, Aetna Life Insurance Company.
Too Well Done — Tan Gradually, National Safety Council.
Which One Is a Fake?, American Cancer Society.

e. Charts

Bone Structure, National Livestock and Meat Board.
Cancer Wall Chart (3' × 4'), Eli Lilly and Company.
Heart Charts (12), American Heart Association.
How Tall, The Travelers Insurance Company.
Human Body (kit), Owen Publishing Company, Danville, N.Y.
My Growth Record, National Dairy Council.
Physical Growth Record for Boys, American Medical Association.
Physical Growth Record for Girls, American Medical Association.
Your Heart and How It Works, American Heart Association.

f. Transparencies

Physiology of the Heart, Media Visuals, Inc.
Physiology of the Nervous System, Media Visuals, Inc.

g. Records

Childhood Rhythms for Intermediate Grades (Evans CHR-3), Stanley Bowmar Company.
Childhood Rhythms for Lower Grades (Evans CHR-1), Stanley Bowmar Company, Valhalla, N.Y.
Creative Rhythm Album (Burns-Wheeler), Stanley Bowmar Company.
My Heart and I, American Heart Association.

h. Models

Plastic Anatomical Reproductions, Medical Plastics Laboratory, Gatesville, Texas, 76528.
The Heart and Circulation, American Heart Association.

j. Selected Stories for Children
(P) Primary Level, (I) Intermediate Level

A Baby Is Born (P), L. I. Mitton and J. N. Seligmann (Simon & Schuster).
A Baby Starts to Grow (P), Paul Showers (Crowell).
A Drop of Blood (P), Ellen Raskin (Atheneum-Aladdin).

All About Eggs (P), Selsan Millicent (W. R. Scott).
All About the Human Body (I), B. Glemser (Random).
All About Us (I), Eva Evans (Capital).
All Kinds of Babies and How They Grow (P), Selsan Millicent (W. R. Scott).
Brave Gives Blood (I), Philip and Mirina Eisenburg (Messner).
Do You Know What I Know? (P), Helen Borten (Abelard).
Freddie Found a Frog (P), James Napjas (Van Nostrand).
Growing Story (P), Ruth Krauss (Harper).
Growing Up (P), Karl DeSchweintz (Macmillan).
How We Grow (I), P. O'Keefe and C. H. Maxwell (Winston).
How Your Body Works (I), H. Schneider (W. R. Scott).
Linda Goes to the Hospital (I), Nancy Dudley (Coward-McCann).
My Five Senses (I), Aliki (Crowell).
Oxygen Keeps You Alive (P), F. M. Branley (Crowell).
Patrick Will Grow (P), Gladys Baker Bond (Whitman).
Push and Pull (I), P. Blackwood (McGraw-Hill).
The Ear Book (I), Al Perkins (Random).
The Eye Book (I), Theodore LeSieg (Random).
The Smallest Boy in the Class (I), J. Beim (William Morrow).
What's Inside of Me? (I), Herbert S. Zim (Morrow).
What's Inside of Me? (P), Herbert S. Zim (Morrow).
When I Am Big (P), R. P. Smith (Harper).
Wonders Inside You (P), L. Cosgrove (Dodd).
Wonders of the Human Body (I), A. Ranelli (Viking).
Your Body and How It Works (I), P. Lauber (Random House).
Your Bones Are Alive (P), S. Kalina (Lothrop).
Your Heart and How It Works (I), H. Zim (Morrow).

6. Prevention and Control of Disease

a. Pamphlets or Leaflets

A Hot War Against the Common Cold, Kimberly-Clark Corporation.
Colds and Other Respiratory Diseases, Travelers Insurance Company.
Common Cold, U.S. Public Health Service.
Facts About Hay Fever, American Medical Association.
Health Heroes Series, Metropolitan Life Insurance Company.
I Promise Common Sense, Kimberly-Clark Corporation.
Key Facts About Tetanus, American Medical Association.
Louis Pasteur and the Germ Theory of Disease, Metropolitan Life Insurance Co.
Marie Curie and the Story of Radium, Metropolitan Life Insurance Co.
Measles Vaccine, American Medical Association.

Men Against Disease, American Red Cross.
Old King Cold, American Medical Association.
Pick Your Shots, American Medical Association.
Poisonous Plants, National Safety Council.
Poliomyelitis — Teacher's Guide, National Foundation.
The American Red Cross: A Brief Story, American National Red Cross.
The Triad of Infection, Eli Lilly and Company.

b. Films

Avoiding Infections, Encyclopaedia Britannica.
Child With a Cold, Pharmaceutical Manufacturers Association.
Cleanliness and Health, Coronet Instructional Films.
Common Cold, Encyclopaedia Britannica.
Germs and What They Do, Coronet Films.
Goodbye, Mr. Germ, National Tuberculosis Association.
Health: Germs and the Space Visitors, Encyclopaedia Britannica.
Health Heroes: the Battle Against Disease, Metropolitan Life Insurance Co.
House Fly, Encyclopaedia Britannica.
How to Catch a Cold, Walt Disney Productions.
I Never Catch a Cold, Coronet Instructional Films.
Immunization, Encyclopaedia Britannica.
Joan Avoids a Cold, Coronet Instructional Films.
Let's Have Fewer Colds, Coronet Instructional Films.
Life in a Drop of Water, Coronet Instructional Films.
Mr. Galen Comes To Town, Pharmaceutical Manufacturers Association.
Spot Prevention, U.S. Public Health Service.
Story of Dr. Jenner, Teaching Film Custodians.
Story of Louis Pasteur, Teaching Film Custodians.
The Body Fights Bacteria, McGraw-Hill Book Company.
The Fight Against Microbes, International Film Bureau.
The Inside Story, National Tuberculosis Association.
Time for Living, Pharmaceutical Manufacturers Association.
Tiny Water Animals, Encyclopaedia Britannica.
Unmasking the Germ Assassins, International Film Bureau.
Water We Drink, Coronet Instructional Films.
Your Health, Disease and Its Control, Coronet Instructional Films.

c. Filmstrips

Avoiding Infections (Treating a Cold), Encyclopaedia Britannica.
Cancer, the Challenge to Youth, American Cancer Society.
Checking Your Health, Encyclopaedia Britannica.
Common Cold, Encyclopaedia Britannica.
Communicable Diseases, Young America Films.
Controlling Germs, Curriculum Films.
Fighting Disease, Stanley Bowmar Co.
Florence Nightingale, Metropolitan Life Insurance Company.
Germ Invaders, McGraw-Hill Book Company.

Health Heroes, Metropolitan Life Insurance Company.

Helping the Body Defenses Against Disease, McGraw-Hill Book Company.

Infectious Disease: Causes and Defense, Stanley Bowmar Co.

Keeping Ourselves Healthy, Curriculum Films.

Keeping Sickness Away, McGraw-Hill Book Company.

Keeping Well, Young America Films.

Learning About Germs, Encyclopaedia Britannica.

Louis Pasteur and the Germ Theory of Disease, Metropolitan Life Insurance Co.

Madame Curie, Metropolitan Life Insurance Company.

Making Water Safe to Drink, McGraw-Hill Book Company.

Shots for Your Health, National Education Association.

The Little Pink Bottle, National Foundation.

The Water We Drink, Young America Films.

Walter Reed and the Conquest of Yellow Fever (with transcription), Metropolitan Life Insurance Company.

We Have You Covered, Society for Visual Education.

Witchcraft to Modern Medicine, International Education and Training, Inc.

d. Posters

Germs Can Hatch in a Scratch, National Safety Council.

Help Us Fight Infection, National Safety Council.

How to Catch a Cold, Kimberly-Clark Corporation.

How to Cure a Cold, Kimberly-Clark Corporation.

How to Spread a Cold, Kimberly-Clark Corporation.

Protect Them with Shots, National Tuberculosis Association.

Soap Before Soup, Travelers Insurance Company.

We Had Polio Vaccine, National Foundation.

e. Records

Chest X-ray Song, National Tuberculosis Association.

Cover Your Mouth, Educational Activities.

Doctors Make History, American Medical Association.

Health Heroes, American Medical Association.

Keep the Germs Away, Educational Activities.

Rainy Days, National Safety Council.

Shots For Your Health, National Education Association.

The Constant Invader (15 each), Wisconsin Anti-Tuberculosis Association.

f. Charts

Cancer Wall Chart (3' × 4'), Eli Lilly and Company.

I Promise Common Sense, Kimberly-Clark Corporation.

The Good Seed, Eli Lilly and Company.

g. Radio Scripts

(From Bureau of Research in Education by Radio, University of Texas)

Fly Control

Health Living Radio Broadcast (kit of 30 scripts)

Keep Your Cold at Home

Mosquito Control

Safe Water Supply

We Wash Our Hands Before We Eat

h. Selected Stories for Children

(P) Primary Level, (I) Intermediate Level

Conquest of Disease (I), L. Martin (Coward).

Doctors and Nurses: What They Do (I), C. Greene (Harper & Row).

Doctors and What They Do (I), H. Coy (G. P. Putnam's Sons).

Dr. Trotter and His Big Gold Watch (P), H. Gilbert (Abingdon).

Have a Happy Measle, a Merry Mumps and a Cheery Chickenpox (I), J. Bendick (Whittlesey House).

Health Can Be Fun (P), Munro Leaf (Lippincott).

Johnny Goes to the Hospital (P), J. Sener (Houghton).

Linda Goes to the Hospital (P), N. Dudley (Coward).

Modern Medical Discoveries (I), E. Bigland (Criterion).

Moptop (P), D. Freeman (Viking).

Our Insect Friends and Foes (I), W. A. DuPuy (Winston).

The Clean Pig (P), Leonard Weisgard (Scribner).

The First Book of Microbes (I), L. Lewis (Watts).

The Water That Jack Drank (P), William R. Scott (W. R. Scott).

True Book of Health (P), Mary Brockman (Scribner).

What's Inside of Me? (P), Herbert S. Zim (Morrow).

7. Safety and First Aid

a. Pamphlets or Leaflets

About Electricity, National Fire Protection Association.

Artificial Respiration, American Medical Association.

Bicycle Riding Clubs, Bicycle Institute of America.

Bicycle Safety Information Test, National Safety Council.

Bicycle Safety Test, Bicycle Institute of America.

Bicyclists' Safety Rules, Bicycle Institute of America.

Bike Fun, Bicycle Institute of America.

Bike Regulations in the Community, Bicycle Institute of America.

Bike Safety Program, Bicycle Institute of America.

Buckle Down and Stay Safe, American Medical Association.

Children and Matches, National Fire Protection Association.

Emergency First Aid Guide, American Insurance Association.

Fatal Fallacies, The Travelers Insurance Company.

Fire Prevention Guide, Intermediate, American Red Cross.

Fire Prevention Guide, Primary, American Red Cross.

First Aid Now! Pharmaceutical Manufacturers Association.

First Aid (Programmed instruction), Behavioral Research Laboratories.

First Aid Facts, Johnson & Johnson.

First Aid Guide, Johnson and Johnson.

How Are You Fixed For Poisons?, American Medical Association.

How to Bandage, Johnson and Johnson.

How to Restore the Breath of Life, Metropolitan Life Insurance Co.

In Case of Fire, National Fire Protection Association.

It All Adds Up to Saving Lives, American National Red Cross.

Junior Bicycle Courts, Bicycle Institute of America.

Learn Safe Boating, American National Red Cross.

Learn to Swim, American National Red Cross.

Let's Learn About Safety, Eli Lilly and Company.

On Your Own — With Safety, Metropolitan Life Insurance Co.

Panic and Its Control, American Insurance Association.

Poison Isn't Kid Stuff, American Association of Poison Control Center.

Poisonous Plants, National Safety Council.

Read the Label, National Fire Protection Association.

Rescue Breathing, Aetna Life and Casualty Company.

Safe Play to Save Sight, National Society for the Prevention of Blindness.

Seat Belts Save, American Medical Association.

Standard Rules for School Safety Patrols, National Safety Council.

Ten Little Tasters, U.S. Public Health Service (Food and Drug Administration).

The Open and Shut Case For Safety Belts, Aetna Life and Casualty Company.

The Safest Route to School, American Automobile Association.

Your Clothing Can Burn, National Fire Protection Association.

b. Films

A Monkey Tale (Bicycle Safety), Encyclopaedia Britannica.

Bicycle Rules of the Road, Aims Instructional Media Services.

Bicycle Safety Skills, Coronet Instructional Films.

Children at Play with Poison, U.S. Public Health Service (Food and Drug Administration).

Drugs, Drinking and Driving, Aims Instructional Media Services.

Emergency 77, Metropolitan Life Insurance Company.

Fifty Thousand Lives, Johnson & Johnson.

Fire Exit Drill at Our School, Coronet Instructional Films.

Fireman, Encyclopaedia Britannica.

First Aid Now, Johnson and Johnson.

Health: Eye-Care Fantasy, Encyclopaedia Britannica.

Help Prevent Fires, National Fire Protection Association.

Help Wanted, Johnson & Johnson.

If Bicycles Could Talk, Aetna Life and Casualty Company.

I'm No Fool as a Pedestrian, American Automobile Association.

I'm No Fool with a Bicycle, American Automobile Association.

Mouth-to-Mouth Resuscitation, American Heart Association.

Playground Safety (2nd ed.), Coronet Instructional Films.

Primary Safety: In the School Building, Coronet Instructional Films.

Read the Label and Live, National Fire Protection Association.

Safe Living at Home, Coronet Instructional Films.

Safe Living at School, Coronet Instructional Films.

Safe Living in Your Community, Coronet Instructional Films.

Safe Through Seat Belts, International Film Bureau, Inc.

Safety: The Helpful Burglars, Encyclopaedia Britannica.

Safe Use of Tools, Coronet Instructional Films.

Safest Way, American Automobile Association.

Safety Begins at Home, Young America Films.

Safety Belts for Susie, Charles Cahill and Associates.

Safety in Winter, Coronet Instructional Films.

Safety on the Playground, Encyclopaedia Britannica.

Safety on the Streets, Encyclopaedia Britannica.

Safety on the Way, Coronet Instructional Films.

Safety with Fire, Coronet Instructional Films.

School Bus and You, Progressive Films.

School Rules — How They Help Us, Coronet Instructional Films.

Singing Wheels, Bicycle Institute of America.

Sniffy Escapes Poisoning, Henk Wewenhouse Films.

Stop, Look, and Think, Charles Cahill and Associates.

Water Safety, Young America Films.

You and Your Bicycle, Progressive Films and Employers Mutuals of Wausau.

c. Filmstrips

Be a Better Pedal Pusher, Society for Visual Education.

Bicycle Safety, Curriculum Films.

Controlling Fire, McGraw-Hill Book Company.

Electrical Hazard, Stanley Bowmar Company.

Happy Hollow Makes the Honor Roll, Society for Visual Education.

Home Safety, Encyclopaedia Britannica.

I'm No Fool Having Fun, McGraw-Hill Book Company.

I'm No Fool with a Bicycle, McGraw-Hill Book Company.

I'm No Fool with Fire, McGraw-Hill Book Company.

Keeping Food Safe to Eat, McGraw-Hill Book Company.
Little Children and Big Poisons, American Association of Poison Control Center.
Play Safety, Encyclopaedia Britannica.
Playing in City Streets, Curriculum Films.
Safe and Sure with Electricity, McGraw-Hill Book Company.
Safety at School, Curriculum Films.
Safety Helpers, Encyclopaedia Britannica.
Safety in the Summer, Curriculum Films.
School Safety, Encyclopaedia Britannica.
Street Safety, Encyclopaedia Britannica.
Vacation Safety, Encyclopaedia Britannica.
Wintertime Safety, McGraw-Hill Book Company.

d. Posters

Accidents Occur When Least Expected, National Safety Council.
A Clean House Seldom Burns, National Fire Protection Association.
Always Use Bike Hand Signals, Bicycle Institute of America.
ARC Safety Posters, 1446 and 1447, American National Red Cross.
Be Extra Careful, National Safety Council.
Be Sure Your Bike Is Ready to Go, Bicycle Institute of America.
Bicyclists Use Your Hand Signals, Bicycle Institute of America.
Bike Route, Bicycle Institute of America.
Bike Safety Aids, Bicycle Institute of America.
Exit: Plan Your Way Out, National Fire Protection Association.
Get First Aid Promptly, National Safety Council.
Little People Don't Read Labels, American Association of Poison Control Center.
Look Both Ways at School, Bicycle Institute of America.
Poison-Ivy-Oak, National Safety Council.
Prevent Fire, National Fire Protection Association.
Protect Your Eyes, National Safety Council.
Safety Is Always In Season, National Safety Council.
Safety Is a Year Round Job, National Safety Council.
Seat Belts, American Medical Association.
See, Be Seen, Bicycle Institute of America.
Show-offs Get Hurt, National Safety Council.
Sports Accidents, American Medical Association.
Stop Fires, Save Lives, American Insurance Association.
Take It Easy on Your Vacation, National Safety Council.
Wait on the Curb for Your Go Signal, American Automobile Association.

e. Charts

First Aid, Metropolitan Life Insurance Company.
First Aid Wall Chart, Johnson and Johnson.
Home Fire Safety Check List, National Fire Protection Association.
Six Month Inspection, Bicycle Institute of America.
Stop-Dial, Aetna Life & Casualty Company.

f. Records

Buckle Your Seatbelt, Educational Activities.
Fire on Thunder Hill, American Forest Products Industries, Inc.
Safety Through Music, Educational Activities.

g. Comics

Dennis the Menace Takes a Poke at Poison, U.S. Public Health Service.
Early Man and Fire, National Fire Protection Association.
Hello, I Am Fire!, National Fire Protection Association.
Man Learns More about Fire, National Fire Protection Association.
Sparky, National Fire Protection Association.
Sparky Makes a Home Fire Inspection, National Fire Protection Association.

h. Radio Scripts

Benny, the Matchstick, National Safety Council.
Bobby Grows Up, National Safety Council.
Carl, the Bear Cub, National Safety Council.
Child Safety Stories, National Safety Council.
Danger, Children at Play, National Safety Council.
Fire Prevention, Bureau of Research in Education by Radio, University of Texas.
Fire Safety, National Safety Council.
Happy and Safe Thinking, National Safety Council.
Lady from Safety Land, National Safety Council.
Louis Agazzi Fuertes, National Safety Council.
Make Your City Safer, National Safety Council.
Mary and the Broken Glass, National Safety Council.
Needles and Pins, National Safety Council.
On a Bicycle Not Built for Two, National Safety Council.
Our Animal Show, National Safety Council.
Out of the Night, National Safety Council.
Safe Water Supply, Bureau of Research in Education by Radio, University of Texas.
The Bat Blinky, National Safety Council.
The Safety Elf, National Safety Council.
The Twins Have Safety Trouble, National Safety Council.
To Walk in the Night, National Safety Council.
Worrying Bike, National Safety Council.

i. Loop Films

Preventing Slips and Falls, Encyclopaedia Britannica.
Safety with Pets, Encyclopaedia Britannica.

j. Selected Stories for Children
(P) Primary Level, (I) Intermediate Level

Andy and the School Bus (P), J. Beim (Morrow).
Big Fire (P), E. Olds (Houghton).
Binkey's Fire (P), Sally Scott (Harcourt).
Country Fireman (P), J. Beim (Morrow).
Dr. Squash, the Doll Doctor (P), Margaret Wise Brown (Simon & Schuster).
Fireman for a Day (I), Z. K. McDonald (Messner).
Fireman Fred (P), Jean Barry (Whitman).
First Book of Firemen (I), Mary Elting (Watts).

Forest Fireman (P, I), Bill and Rosalie Brown (Coward).

Going to Blazes (I), R. V. Masters (Sterling).

Hercules, Story of an Old Fashioned Fire Engine (P), Hardie Gramatsky (Putnam).

I Want to Be a Policeman (P), C. Greene (Children's Press).

Johnnie Wants to Be a Policeman (I), W. J. Granberg (Aladdin).

Let's Find Out about Safety (I), M. Shapp (Watts).

Mountain Courage (I), D. Hawkins (Doubleday).

Pat and Her Policeman (I), F. Friedman (Morrow).

Rags, the Firehouse Dog (P), E. Morton (Winston).

Red Light, Green Light (P), Margaret Wise Brown (Doubleday).

Safety Can Be Fun (P), Munro Leaf (Lippincott).

The Bike Lesson (P), S. and J. Berenstain (Random House).

The Firefighter (I), H. B. Lent (Macmillan).

The Little Igloo (P), L. Beim (Harcourt Brace).

The New Fire Engine (P), Jay Barnum (Morrow).

Time and the Brass Buttons (P, I), Ruth Tooze (Messner).

Try It Again Sam: Safety When You Walk (P), Judith Viorist (Lothrop).

Walkabout Down Under (I), K. S. Foote (Scribner).

Watch Out (I), Norah Smaridge (Abington).

8. Mental Health

a. Pamphlets or Leaflets

A Happy Day, National Dairy Council.

Children of the Evening, Hogg Foundation for Mental Health.

Emotional Health in Work and Play, American Medical Association.

Getting Along with Brothers and Sisters, Child Study Association of America.

How Teachers Can Build Mental Health, American Medical Association.

Mental Hygiene in the Classroom, American Medical Association.

Stress and Your Health, Metropolitan Life Insurance Co.

Teachers Listen, the Children Speak, U.S. Children's Bureau.

Three Cheers for a Big Smile, National Dairy Council.

What Is Mental Illness? U.S. Public Health Service.

b. Films

Act Your Age, Coronet Instructional Films.

Adventuring Pups, Young America Films.

Are You Popular?, Coronet Instructional Films.

Attitudes and Health, Coronet Instructional Films.

Curious Alice, National Institute of Mental Health.

Don't Be Afraid, Encyclopaedia Britannica.

Face Yourself, Aetna Life and Casualty Company.

Feeling Left Out, Coronet Instructional Films.

Getting Along With Others, Coronet Instructional Films.

Good Sportsmanship, Coronet Instructional Films.

Growing Up, Coronet Instructional Films.

How Do You Do, Young America Films.

How Friendly Are You? Coronet Instructional Films.

How Honest Are You? Coronet Instructional Films.

If These Were Your Children (Adult), Metropolitan Life Insurance Company.

Jimmy Rabbitt, Bailey Films.

Let's Play Fair, Coronet Instructional Films.

Making Life Adjustments, McGraw-Hill Book Company.

Mental Health, Encyclopaedia Britannica.

Other Fellow's Feelings, Young America Films.

Out of Orbit, National Council on Alcoholism.

Overcoming Worry, Coronet Instructional Films.

Planning for Success, Coronet Instructional Films.

Sky Guy, Coronet Instructional Films.

The Outsider, Young America Films.

The Ugly Duckling, Coronet Instructional Films.

To See Ourselves, Aetna Life and Casualty Company.

To Your Health, World Health Organization.

Understanding Stresses and Strains, Walt Disney Productions.

Ways to Good Habits, Coronet Instructional Films.

What To Do About Upset Feelings, Coronet Films.

What Do Drugs Do?, National Institute of Mental Health.

You and Your Family, Association Films, Inc.

You and Your Friends, Association Films, Inc.

You and Your Time, Association Films, Inc.

c. Filmstrips

Getting Acquainted, McGraw-Hill Book Company.

Health Helpers, Encyclopaedia Britannica.

Keeping Children Happy, McGraw-Hill Book Company.

Learning To Make Friends, Society For Visual Education.

Let's Have a Party, Society for Visual Education.

Lonely Boy, Stanley Bowmar Co.

Mental Health, Image Publishing Corporation.

Mike Finds out about Friendship, Society for Visual Education.

Orphan Willie, Canadian National Film Board.

Promises Are Made to Keep, Encyclopaedia Britannica.

Reflection, Image Publishing Corporation.

Sense and Nonsense, Popular Science.

Share the Sandpile, Society for Visual Education.

Sharing with Neighbors, Encyclopaedia Britannica.

Talk About Good, Talk About Bad, American Cancer Society.

The Little Cloud, Society for Visual Education.

The Nervous System, Encyclopaedia Britannica.

The Raggedy Elf, Society for Visual Education.

Thinking for Yourself, Encyclopaedia Britannica.

We Play Together, Stanley Bowmar Co.
We Work Together, Stanley Bowmar Co.
Working and Playing Together, McGraw-Hill
  Book Company.

d. Posters

Helping Brothers and Sisters, David C. Cook.
Mother Helps At Home, David C. Cook.
Sharing Toys, David C. Cook.

e. Plays
(From Mental Health Materials Center)

The Daily Special
What Did I Do?

f. Records

Getting To Know Myself, Educational Activities.
Won't You Be My Friend, Educational Activities.

g. Selected Stories for Children
(P) Primary Level, (I) Intermediate Level

A Friend Is Someone Who Likes You (P), J. Walsh
  (Harcourt Brace).
A Name for Obed (P), E. C. Phillips (Houghton).
A Race for Bill (I), M. N. Wallace (Nelson).
Ann and the Sand Dobbies (I), John Colburn (Sea-
  bury Press).
"B" Is for Betsy (P), Carolyn Haywood (Har-
  court).
Ben And Me (I), Robert Lawson (Walt Disney).
Child of the Silent Night (I), Edith Hunter
  (Houghton Mifflin).
David's Bad Day (P), Ellen McKean (Vanguard).
Even Steven (P), W. Lipkind (Harcourt).
Fair Play (P), Munro Leaf (Lippincott).
Finders Keepers (P), W. Lipkind (Harcourt).
Grandfather and I (P), Helen Buckley (Lothrop,
  Lee, Shepherd).
Granite Harbor (I), D. Bud (Macmillan).
Growing Story (P), Ruth Krauss (Harper).
Growing Up (P), Karl DeSchweintz (Macmillan).
Here's a Penny (P), Carolyn Haywood (Harcourt).
How to Behave and Why (I), Munro Leaf (Lippin-
  cott).
How To Stand Up for What You Believe (I), H.
  Detwiler (Association Press).
I Like To Be Me (P, I), Barbara Bel Geddes (Vik-
  ing).
I Like You (P), Sandel Warburg (Houghton Mif-
  flin).
Jerry at School (P), Kathryn Jackson (Simon &
  Schuster).
Judy's Journey (I), Lois Lenski (Lippincott).
Just Me (P), Marie Hall ETS (Viking).
Let's Do Better (P, I) Munro Leaf (Lippincott).
Liam's Catch (P), D. D. Parker (Viking).
Love Is a Special Way of Feeling (P), J. Walsh
  (Harcourt Brace).
Manners to Grow on (P), T. Lee (Doubleday).
Mine for Keeps (P), Jean Little (Little, Brown).
My Brother Stevie (I), Eleanor Clymer (Holt).
My Friend Johnny (P), Vane Earle (Lothrop).
Noise in the Night (I), A. Alexander (Rand).
North Fork (I), Doris Gates (Viking).
Old Can and Patrick (I), Ruth Sawyer (Viking).
Out to Win (I-Boys), M. G. Bonner (Knopf).

Peter's Chair (P), E. J. Keats (Harper and Row).
Peter's Treasure (I), C. I. Judson (Houghton).
Petunia (P), Roger Duvoisin (Knopf).
Play Fair (P, I), Munro Leaf (Lippincott).
Sad Day — Glad Day (P), Vivian Thompson (Holi-
  day House).
Shaken Days (I), Doris Gates (Viking).
Something to Live By (I), Dorothea Kopplin
  (Doubleday).
Switch on the Night (P), R. Bradbury (Pantheon).
Tales of A Fourth Grade Nothing (I), Judy Blume
  (Dutton).
The Elephant Who Liked To Smash Small Cars
  (P), Jean Merrill (Pantheon).
The Lion Twins (P, I), Elizabeth Stewart (Athen-
  eum).
The Night the Storm Came (P), G. Relyea (Alad-
  din).
The Secret Name (I), Barbara Williams (Har-
  court).
The Smallest Boy in the Class (I), M. Wohlberg
  (Morrow).
The Ugly Duckling (I), Hans C. Anderson (Har-
  court).
The Very Little Girl (P), P. Krasilovsky (Double-
  day).
The Wonderful Year (I), Nancy Barnes (Messner).
Timid Timothy (P), G. Williams (W. R. Scott).
Understood Betsy (I), C. L. Judson (Houghton).
What Do They Say? (P), Ellen McKean
  (Vanguard).
What Is She Like? (I), Mary Brockman (Scribner).
What Mary Jo Shared (P), Jamie May Udry (Al-
  bert Whitman).
What's That Noise? (I), L. Kauffman (Lothrop).
Who Are You? Joan Bradfield (Whitman).

9. Sex and Family Living Education

a. Pamphlets or Leaflets

A Baby Is Born (Teacher), American Social Health
  Association.
A Story about You, American Medical Associa-
  tion.
Accent on You, Tampax Incorporated.
Are You in the Know?, Kimberly-Clark Corpora-
  tion.
*At What Age Should a Girl Be Told about Men-
  struation?* Kimberly-Clark Corporation.
Boy and His Physique, National Dairy Council.
Boys Want to Know, American Social Hygiene
  Association.
From Fiction to Facts, Tampax Incorporated.
Girl and Her Figure, National Dairy Council.
Growing Up and Liking It, Personal Products
  Company.
Growing Up Young, Kimberly-Clark Corporation.
How Shall I Tell My Daughter? Personal Prod-
  ucts Corporation.
It's Time You Knew, Tampax Incorporated.
Life with Brothers and Sisters, American Social
  Hygiene Association.
Off to a Beautiful Start, Scott Paper Company.

Sex Education for the Ten Year Old, American Medical Association.

Some Questions and Answers about V.D., American Social Health Association.

The Doctor Answers Some Practical Questions on Menstruation, American Association For Health, Physical Education and Recreation.

The Gift of Life, American Social Health Association.

The Heart of the Home, American Heart Association.

The Human Story, Scott, Foresman, and Co.

The Miracle of You, Kimberly-Clark Corporation.

The Story of Life, American Medical Association.

The World of a Girl, Scott Paper Company.

Very Personally Yours, Kimberly-Clark Corporation.

What to Tell Your Children about Sex, Child Study Association of America.

Why Girls Menstruate, American Medical Association.

Your Own Story, American Social Health Association.

You're a Young Lady Now, Kimberly-Clark Corporation.

Your Years of Self-Discovery, Kimberly-Clark Corporation.

b. Films (P) Primary Level, (I) Intermediate Level

Animals Hatched From Eggs (P), Coronet Films.

A Happy Family (P), Classroom Film Distributors. Family relations between a seven year old girl, her younger brother, older sister, and their parents. Depicts how members of the family have learned to live together.

Baby Animals (P), McGraw-Hill Book Company. Elementary.

Birth of a Colt (I), Thorne Films.

Birth of Puppies (P), Coronet Films.

Farmyard Babies (P), Coronet Films.

Farm Babies and Their Mothers (P), Film Associates.

Friendship Begins at Home (P), Coronet Instructional Films.

Growing Up (P), Coronet Instructional Films. Elementary material.

Growing Up Day by Day (P), Encyclopaedia Britannica. Explains the principles of physical, mental, social, and emotional growth to children by comparing members of a group of eight year olds at a birthday party. Explains that actions should vary at different ages and that, as a child grows older, he should learn to do more for himself and others.

Human and Animal Beginnings (P), E. C. Brown Trust. 22 minutes in color. Young children express their beliefs about origin of human life in drawings. Starts with newborn baby and compares with animal babies. Reviews egg development (human and animal) at one month, four months, six months, and nine months.

Kittens—Birth and Growth (P), Bailey Films. Robin and Billy are present when their cat "Mil-
lie" gives birth to four kittens. Shows the kittens nursing, crawling, playing, and being weaned. Emphasizes the care the children give to the kittens.

Mike Finds out about Growing (P), Society for Visual Education. Elementary.

Mother Hen's Family (The Wonders of Birth) (P), Coronet Instructional Films. 10 minutes. Depicts how eggs are hatched by hens. Shows a small boy, with the help of his father, following the process from the laying of the eggs to the hatching of the chicks. The boy charts on a calendar the time of setting to the day of the hatching.

Our Family Works Together (P), Coronet Instructional Materials.

Tabby's Kittens (P), Kindergarten.

What Do Fathers Do? (P), Churchill Films. Develops father's image of providing for family's needs. Tells of importance of being on time to work, of cooperation with others, and how happy people are who like their work and perform it well. (Fourth grade.)

Your Family (P), Coronet Instructional Films.

Boy to Man (I), Churchill Films. 16 minutes in color. Depicts the physical changes of the adolescent as well as complete glandular development. For boys 11–14; may also be used with girls. (Excellent for sixth or seventh grade.)

Everyday Courtesy (I), Churchill Films. Pupils arrange and present an exhibit on courtesy. Invitations are written by children to their parents and guests. Regards courtesy in connection with invitations, telephone conversations, introductions, and entertaining guests.

Growing Girls (I), Encyclopaedia Britannica.

Growing Up (Preadolescence) (I), McGraw-Hill Book Company. 10 minutes in color. Silhouette and animal photography regarding the development of twins. Discusses irregular growth, glands involved in growth, sex differences in growth. Emphasizes diet, relaxation, recreation, and rest.

Human Growth (I), Wexler Film Productions. 20 minutes, 16 mm., color. Shows a seventh grade class viewing and discussing animated film that traces human growth from conception to adulthood. Differences in male and female structural development are emphasized. (Revised.)

Human Reproduction (I), McGraw-Hill Book Company, 22 minutes, 16 mm. Stresses the biological normalcy of human reproduction. Models and animated drawings depict the anatomy and physiology of the male and female reproductive organs.

It's Wonderful Being a Girl (I), Personal Products. 20 minutes in color. This is an excellent film on menstruation. It presents a fine philosophy of being a girl.

Molly Grows Up (I), Personal Products. Upper elementary—junior high.

Story of Menstruation (I), Kimberly-Clark Corporation. 10 minutes in color. Animated drawings and diagrams present, in a direct and scientific way, the story of this natural phenomenon.

The Day Life Begins (I), Carousel Films. 23 minutes.

The Endocrine System (I), Encyclopaedia Britannica.

VD — Name Your Contacts (I), Coronet Instructional Materials.

The Menstrual Cycle (I), Eli Lilly and Company.

The Story of Menstruation (I), Walt Disney Productions.

Tomorrow's Children (I), E. C. Brown Foundation.

You and Your Five Senses (I), Walt Disney Productions. Jiminy Cricket develops theme "All your pets are smart, but the only thinking animal is you. You use thought and reason with your five senses. Animals use their senses entirely by instinct."

You and Your Parents (I), Coronet Instructional Films.

Your Body During Adolescence (I), McGraw-Hill Book Company. Shows the seven glands that regulate human life and growth with emphasis on the pituitary and sex glands. Outlines changes that take place in the bodies of boys and girls.

c. Filmstrips

About Your Life, Denver Public Schools. Denver, Col. (Grade 5).

After School Hours, Popular Science.

Becoming A Woman/Becoming A Man (I), Guidance Associates.

Confidence Because . . . You Understand Menstruation, Personal Products Corporation.

Families Around the World, Encyclopaedia Britannica.

Family Fun, Encyclopaedia Britannica.

Finding Out How Animals Grow, Society for Visual Education.

Fun at the Beach, McGraw-Hill Book Company.

Fun on a Picnic, Curriculum Films.

Getting Ready for School, Popular Science.

Growing Into Womanhood/Growing Into Manhood (I), Guidance Associates.

How Babies Are Made, Creative Scope Inc. (Grades K-3).

Janet Helps Mother, Curriculum Films.

Let's Visit Our Friends, Society for Visual Education.

Miss Brown's Class Goes to the Zoo, Eye Gate House (Grades 2–3).

Reproduction in Flowers, Eye Gate House (Grades 4–6).

The Me I Want To Be, Kimberly-Clark Corporation.

d. Posters

What Happens During Menstruation? Personal Products Corporation.

e. Charts

Baby's Bath, Scott, Foresman and Company.

Beginning the Human Story: A New Baby in the Family, Scott, Foresman and Co.

Father, David C. Cook.

Female Anatomical Charts, Tampax, Incorporated.

How Baby Grows, Johnson and Johnson.

Mother, David C. Cook.

Physiology Chart, Kimberly-Clark Corporation.

What Happens During Menstruation? Personal Products Corporation.

f. Records

Talks With Growing Boys, Stanley Bowmar Co.

Talks With Growing Girls, Stanley Bowmar Co.

The Story of Growing Up, Stanley Bowmar Co.

g. Slides

How Babies Are Made, Creative Scope, Inc., 509 5th Avenue, New York, N.Y., 10017.

Happy Vacation (H56), New York State University College of Agriculture, Cornell University.

House of Darkness, National Safety Council.

Human Reproduction, Guidance Associates.

Stop — Look — Listen (H70), New York State University College of Agriculture, Cornell University.

The Story of Growing Up (Girls), Stanley Bowmar Co.

What It Means to Grow Up (Boys), Stanley Bowmar Co.

h. Transparencies

Babies From Eggs, 3M Company.

Frog's Life Cycle, 3M Company.

Mammal Babies, 3M Company.

Moth's Life Cycle, 3M Company.

Problems of Venereal Disease, Lansford Pub. Co., San Jose, Calif. 95125.

Venereal Disease, Popular Science.

i. Selected Stories for Children
(P) Primary Level, (I) Intermediate Level

A Baby Is Born (P), M. I. Levine and J. H. Seligmann (Golden Press).

A Baby Starts to Grow (P), Paul Showers (Crowell).

A Chimp in the Family (P), Charlotte Beeker (Messner).

A Doctor Talks to 5 to 8 Year Olds (P), D. Meilach (Budlong Press).

A Doctor Talks to 9 to 12 Year Olds (I), M. U. Lerrigo and M. Cassidy (Budlong Press).

A Story about You (I), M. O. Lerrigo and M. J. Senn (American National Association).

About Eggs and Creatures That Hatch from Them (I), M. Uhl (Melmont).

All About Eggs and How They Change into Animals (P), Millicent Selsam (W. R. Scott).

All Kinds of Babies and How They Grow (P), S. E. Millicent (W. R. Scott).

Animal Babies (P), Ylla (Harper).

Animals As Parents (P), M. Selsam (Morrow).

Animal Daddies and My Daddy (P), Barbara Sheek Hazen (Golden Press).

Baby Sister for Francis (P), R. Hoban (Harper & Row).

Bees and Beehives (P), Judy Hawes (Crowell).

Big Lion, Little Lion (P), M. Schlein (Albert Whitman & Co.).

Birthday of Obash (P), A. Chalmers (Viking).

Boo, Who Used to Be Scared of the Dark (P), Munro Leaf (Random House).

Daddies (P), L. Carton (Random House).

Daddy and Me (P), Monte Stein Jonathan (Scribner).

Daddy Is Home (P), D. Blomquist (Holt, Rinehart Winston).

Exploring Home and Family Life (I), H. Fleck (Prentice-Hall).

Facts of Life for Children (I), (Child Study Association).

Finding Yourself (I), M. O. Lerrigo (American Medical Association).

Fine Eggs and Fancy Chicks (P), M. Marks (Dial).

Growing Up (I), K. DeSchweitz (Macmillan).

Happy Little Family (P), R. Candill (Winston).

Holiday on Wheels (I), C. Wooley (Morrow).

How a Seed Grows (I), Helen Jordon (Crowell).

How Animals Live Together (I), M. Selsam (Morrow).

How Babies Are Made (P), A. Andry (Time-Life).

How Life Is Handed on (I), C. Beck (Harcourt Brace).

How We Are Born (I), Julian May (Follett).

Hush Jon! (P), Joan Gill (Doubleday).

I Like to Be Me (P), Barbara Bel Geddes (Viking).

Johnny Jack and His Beginnings (P), Pearl Buck (John Day).

Kid Brother (P), J. Beim (Morrow).

Laurie's New Brother (P), M. Schlein (Abelard-Schuman, Ltd.).

Living Things and Their Young (I), Julian May (Follett).

Man and Woman (I), Julian May (Follett).

Mommies (P), L. Carton (Random House).

Mommies Are for Loving (P), R. Penn (Putnam's Sons).

Mommies at Work (P), J. Marian (Alfred A. Knopf).

Peter and Caroline (P), S. Hegeler (Abelard-Schuman Ltd.).

Possum (P), R. McClung (Morrow).

Red Bantam (P), L. Fatio (McGraw-Hill Book Company).

Sam (I), Ann Scott (McGraw-Hill).

Seeds Are Wonderful (I), W. Foster and P. Queree (Melmont).

Sigurd and His Brave Companions (I), S. Undset (Knopf).

Sky Bed, a Norwegian Christmas (I), T. T. Grundrun (Scribner).

Squirrels in the Garden (P), O. Earle (Morrow).

Stepsister Sally (P), H. F. Daringer (Harcourt).

The Beginning of Life (I), Eva Knox Evans (Collier-Macmillan).

The Best Birthday (P), Quail Hawkins (Doubleday).

The Chosen Baby (P), V. P. Wasson (Lippincott).

The Growing Story (I), Ruth Grauss (Harper).

The Human Story (I), S. Hoftein (Scott-Foresman).

The Little Girl and Her Mother (P), Beatrice DeRiginier (Vanguard).

The New Pet (P), Marjorie Flack (Doubleday).

The People Upstairs (I), Phyllis Cote (Doubleday).

The Stork Didn't Bring You (I), Lloyd Pemberton (Thomas Nelson & Sons).

The Story of Life (I), M. O. Lerrigo and M. J. Senn (American National Association).

The Wonder of Life (I), M. I. Levine and J. H. Seligmann (Simon & Schuster).

The Wonderful Story of How You Were Born (P), J. Gruenberg (American Social Hygiene Association).

The Wonderful Year (I), Nancy Barnes (Messner).

True Book of Health (P), O. V. Haynes (Children's Press).

Two Little Birds and Three (P), J. Kepes (Houghton).

Wait and See (P), C. Georgion (Harvey House).

What Makes Me Tick? (I), H. Ruchlis (Harvey House).

What's Inside of Animals? (P), H. S. Zim (Morrow).

When Animals Are Babies (P), Elizabeth and Charles Schwartz (Holiday House).

When An Animal Grows (I), Millicent Selsam (William Morrow).

When Boy Likes Girl (I), A. Stowe (Random House).

Whitefoot—the Story of a Wood Mouse (I), R. McClung (Morrow).

Window into An Egg: Seeing Life Begin (P), G. Lux Flanagan (W. R. Scott).

You and the World Around You (P), M. Selsam (Doubleday).

Young Man of the House (P), Mabel L. Hunt (Lippincott).

10. Environmental Health

a. Pamphlets or Leaflets

Bicycle Riding Clubs, Bicycle Institute of America.

Bike Regulations in the Community, Bicycle Institute of America.

Clean Water, U.S. Public Health Service.

Crusade of the Christmas Seal, National Tuberculosis Association.

Hot Tips on Food Protection, U.S. Public Health Service.

Medical Uses of Blood, American Red Cross.

Some Facts . . . Why Blood Is Needed, American Red Cross.

Suggestions on What to Teach about Cancer, American Cancer Society.

The Doctor Is Your Friend, National Tuberculosis Association.

The Long Adventure, National Tuberculosis Association.

Your Friend the Doctor, American Medical Association.

b. Films

Adventuring in Conservation, Indiana University Audio-Visual Center.

Bulldozed America, Carousel Films.

Choosing a Doctor, McGraw-Hill Book Company.
Communities Keep Clean, Coronet Instructional Films.
Community Health Is Up to You, McGraw-Hill Book Company.
Conservation and the Balance of Nature, International Film Bureau.
Defending the City's Health, Encyclopaedia Britannica.
Farm Animals, National Dairy Council.
Fun on the Playground, Encyclopaedia Britannica.
Little Man, Big City, Center for Mass Communications, Columbia University Press.
Man's Natural Environment, Guidance Associates.
Mosquito, Encyclopaedia Britannica.
Policemen—Day and Night, Charles Cahill and Associates.
The Doctor, Encyclopaedia Britannica.
The Endless Chain, Tribune Films, Inc.
The Fireman, Encyclopaedia Britannica.
The Ravaged Land, John Wiley & Sons, Inc.
The Water We Drink, Coronet Instructional Films.
To Live and Breathe, Aetna Life and Casualty Company.
Uncle Jim's Dairy Farm, National Dairy Council.
Vegetables for All Seasons, Arthur Barr Productions, Inc.
Your Friend the Doctor, Coronet Instructional Films.
Your Health in the Community, Coronet Instructional Films.

c. Filmstrips

Community Sanitation, Young America Films.
Environmental Crisis, American Association for Health, Physical Education and Recreation.
Fun at the Beach, McGraw-Hill Book Company.
Health Heroes (with transcription), Metropolitan Life Insurance Company.
Keeping Sickness Away, McGraw-Hill Book Company.
Maintaining Community Health, Young America Films.
Making Water Safe to Drink, Popular Science.
On the Road to the Country, Curriculum Films.
Our Health Department, Encyclopaedia Britannica.
Safeguarding Our Food, Young America Films.
Safety in the Community, Young America Films.
Sewage Disposal, McGraw-Hill Book Company.
The School That Learned to Eat, General Mills, Inc.
The Water We Drink, Young America Films.
Tommy and His Health Department, Educational Activities, Inc.
Tree Man: A First Adventure In Ecology, Coronet Instructional Films.
Vacation in the City, Curriculum Films.
Walter Reed and the Conquest of Yellow Fever (with transcription), Metropolitan Life Insurance Company.
Waste Disposal for the Community, Encyclopaedia Britannica.
Water and How We Use It, Coronet Instructional Films.

Water for the Community, Encyclopaedia Britannica.

d. Comics

Alfie Looks for Fire Trouble, National Fire Protection Association.
Sparky, National Fire Protection Association.
Sparky's Coloring Book, National Fire Protection Association.

e. Records

Fire on Thunder Hill, American Forest Products Industries, Inc.
The Constant Invaders, Wisconsin Anti-Tuberculosis Association.
Tommy and His Health Department, Educational Activities, Inc.

f. Radio Scripts

Fly Control, Bureau of Research in Education by Radio, University of Texas.
Home Safety, National Safety Council.
Keep Your Cold at Home, Bureau of Research in Education by Radio, University of Texas.
Know Your Traffic Laws, National Safety Council.
Make Your City Safer, National Safety Council.
Safe Water Supply, Bureau of Research in Education by Radio, University of Texas.
Swimming and Water Safety, Bureau of Research in Education by Radio, University of Texas.
To Walk in the Night, National Safety Council.

g. Slides

Urban Slum Problems, J. Weston Walch, Publisher.
Water Conservation, J. Weston Walch, Publisher.
Water Pollution, J. Weston Walch, Publisher.

h. Selected Stories for Children
(P) Primary Level, (I) Intermediate Level
A Chimp in the Family (P), Charlotte Beeker (Messner).
ABC's of Ecology (I), Isaac Asimov (Walker).
About the Nature of Air (I), Harry Sootin (W. W. Norton).
And It Rained (I), Ellen Raskin (Atheneum).
A Walk in the City (P), Rosemary Dawson (Viking).
Boating Is Fun (I), R. Brindze (Dodd).
Brave Gives Blood (I), Philip and Mirina Eisenburg (Messner).
Camp-in-the-Yard (P), V. Thompson (Holiday).
Come to the City (P), Ruth Tensen (Pertly & Lee).
Dangerous Air (I), Lucy Kavaler (John Day).
Experiences With Living Things for Five to Eight Year Olds (P), Katherine Wensberg (Beacon).
Fireman for a Day (I), Z. K. MacDonald (Messner).
First Book of Nurses (I), M. Etting (Watts).
Johnny Goes to the Hospital (P), J. Sever (Houghton).
Johnny Wants to Be a Policeman (P, I), W. J. Granberg (Aladdin).
Let's Go Fishing (I), Lee Wulff (Lippincott).
Let's Go to Stop Air Pollution (I), Michael Chester (G. P. Putnam's Sons).

Little Town (P), Bertrand Elmer Hader (Macmillan).

Our Insect Friends (I), W. A. DuPuy (Winston).

Our Polluted World (I), John Perry (Franklin Watts).

Pat and Her Policeman (I), F. Friedman (Morrow).

Poems and Verses about the City (I), Nancy Varrick (Garrard).

Rain, Rain, River (P), Uri Shulevitz (Farrar).

Smoke (P), Ab Spang Olsen (Coward).

Strange Companions in Nature (I), I. Smith (Morrow).

Su-Mei's Golden Year (I), M. H. Bro (Doubleday).

The City Book (P), L. Corcos (Golden).

The Discontented Village (I), Rose Dobbs (Coward-McCann).

The Fight to Save America's Water (I), U.S. Public Health Service.

The Last Free Bird (P), A. Harris Stone (Prentice-Hall).

The Life in the Forest (I), Jack McCormick (McGraw-Hill).

The Water That Jack Drank (P), William R. Scott (W. R. Scott)

The Wonderful Farm (P), M. Ayme (Harper).

There Is a Seal in My Sleeping Bag (I), Lyn Hancock (Alfred A. Knopf).

This Vital Air (I), Thomas Hylesworth (Rand McNally).

Tim and the Brass Buttons (P), Ruth Tooze (Messner).

True Book of Policemen and Firemen (P), I. Miner (Children's Press).

Water (I), Luna Leopold (Time-Life).

Water, the Vital Essence (I), Peter Briggs (Harper & Row).

Weather (I), P. Thompson (Time-Life).

Where the Lilies Bloom (I), Vera and Bill Cleaver (Lippincott).

While Susie Sleeps (P), N. Schneider (W. R. Scott).

11. Tobacco, Alcohol and Drugs

a. Pamphlets or Leaflets

A Light on the Subject of Smoking, U.S. Children's Bureau.

About Alcohol and Narcotics, Licensed Beverage Industries, Inc.

Alcoholism, Metropolitan Life Insurance Co.

Alcohol, Science and Society, Center for Alcohol Studies, Yale University.

Alcoholics Anonymous — 44 Questions, Alcoholics Anonymous.

Charlie's Party, Connecticut State Department of Mental Health, Hartford, Conn.

Cigarette Smoking and Cancer, American Cancer Society.

Drugs and Driving, U.S. Food and Drug Administration.

Facts about Alcohol, Connecticut State Department of Mental Health, Hartford, Conn.

How Alcohol Affects the Body, Connecticut State Department of Mental Health, Hartford, Conn.

I'll Choose the High Road, American Cancer Society.

Marihuana, U.S. Government Printing Office.

Marihuana and Health, U.S. Public Health Service.

Marihuana Questions and Answers, U.S. Public Health Service.

My Dear, This'll Kill You! National Tuberculosis Association.

Smoking — It's up to You, Health Education Service.

Smoking and Illness, National Clearinghouse for Smoking and Health.

The Most Frequently Asked Questions About Drug Abuse, The White House, Washington, D.C. 20506.

Thirteen Steps to Alcoholism, National Council on Alcoholism.

Tips on Drug Abuse Prevention, National Institute of Mental Health.

To Your Health, American Medical Association.

What the Body Does With Alcohol, Licensed Beverage Industries, Inc.

What to Tell Your Parents about Smoking, American Heart Association.

Why Nick the Cigarette Is Nobody's Friend, U.S. Children's Bureau.

b. Films

Alcohol, General Services Administration.

Alcohol — a New Focus, American Educational Films.

Alcohol in the Human Body, Sid Davis Productions.

Alcoholism, Encyclopaedia Britannica.

Alcoholism, the Hidden Disease, National Council on Alcoholism.

Barney Butt, American Heart Association.

Breaking the Habit, American Cancer Society.

Curious Alice, General Services Administration.

Drug Abuse — Everybody's Hang-up, American Association for Health, Physical Education and Recreation.

Drug Addiction, Encyclopaedia Britannica.

Drug Education at the Elementary Level, General Services Administration.

Drugs: A Primary Film, Arthur Barr Productions.

Drugs and the Nervous System, Churchill Films.

Drugs, Drinking and Driving, Aims Instructional Media Services.

Drugs — Use or Abuse, Instructional Media Services.

Drunk Driving, Teaching Film Custodians.

Flagged for Actions, National Film Board of Canada.

Focus on Drugs, American Educational Films.

From One Cell, American Cancer Society.

Huffless, Puffless Dragon, American Cancer Society.

Is Smoking Worth It? American Cancer Society.

Narcotics — Why Not? Charles Cahill and Associates.

One Day's Poison, National Film Board of Canada.

Out of Orbit, National Council on Alcoholism.

Rick—File X-258375, General Services Administration.

Should You Drink? McGraw-Hill Book Company.

Smoking: A New Focus, American Educational Films.

Smoking and You, American Heart Association.

Smoking and Your Oral Health, American Dental Association.

The Drug Dilemma: A New Day Dawning, Coronet Instructional Materials.

The Tobacco Problem: What Do You Think? Encyclopaedia Britannica.

Tobacco and the Human Body, Encyclopaedia Britannica.

To Smoke or Not to Smoke, American Cancer Society.

To Your Health, Ideal Pictures.

Traffic with the Devil, Teaching Film Custodians.

What about Drinking? McGraw-Hill Book Company.

What Should I Do? Walt Disney Productions.

c. Filmstrips

Alcohol and Children (Gr 4–8), Educational Activities, Inc.

Alcohol and You, McGraw-Hill Book Company.

Alcohol and You, Young America Films.

Alcohol and Your Health, Society for Visual Education.

Algernon, the Ambulance, International Education and Training, Inc.

Danger of Narcotics, Popular Science.

Drugs and Children (Gr 4–8), Educational Activities, Inc.

Drugs Helpful and Harmful, Wexler Film Productions.

Drug Misuse and Your Health, Society for Visual Education.

Drugs, Poisons and Little Children, Stanley Bowmar Co.

I'll Choose the High Road, American Cancer Society.

Junkie, Educational Activities.

Me, Myself—And Drugs, Guidance Associates.

Narcotics and You, Young America Films.

Nature's Filter, National Tuberculosis Association.

Only Sick People Need Drugs (K-3), Educational Activities, Inc.

Smoking and Children (Gr 4–8), Educational Activities, Inc.

The Champion, Image Publishing Corporation.

Tobacco and Alcohol, Guidance Associates.

Tobacco and Your Health, Society for Visual Education.

To Smoke or Not to Smoke, American Cancer Society.

d. Posters

Best Time to Stop Smoking, American Medical Association.

Best Tip Yet—Don't Start, American Cancer Society.

Break the Habit, American Medical Association.

I Don't Smoke Cigarettes, American Cancer Society.

100,000 Doctors Have Stopped Smoking, U.S. Public Health Service.

This Chimp is No Chump . . . Don't Smoke, American Heart Association.

This Is a Dumb Bunny, U.S. Public Health Service.

e. Records

The Drugs You Use, American Medical Association.

The Most Frequently Asked Questions about Drug Abuse (3), The White House, Washington, D.C. 20506.

f. Comics

Dennis the Menace Takes a Poke at Poisons, U.S. Government Printing Office.

It's Best to Know, Connecticut State Department of Mental Health.

Where There Is Smoke, American Cancer Society.

g. Charts

Dial a Drug, Spenco Medical Corporation.

Drug Abuse Reference Chart, Pharmaceutical Manufacturers Association.

Facts about Drugs, David C. Cook Pub. Co., Elgin, Ill., 60120.

h. Slides

The Problem of Drug Abuse, Pharmaceutical Manufacturers Association.

i. Kits

Drug Abuse Information Kit, Pharmaceutical Manufacturers Association.

Drug Education Package, Spenco Medical Corporation.

Drug Information Center (Kit), Channing L. Bete Co., Greenfield, Mass. 01301.

Smoking Education Package, Spenco Medical Corporation.

j. Selected Stories for Children
(P) Primary Level, (I) Intermediate Level

About Drugs (I), H. L. Bowen and L. Landen (Fearon).

Alcohol Talks from the Laboratory (I), H. Hamlin (The author, Columbus 12, Ohio).

Facts about Alcohol (I), Raymond McCarthy (Yale Center of Alcohol Studies).

Facts about Narcotics (I), V. A. Vogel (Science Research Associates).

Modern Medical Discoveries (I), I. Eberle (Crowell).

What You Should Know about Drugs (I), S. Christian (Harcourt).

12. Consumer Health

a. Pamphlets or Leaflets

Chiropractic: The Unscientific Cult, American Medical Association.

Consumer Protection—Drugs and Cosmetics, U.S. Food and Drug Administration.

Consumer Protection—Foods, U.S. Food and Drug Administration.

Facts on Quacks, American Medical Association.
Folklore and Fallacies in Dentistry, American Dental Association.
Food Values in Common Portions, U.S. Department of Agriculture.
Health Quackery, American Medical Association.
Hot Tips on Food Protection, U.S. Food and Drug Administration.
How Safe Is Our Food? U.S. Food and Drug Administration.
Key Facts about the Drug Industry, Pharmaceutical Manufacturers Association.
Mail Fraud, American Medical Association.
Make the Most of Your Food Money, Evaporated Milk Association.
Medical Quackery, American Medical Association.
Read the Label, U.S. Food and Drug Administration.
Read the Label, National Fire Protection Association.
Safe New Drugs, U.S. Food and Drug Administration.
The Medicines Your Doctor Prescribes, Pharmaceutical Manufacturers Association.
The Merchants of Menace, American Medical Association.
TV and Your Eyes, National Society for the Prevention of Blindness.
Your Clothing Dollar, Money Management Institute.
Your Food Dollar, Money Management Institute.
Your Health and Recreation Dollar, Money Management Institute.
Your Money and Your Life, American Medical Association.

b. Films

An Ounce of Prevention, Pharmaceutical Manufacturers Association.
Choosing a Doctor, McGraw-Hill Book Company.
Dress for Health, Encyclopaedia Britannica.
Folks, Facts, and Pharmacy, Lederle Laboratory.
Horizons of Hope, American Cancer Society.
How to Select Florida Oranges, Florida Citrus Commission.
I Have a Secret Cure for Cancer, American Cancer Society.
Medicine Man, American Medical Association.
More Food for Your Money, National Dairy Council.
Pork Around the Clock, National Livestock and Meat Board.
Pressure Steam Sterilization, Ideal Pictures.
Quacks and Nostrums, McGraw-Hill Book Company.
Read the Label and Live, Hank Newenhouse Films.
The Best Way to Eat, Florida Citrus Commission.
The Meanest Crime, U.S. Food and Drug Administration.
To Your Health, National Council on Alcoholism.
When It Comes to RX Medicines, Pharmaceutical Manufacturers Association.
Your Friend the Doctor, Coronet Instructional Films.

c. Filmstrips

Be a Balanced Wheel, National Dairy Council.
Buyer Beware, Guidance Associates.
FDA: A Nation's Watchdog? Guidance Associates.
Health Helpers, Encyclopaedia Britannica.
Merchandising Beef, National Livestock and Meat Board.
Project A.M., Cereal Institute.
Spending Your Food Dollars, Money Management Institute.
Tale of a Toothache, Society for Visual Education.
The Little Pink Bottle, National Foundation.
Tommy and His Health Department, Educational Activities, Inc.
You the Shopper, Money Management Institute.

d. Posters

What You Eat Can Make a Difference, Florida Citrus Commission.

e. Selected Stories for Children
(P) Primary Level, (I) Intermediate Level
Doctor John (P), F. Thompson (Melmont).
Doctors and What They Do (I), H. Coy (Watts).
Habits, Healthful and Safe (I), W. Charters (Macmillan).
Health Can Be Fun (P), M. Leaf (Stokes).
How Hospitals Help Us (P), A. Meeker (Benefic Press).
Linda Goes to the Hospital (P), N. Dudley (Coward).
Magic Bullets (I), L. Sutherland (Little).
The Hospital (P), M. Pyne (Houghton Mifflin).
We Went to the Doctor (P), C. Memling (Abelard-Schuman Ltd.).

ADDRESSES OF FILM SOURCES

Aims Instructional Media Services, P.O. Box 1010, Hollywood, Calif., 90028.
American Educational Films, 331 North Maple Drive, Beverly Hills, California, 90210.
Arthur Barr Productions, Inc., P.O. Box 7-C, Pasadena, California, 91104.
Association Films, Inc., 25358 Cypress Avenue, Hayward, California.
Avis Films, 2408 W. Olive Avenue, Burbank, Calif., 91506.
Bailey Films, Inc., 6509 De Longpre Avenue, Hollywood, Calif., 90028.
Canadian National Film Board, 680 5th Avenue, New York, N.Y., 10019.
Carousel Films, 1501 Broadway, New York, N.Y., 10036.
Center for Mass Communication, Columbia University Press, 562 West 113th St., New York, N.Y., 10025.
Charles Cahill and Associates, P.O. Box 3220, Hollywood, Calif., 90028.
Churchill Films, 622 No. Robertson Blvd., Los Angeles, Calif., 90069.

Classroom Film Distributors Inc., 5620 Hollywood Boulevard, Los Angeles, Calif.

Coronet Instructional Materials, 65 E. South Water Street, Chicago, Ill., 60601.

E. C. Brown Foundation, 1825 Willow Rd., Northfield, Illinois, 60093.

Encyclopaedia Britannica Educational Corporation, 425 North Michigan Ave., Chicago, Ill., 60611.

Eye Gate House Inc., 146 Archer Avenue, Jamaica, N.Y., 11435.

Films Incorporated, 1144 Wilmette Ave., Wilmette, Ill., 60091.

Guidance Associates, Pleasantville, New York

Hank Newenhouse Films, 1825 Willow Rd., Northfield, Ill., 60093.

Ideal Pictures Corporation, 321 W. 44th Street, New York, N.Y., 10036.

Image Publishing Corporation, P.O. Box 14 North Station, White Plains, New York, 10603.

International Film Bureau, Inc., 322 S. Michigan Avenue, Chicago, Ill., 60604.

Knowledge Builders, 625 Madison Avenue, New York, N.Y.

McGraw-Hill Book Company, Inc., 330 West 42nd Street, New York, N.Y., 10036.

Media Visuals, Inc., 342 Madison Ave., New York, N.Y., 10017.

Modern Talking Picture Service, 45 Rockefeller Plaza, New York, N.Y.

Moody Institute of Science, 12000 E. Washington Boulevard, Whittier, Calif., 90606.

Popular Science, 330 West 42nd Street, New York, N.Y.

Sid Davis Productions, 2429 Ocean Park Blvd., Santa Monica, Calif., 90405.

Society for Visual Education, Inc., 1345 Diversey Park, Chicago, Ill., 60614.

Teaching Film Custodians, 25 West 43rd Street, New York, N.Y.

Thorne Films, 1229 University Ave., Boulder, Col., 80302.

Tribune Films, Inc., 38 West 32nd St., New York, N.Y., 10001.

United World Films, 221 Park Avenue, South, New York, N.Y.

Walt Disney Productions, 800 Senora Avenue, Glendale, Calif., 91201.

Wexler Film Productions, 801 N. Seward Street, Los Angeles, Calif., 90038.

Young America Films, 330 W. 24th Street, New York, N.Y.

EVALUATION IN HEALTH EDUCATION

11

Prove all things; hold fast to that which is good.

Thessalonians I:5:21

In an indictment of American education, a United States Senate committee condemned the schools for failing to properly educate millions of children. The dollar loss to the nation because of these children, said the 1973 study, was estimated at 77 billion dollars annually in tax revenue, welfare and crime costs, attributable to inadequate education. Obviously, educators stand accused of literally shortchanging the taxpayer. Although they have many successes, they have nevertheless failed to turn out a "product" that is in keeping with the specifications — the preconceived general and specific educational objectives. In the health area alone — where the health goals have been clearly stated for years — students have graduated into adulthood with only a minimum of health understanding, awareness and behavior change. In the company of their colleagues they suffer from poor mental health, drink and smoke to excess, and do little or nothing to identify and practice a way of living that will prevent coronary heart attacks, overweight, emphysema, and a myriad of lesser diseases of the flesh and spirit. Is it not past time, therefore, to do more than talk about accountability in education? Is it not time

to act — to prove all things and to hold fast to that which is good?

Purposes of Evaluation in Health

To profess to have an aim, said John Dewey, and then neglect the means of execution is self-delusion of the most dangerous sort. When we take ends without means, we degenerate into sentimentalism. In the ideal we fall back upon merely luck and chance. It is for this reason that some measurement in health education is necessary. Classroom teachers of health want to know if their pupils are really improving in health practices and attitudes. An uncertain knowledge as to whether a health program is successful or not actually frustrates the conscientious teacher. Only through a continuous appraisal of the results of teaching can information be obtained which will relieve frustration and doubt.

Evaluation does several things when properly implemented:

It determines the health status of pupils. Learning in any area is limited by the presence of organic strains and drains, defects, and poor mental health.

It may be used to classify pupils for school activities. Pupils with chronic fatigue, faulty posture, or malnutrition often need a modified program.

It measures the efficiency of the total health program. The effective health services department, the healthful school environment, and the health teaching program all share in influencing the health status as well as the health practices of each pupil.

It measures teacher efficiency. Even the most elaborate health curriculum depends for its success on techniques and aids employed by the individual teacher.

It provides a basis for grading pupils in the instructional program; it is a means of reporting individual pupil achievement.

It contributes useful information relative to student knowledges, attitudes, and practices which may be of value when the curriculum or course of study is being updated.

EVALUATING THE TOTAL SCHOOL HEALTH PROGRAM

It is a major undertaking to appraise the effect of the total elementary school health education effort. The combined activity of many people is involved. The contributions of the classroom teacher are supplemented by those of the guidance and physical education personnel. In larger schools it involves not only the physician and nurse but also often involves a school dentist, school nutritionist, and psychiatrist actively engaged in promoting child health. There may also be an active health council. These persons work in the three areas of health education: health services, healthful school environment, and health instruction. Any measure of pupil improvement in health understanding, awareness and behavior must, therefore, relate to the cooperative efforts of several forces within the school.

As previously indicated in Chapter 3, there are many ways a pupil's health status can be appraised. Much of this appraisal, when understood by the student, has a beneficial effect on health attitudes and practices. By the same token, the example of a healthful school environment does much in a quiet, even subtle, way to influence the formation of desirable health behavior (Chap. 4). Usually, any formal health effort beyond this becomes one of specific instruction in the classroom.

It is sound educational practice to periodically evaluate the total elementary school program in health education. This may be accomplished every two or three years by employing a specially prepared evaluation instrument. Several such instruments are available for the use of elementary school administrators. Two of the more complete ones are as follows:

Criteria for Evaluating the Elementary Health Program (California State Department of Education, Sacramento, Calif.). This form is used to evaluate: Administration, Health instruction, Health services, and Healthful school environment. Each of the criteria are set forth as desirable practices. The quality of each practice is judged for a particular school on a four-point scale: excellent, good, fair, and poor.

An especially thorough instrument is the *Evaluative Criteria, Health Education* (NSSSE) prepared by the American Council On Education, 1785 Massachusetts Avenue, N.W., Washington, D.C., 20036. Health education criteria are presented in checklist form so that they may easily be applied to local health education programs as a self-testing activity or by an evaluating agency. Searching questions are raised about the extent of the instructional program.

Today the total school health program is focused on *output*—on achievement—on demonstrated results. We have moved from input to output. Thus the health services, curriculum content, materials and grade placement of learning activities are viewed in terms of student output. How well is he now as compared with before, and how does he feel and act?

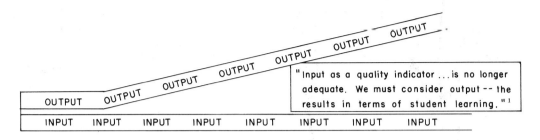

"Input as a quality indicator ... is no longer adequate. We must consider output -- the results in terms of student learning."[1]

PROBLEMS IN EVALUATING THE HEALTH INSTRUCTION PROGRAM

While health is not in itself the flower of life, it is the soil from which the finest flowers grow.

—Duncan Spaeth

The very meaning of the above quotation suggests that the effect of good health teaching on human activity may be difficult to measure. This is true for several reasons:

The power of the human organism to adapt to the physical and psychological stresses placed upon it is most remarkable. All too often the apparently healthy person is harboring one or more potential killers. Heart disease, cancer, respiratory congestion, and kidney malfunction are all about us. The diseases of stress and the shades of malnutrition do not always manifest themselves so that they are easily observed. The line between adjustment and maladjustment is not always defined. Even "normality" is relative.

There is a "sleeper effect" in health teaching. What is learned today in terms of factual knowledge may not be applied until months or years later. Improved attitudes and practices make themselves known at a time when they do not seem to be directly related to anything—least of all to a health course taken at an earlier time.

This chapter is chiefly concerned with appraising the *health instruction* aspects of health education. There is, here, a manifest interest in healthful behavior that is the result of health teaching in the classroom. The one big question raised is "Just how effective is health teaching?" Once the teacher secures the answer to this question she is in a better position to fulfill one of the major purposes of evaluation—that of program improvement. Deciding on health instruction objectives and selecting measuring instruments is not enough. One must appraise and interpret the results of measurement. The findings are then applied toward the improvement of the health instruction program.

Even under the most favorable conditions it will be difficult to fully appraise the health instruction program. Not all of the ramifications of a health lesson are statistically measurable. Very often health instruction goes far beyond the pupil and affects the behavior of his parents and other members of the community. Frequently the support which the public gives to a health project is at least partially the result of effective school health teaching. Even such community items as improved disease reporting, increased circulation of health literature in public libraries, reduced water pollution, the further installation of sanitary facilities, the increase in dental and physical examinations, and even the increase in newspaper editors who speak out on consumer health—all of these may be related to the efforts of the classroom teacher.

An accurate measurement of health attitudes and practices is difficult under the best of circumstances. It has always been rather simple to test for health facts, and considerably more difficult to sample attitudes or beliefs, or ascertain whether a pupil has shown the ability to apply health information in an effective manner.

Too many teachers through the years have simply handed out facts to their pupils and have received the facts back at examination time. Thousands of schoolchildren can spell, write, and recite the names of the vitamins and minerals found in specific foods; they can name the teeth, and diagram how the blood circulates in the body. Yet many of them do not choose foods wisely; they do not own a toothbrush, or appreciate the relationship of adequate rest and sleep to personal well-being in work and play. In short, they are rated as good students of health because they have given the teacher what she wanted to hear—health facts and figures.

These statements are not meant to imply that facts are unimportant in health teaching. Quite the opposite is true, for facts are always of value when it comes to specific knowledge and intelligent behavior. The quarrel comes when mere facts by themselves are the meat of the teaching and testing program. Personal involvement must be added. Students who *act* on facts during the teaching program are more apt to *behave* differently when habits and attitudes are appraised at a later date. Appraisal, therefore, involves pupil behavior and attitudes as well as a number of noteworthy facts. One of the specific findings in the Los Angeles study was that "how people *feel* toward health education" determines to a great extent what they do about their health behavior. It takes time and a concentration of effort in school to develop *feelings* toward health. Research supports this view by showing that direct teaching is superior to integrated and correlated instruction.

The classroom teacher will evaluate health instruction by noting such concrete items as the increase in children having dental work completed, the number of improved practices relative to milk drinking, cleanliness, posture, and appearance, the increase in the sale of nutritious foods at the cafeteria, the reports on changed behaviors made by parents, the increase in the number of parents attending school health examinations of their children, the increase in the percentage of physical defects remedied, and many more such specific items.

There is a shortage of valid and useful elementary health education tests, scales, and other appraisal devices. While local knowledge tests are not difficult to construct, homemade tests of attitudes and practices are harder to come by. Even when there are fairly good tests, their usefulness is reduced by the fact that many teachers fail to determine what a pupil or class knows about a health topic at the beginning of the study. In other words, some *pretesting* or early appraisal is necessary before a particular unit of work is started. The teacher's objective is simply to find out what the class knows and how it feels about the topic *before* instruction begins. There is tremendous variation in initial health knowledge, not only between individuals, but also between classes and between schools. Pre-testing provides the teacher with information relative to pupil inadequacies and strengths, and thus makes possible the selection of the most appropriate subject matter and the placement of emphasis to meet individual pupil shortcomings. In this connection, the selection of appropriate subject matter involves *action research*—a kind of on-the-spot evaluation process that appraises immediate classroom situations by setting up simple designs to get at real problems without carrying on a thorough research project. Parents, for instance, may be interviewed to discover what children are doing or where the learning difficulties are. Classroom teaching techniques may be balanced against other school-community influences.

APPRAISAL METHODS IN THE CLASSROOM

Health appraisal is not something that is done after the instruction has been completed; it occurs simultaneously with teaching and learning. Evaluation is much broader than organized testing which takes place at specific intervals prior to sending report cards home. It is something that occurs whenever pupils are within the observation of the teacher. This permits the teacher to evaluate both the pupils and herself. In this way teaching techniques may be modified or better ones employed without too much delay.

Bloom, Hastings and Madaus have done much to advance the concept of concurrent teaching and appraising by stressing the need to broaden cognitive evaluations and *measure progress by the degree to which individual behavior conforms to the prearranged behavioral objectives.*[2] In keeping with what Bloom had done earlier in his *Taxonomy of Educational Objectives*, a considerable amount of attention is directed toward the application of knowledge. The student who is able to apply his knowledge uses abstractions in various situations. These may be in the form of general ideas, rules of procedure, or they may involve technical principles and theories. Bloom feels that if the student learns well it is partly due to the fact that the item learned is so serviceable—somehow important to the individual.

In his original work, Bloom set up six educational objectives in the *cognitive domain* that bear examining from the point of view of health education.[3]

No. 1 Knowledge
This is the recall of specifics—methods, processes, theories, structures or settings. Here one would test for knowledge relative to health terminology, definitions and trends.
    Example: Which of the following is employed to prevent night blindness?
        1. Vitamin C
        2. Vitamin B

        3. Vitamin A
        4. Iron compound

No. 2 Comprehension
The lowest level of understanding, where the individual can make use of something without necessarily relating it to other things.
    Included in this category is the ability to *translate* or paraphrase a communication
    Example: While listening to the teacher you have heard the following terms frequently used: "alcohol," "drug," "alcoholic," "proof," and "social drinking." In a short paragraph tell in your own words what these terms mean to you.

No. 3 Application
Using abstractions or technical principles, ideas, and theories in some way. There is sufficient student understanding here in order to select and apply the abstraction. Application questions call for a show of practical ability where the student is able to match some already acquired concept with the phenomenon being considered.
    Example: a. Will this lightweight coat keep me comfortably warm in Alaska in the winter?
           b. Choose two pictures of automobile accidents from the local newspaper and compare them in terms of their being representative of what is happening on the highways today.

No. 4 Analysis
The examining of an idea, concept or structure by breaking it down into its elements or parts so that the *relationship* between elements is clear.
    Example: The husband of a woman who died of lung cancer claimed that the physician did not provide proper medical care during the several months in which he had the woman as a patient. Why is this accusation unfair?
        1. The woman was told several times by the physician to stop smoking, but she paid no attention.
        2. Lung cancer cannot be cured unless the lungs are removed.
        3. The woman went to the physician too late for the

---

[2] Bloom, Benjamin S., Hastings, J. Thomas and Madaus, George F., *Handbook on Formative and Summative Evaluation of Student Learning*, New York: McGraw-Hill Book Company, 1971.
[3] For a fine elaboration on this see Solleder, Marion K., "Evaluation in the Cognitive Domain," *Journal of School Health*, 42:16–20, January 1972.

cancer to be brought under control.

4. The cancer appeared suddenly in the woman the week before she died.

No. 5 Synthesis

The bringing together of all parts and elements to form a whole. The student is able to work with pieces and make arrangements in such a manner as to create a structure or pattern not there before. Theorizing or making a firm statement on the basis of data on hand demonstrates the ability to synthesize.

Example: Prepare an essay in which you consider the relationship between man and his plant-animal world, and how this has a bearing on his general health and well-being. This is explained in the Guidance Associates filmstrip, *Man's Natural Environment.*

The filmstrip will be shown to you once as you begin to think about the assignment, and once again ten minutes later. It is suggested that after the first showing you spend about ten minutes planning your remarks.

No. 6 Evaluation

This involves the making of judgements relative to the worth of materials, methods and ideas.

Example: Which of the following frequently is responsible for skin disorders in young people?
1. Eating too many acid-type foods.
2. Washing the skin too often.
3. Changes in the chemistry of the body.
4. Overexercise and extreme body fatigue.

In constructing health education tests the *affective domain* is also important. Bloom points out that each cognitive behavior has an affective behavior and vice versa. The five part progression is as follows:

1. *Receiving:* Here there is a willingness on the part of the pupil to "tune in" and receive—to become *aware.*
2. *Responding:* This is active attending— doing something with the phenomena, and not just being aware of it.

3. *Valuing:* The concept of worth becomes part of the individual—consistent enough to take on the characteristics of a belief or an attitude. There is a commitment.
4. *Organization:* The internalized values become organized into the individual's value system and are related to other values.
5. *Characterization:* The organization of values into a total philosophy or world view. The peak of the internalization process.

Example (Through questioning):

Student Objective: Attain relaxation and enjoyment in working and playing with others.

Receiving:
Would you be interested in joining a group of people like yourself which meets occasionally to talk about a happy mental state and how to attain it?

Responding:
Do you find it difficult to talk with others for quite a while without getting tired or even bored?

Valuing:
Do you often become so interested in what you are talking about in a group that you are almost unaware of what is going on around you?

Organization:
Has your thinking about how you would get along with others led you to make a judgement about people who like to discuss topics in a group setting?

Characterization:
Do you find that you can be more effective as a person by talking things over in small groups?

The *action domain* is the culminating part of the whole process of looking at pupil learnings and evaluation. It is because of the significance of this domain that stress has been put on behavioral objectives. It is true that when behaviors are objectified in terms of the verb "to do," clearly defined actions are set forth and can be readily observed throughout the formal and informal activities of the

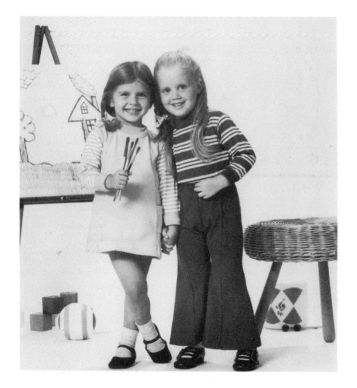

Figure 11–1 How would you evaluate this situation? (Courtesy Gerber Baby Foods.)

school day. One can ask almost anytime whether or not a particular student is indeed able to "describe," "analyze," "investigate," "portray," "develop," "demonstrate," "identify," "distinguish," "select," "employ," "choose," "discriminate," etc.

For the teacher who has behavioral objectives on hand during the teaching of a major health topic, there is a reminder to look for changes. Critical observation, therefore, can be a fruitful evaluation technique, especially if the observer has had some experience in deciding what to look for.

Children of all ages have much to communicate if the teacher will simply question and observe. Written tests alone will not provide the answers. Answers to simple behavioral questions may be more enlightening. How do children get along with each other? Is there evidence of happiness? (See Fig. 11–1.) In one first grade the teacher made three face discs (See below) and asked certain students to "choose the disc that tells how you *feel*." It proved to be a fun activity.

Observing how children go about a task, how they work together, how they discuss and share information and ideas,

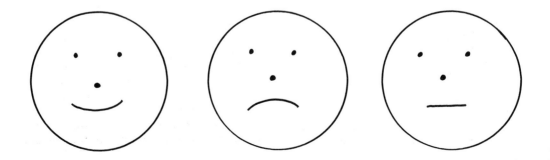

how they report, and how well they manage the transition from one health activity to another — these are examples of situations which may be created to appraise their behavior. Some of the individual pupil items which shed a good deal of light on the application of health knowledge, and may readily be observed by the teacher, are as follows:

Evidence of a cleaner and more attractive school building.

Increased cooperation in helping to maintain a healthful classroom.

Improved personal cleanliness — related to the use of the handkerchief, handwashing and toilet practices, condition of clothing, and eating.

Improved general appearance and posture, mental alertness, enthusiasm.

Better practices of oral cleanliness, e.g., rinsing mouth after meals.

Improved eating practices as observed at lunchtime: Increased consumption of milk during snack and lunch periods. Better lunches brought from home. Less food thrown away at lunchtime.

Evidence of attitude changes with respect to appreciation of the human body and its functions.

Evidence of practices to limit the use of sweets and carbonated drinks for class trips and parties.

Improved practices with regard to working and playing in good light.

Evidence of greater awareness of others, of social adjustment, personal friendliness, more willingness to share materials and to help when help is asked for.

Improved attitudes toward safety patrols, traffic officers, the handling of pets and animals, the handling of scissors, leaving materials and equipment where they may cause falls, and so on.

Improved behavior during safety and fire drills.

Evidence of increasing responsibility for planning a balanced school day by participating in rest, play, lunch, and work periods with decreasing assistance from the teacher.

An observation of an individual or group may be much more revealing if the teacher has something to use as a guide.

It is not difficult to make a list of the more important "behavior" outcomes expected for each unit or health topic. Once such a list has been formulated, however, it is then reworked into a list of expected day-to-day practices and attitudes.

Health Records

In practically every elementary school, health records are available for teachers to look over. Very often the school nurse will be able to interpret the physical examination in such a way that a good deal of meaningful information may be obtained. A review of individual pupil health records will reveal improvement in attendance, the extent to which remediable physical defects have been corrected, and the degree of personal illness. It will also show improvements in growth factors such as height and weight and the results of special screen-

	Always	*Usually*	*Seldom*	*Never*
Are the hands, face, neck, and ears clean?				
Are the fingernails clean?				
Are the clothes neat and clean?				
Is the hair combed?				
Is a handkerchief or tissue carried?				
Are the hands washed before eating?				
Is the shower enjoyed following the physical education period?				
Is the mouth covered during coughing and sneezing?				
Is there good sitting and standing posture?				

ing examinations for vision, hearing, and mental health. Very often there is evidence of improvement of dental health status. Moreover, properly kept health records tell how much "follow-up" has been accomplished as a result of the discovery of organic drains, defects, or poor health habits and attitudes.

The cumulative record or anecdotal record has considerable value when it comes to pupil health evaluation. By making notations from time to time on the progress of a particular pupil, a record of lasting value is accomplished for others to use at a later date. Excellent examples of cumulative health record cards are found in the states of California and New York.

Some classroom teachers prefer to keep a class chart which they call a Pupil Observation Chart. This lists the names of all class members in alphabetical order with space to the right for notations. Each day when the attendance is checked the teacher may make a comment if she feels that it is necessary. Such a chart tends to keep evaluation current with everyday teaching.

Another useful health record is one that may be kept by the pupils themselves and appraised periodically by the teacher. This includes diaries and other autobiographical records of pupils.

Performance Tests

One of the increasingly rewarding ways of appraising health status and health improvement in the elementary grades is to formally measure the *physical performance* of boys and girls. Those pupils who generally demonstrate a high degree of vigor, strength, muscular endurance, and enthusiasm usually possess a high degree of physical fitness. When they appear to "slow down" and become less vigorous and enthusiastic, it is time to check more closely for hidden organic strains and drains, physical defects, poor sleep and food habits, maladjustment, or something else.

In a number of elementary schools, tests of physical fitness are given by physical education teachers in cooperation with school health services personnel. The findings of such tests almost always reveal information of value to the classroom teacher of health. The pupil whose physical performance is substrength and below par is in need of special help, part of which may involve the health instruction program.

A relatively simple screening device for physical fitness should be employed in schools where there is no physical education department, or where the appraisal of physical capacity is a responsibility of the classroom teacher. Such a test can be most revealing in pointing out those pupils who lack the "work capacity" to put in a full day of study and play. Such pupils are frequently underachievers who are existing at a point far below their potential level of intelligence and effort.[4] The classroom teacher should be able to check her boys and girls against the standards of the A.A.U. Junior Physical Fitness Tests. These are adaptable to any school situation and can be used with little motivation as self-testing activities.[5] Ideally, every elementary school pupil should have his level of physical fitness routinely appraised three times during the school year by a regular teacher of physical education who is able to employ more sophisticated measures and work with health service personnel to interpret the findings.

There is one other performance test that is being used more and more in elementary schools. This is a motor skill *test for bicycle safety*. The children bring their bicycles to school and demonstrate how to turn, using appropriate hand signals. In the primary grades they demonstrate the method of getting on a bicycle, the means of guiding it, applying the brake, and the methods of stopping and parking. The National Safety Council

---

[4] Among the better screening tests for elementary school-age physical fitness are the Kraus-Weber, Physical Fitness Index, AAHPER Youth Fitness Test, Indiana Motor Fitness Test, Oregon Motor Fitness Test, and the Washington Elementary School Physical Fitness Test.

[5] Free copies with full directions may be obtained from the Amateur Athletic Union, 233 Broadway, New York, N.Y.

A. A. U. JUNIOR PHYSICAL FITNESS TESTS STANDARDS — BY YEARS

Event	Boys			Girls		
	6–7	8–9	10–11	6–7	8–9	10–11
Required events:						
1. Sprints	40 yd. 9 sec.	40 yd. 8 sec.	50 yd. 8 sec.	40 yd. 9 sec.	40 yd. 8 sec.	50 yd. 9 sec.
2. Walk and Run	1/4 mile 5 min.	1/2 mile 8 min.	3/4 mile 10 min.	1/4 mile 5 min.	1/2 mile 8 min.	3/4 mile 11 min.
3. Sit-ups	8	12	16	8	12	14
4. Pull-ups	(modified) 3	(modified) 7	(regular) 3	(modified) 3	(modified) 7	(modified) 8
5. Standing Broad Jump	3'	4'	5'	3'	4'	4'6"
Choose any one of these events:						
6. Push-ups	(modified) 5	(modified) 8	(modified) 13	(modified) 4	(modified) 7	(modified) 9
7. Playground Ball Throw for Distance	35'	65'	85'	20'	30'	40'
8. Continuous Hike for Distance	1 mile	2 mile	3 mile	1 mile	2 mile	3 mile
9. Running High Jump	1'6"	2'3"	2'9"	1'6"	2'3"	2'6"

has simple test suggestions to teach and appraise bicycle skills. An excellent bicycle skill test which may be set up on any elementary school playground is distributed free, complete with diagrams, by Aetna Life Insurance Company of Hartford, Connecticut. A guide entitled *Bicycle Safety* is also distributed for use with this test. These particular tests offer quite a challenge to youth and are a first-rate appraisal device for the teacher. (See bicycle safety section of Chapter 8, for a diagram of one of these tests. See also the diagrams for four bicycle performance tests widely used in Oklahoma City in *Safety*, February 1967, p. 20.)

Reports

The results of good health teaching may sometimes be demonstrated by the reports of local physicians, ophthalmologists, nurses, and dentists regarding the increase in medical and dental treatment of school-age groups. Through interviews with these professional people it is possible to become aware of the physical defects and other adverse health conditions that have been corrected or improved. Each year in the city of Cincin-

nati, Ohio, the school health director compiles an extensive breakdown of facts and figures relative to the health of the school-age children. This is used in a number of ways to improve health teaching at several grade levels.

Surveys

The survey is a formal approach to the topic of health appraisal. It may be community-wide and involve information secured from parents and others in the community, or it may be limited to the confines of the school. In either case it is an attempt to discover certain useful health information which may be related to health teaching. There may be a survey of the school cafeteria to check on the sale of milk, salads, fruits, whole-grain cereals, and enriched bread, or of a local restaurant, dairy, meat market, or grocery store. There are surveys of the school environment to determine such things as the cleanliness of shower and toilet rooms, and whether there are appropriate rest and relaxation periods for young children. But more important from a health instruction viewpoint is the survey that seeks to determine *pupil be-*

havior. Environmentally, there may be an opportunity to wash the hands before eating, but what does the survey show? How many children using a lavatory actually wash their hands before eating? The survey, therefore, may make known a real need which calls for a different health teaching emphasis.

There are so many excellent items that lend themselves to being surveyed that care should be taken to select the ones most representative of changes in health behavior in a major health area. In surveying the class as a whole, the teacher will ask such questions as the following:

Are the children eating or at least tasting foods they never ate before? Are they eating more leisurely? What are the most popular breakfast cereals purchased in families? How frequent are colds among class members and their families? What is the most common kind of family recreation in the summer? Winter? How many hours of sleep do children average per night? How aware is the class of health news items as evidenced from newsclippings and other information brought to class? How frequently are the teeth brushed?

Does pupil absenteeism due to illness relate in any way to a lack of sleep? Is there any improvement in achievement and adjustment of pupils when sleep habits improve?

Do children willingly wear glasses after the physician recommends them? Is there any indication that children take more precautions regarding the prevention of physical injury to the eyes and ears?

Do children want to stay home from school at early signs of head colds or other illness?

Are there evidences of good manners while playing and sharing with others? Has there been an improvement in the respect shown for the feelings and viewpoints of others?

Is there evidence that the pupils are learning to accept their own limitations?

Is there less daydreaming, crying, timidity, "tattling," and hostility?

Do the results of a bicycle inspection indicate that adequate equipment is being used and that there is proper maintenance such as good brakes, lubricated chains, and proper air pressure in the tires?

How many class members have seen the dentist during the last six months?

It is becoming more and more common to ask pupils what they think about a certain happening or item of learning. When such questions are organized, they frequently take the form of a *pupil opinion survey.* Fifth and sixth graders sometimes have a very definite opinion about the nature of specific health instruction — techniques, materials, content, and whether or not it is effective in changing their attitudes and habits.

Parental Opinions

Very often when boys and girls apply their health knowledge, the alert parents are the first to notice it. Attitudes and practices relative to visits to doctor and dentist, foods, personal cleanliness, appearance, oral hygiene, and rest are concrete items that frequently cause parents a fair amount of concern. When children show increased cooperation along these lines at home, most parents will be aware of it and are happy to pass the information along to the teacher. One teacher in a small upstate New York town made it a point to talk to all 28 mothers of her second grade class. Using a simple check list she asked pertinent questions relative to home improvement in specific areas where health instruction had been given. After reviewing all the evaluation techniques that she had previously used, it was her judgment that the interview with the parents was by far the most fruitful and enlightening. As a specific example, it was found that following several lessons on activity, rest, and relaxation, a rather large number of children willingly gave up television and radio programs that might interfere with their sleep, and went to bed.

In the elementary schools of Los Angeles, California a definite plan has been in operation whereby parents are asked to cooperate with the schools by keeping a check on the health behavior of their children at a very early age (kindergarten). Attached to the cover letter is a form consisting of 40 clear and straightforward questions which may be answered with "Yes" or "No." Here are a few examples selected at random:

	Yes	No
1. Does your child wash his hands before eating?	☐	☐
2. Does your child wash his hands after toileting?	☐	☐
8. Does your child use his own toothbrush?	☐	☐
14. Does your child go to bed at 7 o'clock?	☐	☐
18. Is your child happy at mealtimes?	☐	☐
39. Does your child stay away from strange animals?	☐	☐

Case Studies

Although it takes time to put together several case studies involving individuals and groups of pupils, they are nevertheless very useful when appraising the effectiveness of the health teaching effort. Consider the implications of a report such as the following:

I am a teaching principal in a small school. As we do not have a school nurse to visit us every day, it is my responsibility to take the children home when they are ill, or when they are injured.

My primary teacher sent a small child to my room with a note. She believed the child had head lice. She wished me to check. I examined Linda and found that she did have head lice.

After making the necessary arrangements to leave my room, I drove Linda to her home. There I found the mother sick and in bed. Venice, who was a student in my room, was at home this day. It had been reported that she was ill, however this was not the case. She had stayed at home to care for the mother.

The house contained one room for the four members of the family. The small amount of furniture was old, dusty, dirty, and broken. The beds were not made and the linen was soiled. The table in the center of the room was piled with dirty dishes and food. It seemed to me that the dishes must not have been washed for several days. The sink and cupboard tops were piled high with dirty dishes, garbage was in evidence on the counter top and was splashed on the cupboards and so on to the floor. The room had not been swept recently. The chairs were covered with clothes so that one had to be unloaded so that I might sit down. There were new curtains at the windows.

Venice, (age 12), was playing a game on the floor, oblivious to the condition of the room. The mother did not apologize for the room. She complained to me that her husband was "mad" about her being home, sick. She worked in a laundry and he thought she ought to go to work. (However, she was at home according to the doctor's orders.)

I explained the reason for my bringing Linda home. I gave her instructions for eliminating the lice. After telling her that the nurse would check both girls before they could return to school, I went back to my classroom. Several questions came to me as I was driving back to school. How could people live in such filth? How could that family be healthy? What could I do? How could I help? I had read about deplorable homes, but they were far away. This home life would be duplicated by these two girls if something was not done about the situation. I decided that this would be a good time for a unit on cleanliness. I called the school nurse, giving her the information and she promised to check on the girls.

We studied cleanliness in our classroom, talking about sanitation, clean clothes, clean bodies, and clean homes. The students were given opportunities to sweep and dust the floors. They washed dishes, emptied garbage, put clean linen on the bed in our infirmary. They learned how to scrub the floor using disinfectant in the water.

The mother came to the next Parent Teachers Association meeting. She was fairly clean. She told me that the girls were helping her so much, now. They were washing the dishes and cleaning the house for her before she came home from the laundry.

I visited the home a few days later. The house did have a different look. There was still room for improvement but a wedge had been made. There were no dirty dishes, no garbage to be seen. The beds were made. The floor had been swept.

Later in the year the father came to Parent Teachers Association with the mother. Both were clean and their clothes were neat. The father took an active part in the discussion on school safety. The next afternoon as I entered the sheriff's office to request some signs, I found Mr. "D." there for the same purpose.

The children now come to school with clean clothes. Their hair, which is very long, has been braided and looks neat. The father bought a television set, and is going to buy a new living room suite this summer.

I know these children have benefited from this lesson and I hope that they will continue to strive for better conditions.

FORMAL TESTING IN HEALTH EDUCATION

Since tests are often limited by calling for straight health facts, it is reasonable to expect the better test to measure also some degree of understanding and application. A satisfactory test requires the student to think about the facts and *apply* them in a specific way. In so doing he demonstrates not only his level of comprehension; he also identifies an awareness and feelings so fundamental to his value system and ultimate commitment. In short, unless formal written and oral testing in health education adheres to the Bloom *Taxonomy* very little valid information relative to pupil progress and teaching effectiveness will be determined.

Teacher-Prepared Tests. In view of the above it is important at the local level to consider the formulation of questions which will measure some degree of knowledge, comprehension, application, analysis, synthesis, and evaluation in the cognitive domain. (See pages 376–377.) Also, these should be mixed in with questions in the affective domain where feelings, beliefs and attitudes can be expressed. This means that health instruction has to be concerned with concepts and behaviors rather than facts. How do pupils *feel* about a topic? What does it mean to them? An appropriate examination would be one in which pupils are asked to support certain concepts with their background of factual information. In this respect, the well-worded essay exam has a new potential value in many classrooms. This free-response type of test can be quite objective — particularly if the instructor knows what specific information he wants to get from the examination, and sets the questions up with such action-oriented words as "develop," "show," "define," "choose," etc.

Most elementary schoolteachers prepare their own test questions and ask them in a manner which benefits the local classroom situation. This is justified on the basis of varied pupil needs and individual differences at the local elementary level. However, test validity, reliability, and objectivity are sometimes sacrificed when local tests are employed.

Teacher-made paper and pencil tests fall into two categories: *free-response* and *choice*. The essay question, in which the pupil explains what he knows about something, has already been mentioned. Another example of the free-response question is the short-answer type:

Short-answer question: In a sentence or two, express your understanding of each of the following terms:

alcohol	dentine
wheat germ	bacteria
vitamin A	obesity
sodium fluoride	mental health
calcium	overweight

Choice or guided-response questions are valuable because they do not depend upon skill in expression and handwriting. They provide a relatively wide sampling of knowledge in a short time. Once a key has been prepared, they encourage highly objective scoring.

Multiple choice questions are extremely adaptable and lend themselves to an unusually wide range of use. They have been used in many health knowledge and attitude tests. A carefully formulated multiple-choice question with several alternatives can provide the teacher with a basis for appraising errors in thinking. The following points apply to the construction of multiple-choice test items:[5]

1. Preface the question with a short, clear set of directions.

---

[5]Willgoose, Carl E. *Evaluation in Health Education and Physical Education.* New York: McGraw-Hill Book Company, 1961, p. 41.

2. State a single, definite problem in the lead statement.

3. Include as much of the item as possible in the lead statement.

4. Make the alternatives consistent with the lead.

5. Make the alternatives reasonably similar. The choices open to the student must be very much alike in order for the discriminatory power of the student to be measured. In a five-choice question, at least three choices should be close so that only the student with real knowledge can select the most appropriate or best answer.

Example
Section 1—Multiple choice: Read each question carefully. Select the one item which *best* answers the question. Put the number of the item selected in the space in front of the question.

  18. At what time of year does the weight of schoolchildren increase more rapidly?
    (1) summer
    (2) winter
    (3) spring and late summer
    (4) fall and early winter
    (5) no set period

True-False questions have their limitations. They have been "worked to death" as a means of measuring factual knowledge. A proper true-false question should be written in the language of the pupil. It should be as nearly true or false as it can be made. Sweeping generalizations should be avoided. Directions should be clear.

Example
Section 2—True and False: The letters T and F have been placed before each statement given. Draw a circle around the letter T if the statement is *True* and around the letter F if the statement is *False* or *Partially False.*

  T F 12. Accidents in the community are still the greatest threat to schoolchildren.

Matching questions are another variety of guided-response tests which, if properly prepared, will save the teacher time. The "stimulus" column should appear to the left and the "response" column to the right. There should be some five to 15 items listed with more response items than stimulus items. Directions regarding matching should be clear, preferably preceded by an oral discussion before the examination sheets are distributed. A matching test works quite well with health information.

Example
Section 3—Matching: Match the food elements listed in the left-hand column with the foods listed in the right-hand column. Put the number of the food element in the parenthesis after each item.

1. Vitamin B	a. Roast pork ( )
2. Iron	b. Calves' liver ( )
3. Calcium	c. Bread ( )
4. Carbohydrates	d. Milk products ( )
5. Fats	e. Ham gravy ( )
	f. Onions ( )
	g. Oysters ( )
	h. Cabbage ( )

Standardized Tests. A limited number of standardized health and safety tests are available for elementary school use. Most of these are several years old and need up-dating, both in terms of current health information and the kinds of questions asked. There are no health education measures that embrace all of the Bloom *Taxonomy* requirements. Some are concerned with knowledge only, and there are others which attempt to tie knowledge and its application together. Recommended are the following:

Cooperative Health Education Test (AAHPER) 1972. Form 4. Educational Testing Service, Box 999, Princeton, New Jersey 08540 and American Association for Health, Physical Education and Recreation, 1201 16th St., N.W., Washington, D.C. 20036. Designed for grades 5 and 6 by a committee of health education leaders and test construction specialists from Educational Testing Service. After thorough country-wide testing the 50-multiple-choice item test was distributed. It is a 40-minute test in which knowledge questions make up only about 20 per cent of the total; the others are as follows: aplication, 50 per cent; analysis, 20 per cent; and evaluation, 10 per cent. Questions asked relate to consumer health, community health, international health, disease and disorders, personal health care, growth and development, nutrition, mental health, drug use and abuse, and safety and first aid.

Los Angeles Health Education Evaluation Instruments. Los Angeles City School District, Calif. Excellent instruments for kindergarten and grades two, four, and six are available for the measurement of knowledge and attitudes. Contact Division of Educational Services, Los Angeles City Schools, P.O. Box 3307, Terminal Annex, Los Angeles, Calif.

Yellen, Sylvia. Health Behavior Inventory, Monterey, California: California Test Bureau, 1963. A 40-item picture-question inventory for pupils in Grades 3, 4, 5, and 6 which relates to the major health areas of personal health, personal cleanliness, nutrition, safety, community health, infection and disease, mental health, and dental health.

There are also a few useful tests for seventh grade pupils which may be of interest to sixth grade teachers and others employed in the middle school or the eight year elementary school:

Veenker, Harold C. "A Health Knowledge Test for the Seventh Grade." Research Quarterly, 30:338–348, Revised. The two test forms of multiple-choice items are available from the author at Purdue University, Lafayette, Ind. The recent edition has been put together with the principles of the Bloom Taxonomy in mind.

Colebank, Albert D. Health Behavior Inventory, Monterey, California: California Test Bureau, 1963. A 100-item test for grades seven, eight, and nine covering all major health topics. There are 24 health attitude items, 25 health behavior items, and 50 health knowledge items. All are multiple-choice.

The most complete set of health and safety tests are those developed by the Los Angeles City Schools for their evaluative survey. These were constructed for kindergarten, grades two, four, and six. In grade two, for example, health appraisal is made by means of a picture test — 27 multiple-choice picture items. The teacher reads the item and asks the pupil to put an x on the picture which is the best answer. (A copy of the test pictures may be found in the appendix of the Instructional Guide, Health in the Elementary Schools, Los Angeles City School Publication No. EC-201, Revised.) As a result of using this test schoolchildren were found to be in need of more health instruction relative to sleep and rest, grooming, growth, and disease control. Here is an example of what the teacher says and what the pupils see (See picture at bottom of page.):

Teacher says:
3. Now let's look at the pictures in row 3. On a hot day, we play quietly in the shade, run around in a sweater, or climb a mountain. Mark the best answer and put your pencils up.

In the area of safety education there are some excellent sources of test materials for elementary school use. One test which gets at both understandings and application at the 5th grade level is How Much Do Your Pupils Know About Safety? It is available from the National Safety Council. The 130 questions cover home, traffic, school, playground, sports, bicycle and holiday safety and can be used with classes anywhere from grades four through eight.

Another test, the Bicycle Safety Quiz, is a 20-question true-false test to be used

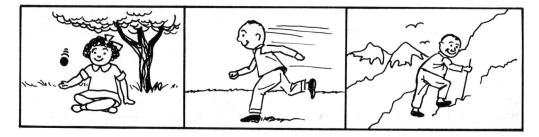

in the classroom. See 20 questions on page 390. The test was originally developed for elementary-age children by Aetna Life and Casualty. The company now distributes (free) a 10-item test in the colorful booklet, *Bicycle Safety*. Acknowledging research findings that two out of three bicycle accidents occur to riders who have failed to follow the rules of the road, the Bicycle Institute of America, Inc. makes available (free) a very thorough *Bike Quiz Guide* which contains 50 in-depth true-false questions, a words test, and a safety matching test. As a public service the National Fire Protection Association distributes free to school personnel their 20-item test for boys and girls relative to home fire inspection appraisal. This is part of the SPARKY program; the questions may be answered "Yes" or "No" and are particularly well written. Here are two examples from the battery:

3. Frayed electric cords often start fires. Are you sure all of the electric cords in your home are in safe condition?
Yes___No___

20. If there is a gas stove or gas heater in your home, do you know that you should call the gas company right away if you ever smell gas?
Yes___No___

The same organization makes available the *Home Fire Safety Quiz* and the *Be-Prepared-For-Fire Quiz*, each of which consists of ten excellent multiple-choice questions for teachers to use in connection with safety education.

Knowledge testing may be made more revealing when the results are combined with teacher observations. The kind of classwork that pupils do—their drawings, projects, photographs, oral reports, and personal questions—provides evidence which, combined with formal test results, frequently gives a good appraisal of the health instruction efforts.

MEASURING ATTITUDES AND BEHAVIORS

As previously indicated, it is both important and difficult to readily appraise student responses in the affective and ac-

tion domains. Where there are large numbers of schoolchildren assigned to teachers it will always be hard to find out how everyone feels about a health issue and what they may be doing about it in their own community. This is perhaps the biggest reason why standardized written tests are created—to elicit a response from the masses. A major problem, however, is one of validity. How much weight can be placed on the answers? How often do students at every age tell teachers *not* what they really feel and do, but what they believe the teachers *want* them to feel and do? This is why Gordon Allport, after decades of wrestling with the subject of human attitudes, concluded that it is most difficult to measure accurately in this area simply because attitudes are so personal, deep-seated, and represent a latent predisposition to act.

Working with smaller groups of children it is possible to explore the affective and action domains by becoming more personally involved. A close relationship is required. Seeking expressions of feelings, convictions, beliefs, values and judgements is much better accomplished on a one-to-one basis than it is in a mob scene. Small groups of children, taking their turn throughout the school year, can provide much evaluative information for the teacher. For example, in working on tobacco smoking and health with fifth, sixth, or seventh grade pupils, it is possible to sit in a small comfortable circle and discuss personal feelings about smoking. Test No. 2 from the U.S. Public Health Service's *Smokers Self-Testing Kit* may be obtained in quantity from the U.S. Government Printing Office. (See Fig. 11-2.)

Again, in the small group exchange it is possible to get solid expressions of behavior by presenting well-defined decision making questions. Three statements that were employed in the experimentations of Schley and Banister were:[5]

---

[5]Schley, Robert A., and Banister, Richard E. "Behavioral Change in an Academic Setting: How It Works." *School Health Review*, 1:13–19, November 1970.

TEST 2

WHAT DO YOU THINK THE EFFECTS OF SMOKING ARE?

For each statement, circle the number that shows how you feel about it. Do you strongly agree, mildly agree, mildly disagree, or strongly disagree?

Important: Answer every question.

	strongly agree	mildly agree	mildly disagree	strongly disagree
A. Cigarette smoking is not nearly as dangerous as many other health hazards.	1	2	3	4
B. I don't smoke enough to get any of the diseases that cigarette smoking is supposed to cause.	1	2	3	4
C. If a person has already smoked for many years, it probably won't do him much good to stop.	1	2	3	4
D. It would be hard for me to give up smoking cigarettes.	1	2	3	4
E. Cigarette smoking is enough of a health hazard for something to be done about it.	4	3	2	1
F. The kind of cigarette I smoke is much less likely than other kinds to give me any of the diseases that smoking is supposed to cause.	1	2	3	4
G. As soon as a person quits smoking cigarettes he begins to recover from much of the damage that smoking has caused.	4	3	2	1
H. It would be hard for me to cut down to half the number of cigarettes I now smoke.	1	2	3	4
I. The whole problem of cigarette smoking and health is a very minor one.	1	2	3	4
J. I haven't smoked long enough to worry about the diseases that cigarette smoking is supposed to cause.	1	2	3	4
K. Quitting smoking helps a person to live longer.	4	3	2	1
L. It would be difficult for me to make any substantial change in my smoking habits.	1	2	3	4

HOW TO SCORE:

1. Enter the numbers you have circled to the Test 2 questions in the spaces below, putting the number you have circled to Question A over line A, to Question B over line B, etc.
2. Total the 3 scores across on each line to get your totals. For example, the sum of your scores over lines A, E, and I gives you your score on *Importance*—lines B, F, and J gives the score on *Personal Relevance*, etc.

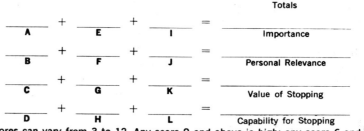

Totals

A + E + I =	Importance
B + F + J =	Personal Relevance
C + G + K =	Value of Stopping
D + H + L =	Capability for Stopping

Scores can vary from 3 to 12. Any score 9 and above is *high*; any score 6 and below is *low*. Learn from Part 2 what your scores mean.

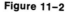

Figure 11-2

1. As a result of studying this unit, my attitude toward the improvement of health practices in this area of health is
(_____better, _____worse, _____unchanged)
2. As a result of studying this topic, my personal actions and/or activities in the area of health with which this topic deals are
(_____better, _____worse, _____unchanged)
3. As a result of studying this topic, I (have, have not) helped someone else improve a personal health practice.

Interestingly, when students are asked to look into their lives for feelings, practices and improvements they begin to illustrate in a number of ways what is actually taking place. Moreover, as the personal approach to evaluation increases confidence, the validity of the process improves.

Self-Testing Activities

When pupils attempt to evaluate their own health improvement, and actually enjoy doing so, there is an opportunity for a more accurate kind of appraisal and a more effective kind of teaching. The student's own immediate problems and how *he* evaluates them is of great interest.

Self-testing activities provide the pupil with a chance to measure progress in terms of his own potential, as well as to compare himself with his classmates. The child as well as the adult wants a certain amount of recognition, status, even prestige—all of which are dependent upon the acquisition of social poise, proper health practices, and mental well-being. He wants these things because his feeling of adequacy, security, and acceptance are contingent upon them.

Adjustment or self-realization cannot be taught, except by providing materials, opportunities, conditions, and experiences whereby, *through self-activity*, the individual reaches the desired goals of achievement. It is not uncommon, therefore, to find that personal health invento-ries and self-rating charts have been used for some time with varying degrees of success. If the chart is one developed by the student himself to measure his own advance toward an accepted goal, or if the chart represents group decisions concerning items to be evaluated, it is likely to be more meaningful to the students involved than a printed or standardized chart.

As younger children learn to read, they help the teacher plan simple rating scales for evaluating group or individual health behavior. Primary grade children evaluate in simple ways, as when they select a food to eat, choose a story to hear, an activity, a color to use in painting. They make such judgments as "We cleaned the room very well today" or "We liked playing with the other children." From such beginnings come standards and expectancies.

Older pupils may discuss the kinds of health tests they need, or develop a set of guides for personal behavior on a bus, field trip, or in the school cafeteria. Later on the same pupils help construct check lists and questionnaires on objective health matters, keep health diaries, and take a critical interest in judging their performance about the school and community.

A pupil may rate himself on posture skills, food habits, attitude toward others, personal appearance, and several other such items. The accompanying check list, simple as it is, was worked out by second graders.

HOW DO I LOOK?		
Do I stand tall?	Yes	No
Do I smile?	Yes	No
Are my hands and face clean?	Yes	No
Are my clothes clean?	Yes	No
Am I happy?	Yes	No
Is there dirt under my fingernails?	Yes	No
Is my hair combed?	Yes	No
Are my teeth clean?	Yes	No

Is your bicycle 100 per cent safe? Take this test and see how you stand:

If your bike has: *Give yourself:*

1. Good brakes .... 20 points
2. A horn or bell that works .... 20 points
3. A light that works .... 20 points
4. A reflector 1-1½ inches in diameter .... 20 points
5. Tight seat and handlebars .... 10 points
6. Solid front and rear fenders .... 5 points
7. No loose spokes on wheels .... 5 points

                                                    Total ....100 points

Bonus Points for:

8. Carrier on back or basket for heavy loads .... 10 points
9. Reflector tape on sides for added protection .... 10 points

---

Check (∨) if statement is True, or False

1. It is safe to learn to ride a bicycle on a busy street. ( ) True ( ) False

2. Bicycles, like autos, should keep to the right side of the road. ( ) True ( ) False

3. Bicycle riders should know and obey all traffic signs and lights. ( ) True ( ) False

4. People who are walking do not have the right-of-way on sidewalks and cross-walks. ( ) True ( ) False

5. Bicycles should be walked across heavily traveled streets. ( ) True ( ) False

6. A bicycle in poor condition is safe if the rider is careful. ( ) True ( ) False

7. It is safe and proper for a bicycle rider to carry a passenger on an ordinary bicycle. ( ) True ( ) False

8. Bicycle riders may hitch to a moving truck if it is traveling less than 20 miles per hour. ( ) True ( ) False

9. Riding in a single line is the sensible thing to do. ( ) True ( ) False

10. Night riding with dark clothing and without a front white light and a rear reflector is dangerous. ( ) True ( ) False

11. When tired, the rider should rest by taking his feet off the pedals. ( ) True ( ) False

12. Bicycle riders should be very careful and give the proper hand signals before making turns or stopping. ( ) True ( ) False

13. It is only necessary to look straight ahead when crossing streets. ( ) True ( ) False

14. The size of the bicycle makes no difference if the rider is skilled. ( ) True ( ) False

15. All bikes should have a horn or bell, rear reflector and front light. ( ) True ( ) False

16. As soon as you can balance your bike you are ready to ride in heavy traffic. ( ) True ( ) False

17. When passing a parked car, you should ride three feet away from it and give a warning with your horn or bell. ( ) True ( ) False

18. When entering a street from a driveway or sidewalk the bicycle rider has the right-of-way. ( ) True ( ) False

19. Bicycle riders should carry books or bundles in one hand if they must be carried on a bicycle. ( ) True ( ) False

20. Bicycles should be kept in good condition at all times and repaired by a mechanic when necessary. ( ) True ( ) False.

NOTE TO TEACHER: { Allow five points for each question. Have each pupil correct any questions he may have answered wrong.

EVALUATING A HEALTH LESSON

There is another kind of evaluation that one should not lose sight of. This applies more to the teacher than it does to the pupils as such. It is concerned with appraising the actual instruction at any one time. The teacher should ask herself some rather definite questions as to whether the health lesson was properly conceived and carried out. Students can be very helpful. Sally Kaizer at the Masconomet Regional School in Massachusetts asks the following probing questions:

1. Do you find my classes
   Boring   Interesting
   Exciting
2. Do you think I do too much talking in class?
   Yes   No
3. Has anything I've done this year made you eager to learn more about the subjects we're studying?
   Yes   No
If your answer was yes, please state that activity which aroused your interest.
4. Do you think I'm
   too strict   easy going
   about right
5. Do you feel comfortable about speaking up in class?
   or are you afraid you'll be laughed at or criticized?
6. Do you think that the material we studied has any use in your life now, or will have any use in the future?
   Yes   No
7. Please check which of the following teaching techniques have been most interesting and helped you the most:
   Lectures or explanations by teacher
   Small group discussions
   Field trips
   Class projects in which the students were involved
   Demonstrations
   Other (Please fill in) _____
8. Would the use of more films, tapes, records, and overhead projectors help you to better understand the course material?
   Yes   No
9. Perhaps I could have helped you to learn more. Do you feel that I have failed you in any of the following ways:
   Didn't give me enough individual help
   Ignored me a lot of the time
   Were too interested in the bright kids in the class
   Other (Please fill in) _____
10. Do you think the textbooks and any other study materials we use are:
    Dull   Hard to read
    Out of date
    Interesting and informative
11. If you were teaching this class would you
    provide more work sheets and other learning aids
    expect students to use more out of class reference materials
    have more class discussion
    provide for more group work

ADVANCING HEALTH — A CONTINUOUS PROCESS

It was Prometheus, that fire-bearing Titan, who sought a "heroic" civilization in which the spirit of man could be expressed. This may be the ultimate state of wellness that emerges from simple search and not-so-simple research.

There is a tendency for some teachers to think of research as a kind of magic done in mythical ivory towers—something strictly divorced from the classroom. This is a species of romantic nonsense. There is no magic in research; nobody waves a wand, and there are no tricks. Research is just plain hard work by competent and dedicated teachers in the fields of their choice. Few elementary schoolteachers are asked to make a significant and scholarly contribution in health, but it is a rare teacher who does not have to ferret out health information, think about it, put it together in a new form, and use it. It is through this kind of activity that health curricula and methods are modified, and programs move in the direction of the preconceived aims and objectives of health education.

Evaluation is an ongoing process. So is education itself. Man and his leaders continually strive to balance his total well-being through a critical appraisal of his physical, mental, social, and emotional health. This is not easy, and it never will be. Yet, as Trow said well over four decades ago:

If enough good food, rest, sunshine, and so forth, are obtainable, so that the physiological organism is strong and healthy, if there is sufficient opportunity for free activity, for strivings for ends which he considers desirable, and for the appreciation of things which are to him beautiful; and if in the eyes of his comrades, there is something of respect for him; and if there are those in whom he can confide and those whom he can in some way serve, man may experience that feeling of happiness which has been the goal of life for untold generations.[7]

---

[7]Trow, W. C. *Educational Psychology.* Boston: Houghton-Mifflin Co., 1931.

QUESTIONS FOR DISCUSSION

1. Why do teachers overlook using health information from school health services, and local physicians, dentists, and public health officials when appraising their health teaching efforts?

2. From your reading, do you see any compelling reason to keep behavioral objectives near-at-hand when teaching in the classroom? What is the relationship between behavioral objectives and instruction?

3. What seem to be the chief values obtained when grade school pupils appraise their own health instruction program? How does this differ from a typical self-testing activity?

4. What is the value of an individual pupil conference in appraising the health instruction program? Would you say that it represents an economical use of time? Would a small group provide better information?

5. Why is learning in health education difficult to measure accurately? Support your answer with specific illustrations.

SUGGESTED ACTIVITIES

1. Many of the sources on the Selected References list have to do with appraising student health behavior, rather than with knowledge by itself. Most authors also point out the *difficulty* involved in evaluating health behavior. Look over some of what has been written and formulate a list of reasons why health practices are so difficult to measure. Later, compare your findings with those of your classmates.

2. Select a major health area in which to appraise pupil health practices. Construct a check list of significant items which should help you identify pupil strengths and weak-nesses. The items included on the check list should be "behavior items"—action evidences of health understandings.

3. In keeping with the Bloom *Taxonomy,* prepare a number of multiple-choice questions on a health topic of your choice.

4. Meet with three or four of your classmates and discuss the difficulties involved in appraising health practices in a given school-community setting. Are the problems any different in an urban setting compared with a rural or suburban location?

5. Ask several elementary school teachers to indicate how effective they believe the school health education program to be. Do they feel that the health service function is worth the money it costs? Are they happy with the results of their own health instruction efforts? Do they really believe they are creating health awareness and behavior change?

SELECTED REFERENCES

Allen, Robert E. "Evaluation of The Conceptual Approach to Teaching Health Education: A Second Look," *Journal of School Health,* 43:293–295, May, 1973.

Anderson, C. L. *School Health Practice,* 4th ed. St. Louis: C. V. Mosby Co., 1968, Chapter 17.

Bloom, B. S. *Taxonomy of Educational Objectives: The Classification of Educational Goals. Handbook 1. Cognitive Domain.* New York: McKay, 1956.

Cornely, P. B., and Bigman, S. K. "Some Considerations in Changing Health Attitudes." *Children,* 10:62, January 1963.

Dalis, Gus. "Effect of Precise Objectives Upon Student Achievement in Health Education," *Journal of Experimental Education,* 39:20–23, Winter 1970.

Fodor, John T., and Dalis, Gus T. *Health Instruction Theory and Application.* Philadelphia: Lea and Febiger, 1966.

Irwin, Leslie W., Cornacchia, Harold J., and Staton, Wesley M. *Health in Elementary Schools*, 2nd ed. St. Louis: C. V. Mosby Co., 1966, Chapter 13.

Larson, Judith K., and Nichols, D. G. "If Nobody Knows You've Done It, Have You. . .?" *Evaluation*, Fall 1972.

Lessinger, Leon M. "Teachers in an Age of Accountability." *Instructor, 80*:19–21, July 1971.

Mayshark, Cyrus, and Foster, Ralph H. *Methods in Health Education*. St. Louis: C. V. Mosby Co., 1966.

Monk, Janice J. "Preparing Tests to Measure Course Objectives." *Journal of Geography, 70*:157–162, March 1971.

Read, Donald A. and Greene, Walter H. *Creative Teaching in Health*. New York: Macmillan Co., 1971, Chapter 18.

Sanders, Norris M. *Classroom Questions—What Kinds?* New York: Harper and Row, 1966.

Silberman, Charles. *Crisis in the Classroom*. New York: Random House, 1970.

Sliepcevich, Elena M. *School Health Education Study: A Summary Report*. Washington, D.C.: School Health Education Study, 1964.

Sollender, Marion K. *Evaluation Instruments in Health Education*. Washington, D.C.: American Association for Health, Physical Education, and Recreation, 1969.

Turner, C. E., Randall, H. B., and Smith, S. L. *School Health and Health Education*, 6th ed. St. Louis: C. V. Mosby Co., 1970, Chapter 20.

Willgoose, Carl E. *Evaluation in Health Education and Physical Education*. New York: McGraw-Hill Book Co., 1961, Chapter 5.

Willgoose, Carl E. *Health Teaching in Secondary Schools*. Philadelphia: W. B. Saunders Company, 1972, Chapter 12.

Willgoose, Carl E. "Providing for Change: New Directions," in Read, Donald A., ed. *New Directions in Health Education*. New York: Macmillan Co., 1971, Chapter 1.

Appendix

GRADUATED LIST OF BEHAVIORAL OBJECTIVES FOR THE MAJOR HEALTH TOPICS, GRADES 1–6

PERSONAL CLEANLINESS AND APPEARANCE

Grade 1

Appears in school clean and well-groomed: hands, nails, face, hair and teeth.
Demonstrates ability to wash hands competently.
Hangs up clothing at school and at home.
Dresses appropriately for the climate and weather for school and play.

Grade 2

Exercises some concern and care for personal articles.
Carries a handkerchief and blows nose properly.
Demonstrates proper toilet practices.
Keeps reasonably clean and washes when dirty without being told.

Grade 3

Relates personal and community cleanliness to disease-control.
Differentiates between being well and being sick.
Explains the necessity for regular bathing.
Evaluates the cleanliness of the skin and nails.

Grade 4

Chooses to keep the school environment clean and attractive.
Is aware of the variety of personal health practices having a bearing on personal
    appearance.
Practices standing, walking and sitting and explains how feelings of the moment are
    reflected in posture.
Prevents skin and scalp infections.

Grade 5

Shampoos the hair and takes frequent baths without being told.
Investigates hair styles for girls and boys.
Explains the relationship of appearance to success in everyday life.
Describes why the wearing of eyeglasses is sometimes necessary.
Takes part in the selection of clothes for durability and style.

Grade 6

Chooses to prevent illness by practicing individual and group cleanliness.
Exercises personal responsibility in maintaining proper health and is able to advise
others.
Describes the process of eliminating body wastes and body odors.
Compares current practices of keeping clean to control disease with the practices in
ancient civilizations.

PHYSICAL ACTIVITY, SLEEP, REST AND RELAXATION

Grade 1

Demonstrates how to play, rest and sleep for proper growth.
Engages in enjoyable activities such as fundamental rhythms, movement
exploration, singing games, dances, stunts, and games of low organization.

Grade 2

Sleeps an appropriate number of hours each night, and acknowledges that parental
guidance is frequently necessary to insure proper sleep and activity practices.
Investigates how sleep and rest as factors help one avoid disease and chronic
fatigue.
Explains and practices appropriate evening recreation, especially before retiring.
Portrays how to exercise for fun and health; demonstrates several stunts, animal
actions, and novelty relay races for fun.

Grade 3

Develops sound reasons for physical strength and endurance.
Demonstrates several different ways of building and maintaining physical fitness:
rhythms, dances, games, rope climbing and jumping, swimming, hiking.
Illustrates through stories and situations the relationship between physical activity
and well-being.

Grade 4

Measures own level of physical fitness in an elemental way.
Explains how vigorous physical exercise may be alternated with rest and
relaxation.
Relates how it feels to be "physically fit."
Describes the place of physical fitness in total health, and the interrelationship of
such variables as exercise, diet, rest, and medical check-ups.

Grade 5

Demonstrates strengthening exercises to improve muscular efficiency for standing,
walking, playing and working.
Explains the several effects of exercise on sleep, rest and the digestion of foods.
Plans recreation to relieve mental fatigue and promote sleep.
Selects activities to promote the wise use of leisure time.
Shows how to develop a wide variety of active and quiet recreational skills.

Grade 6

Employs a number of ways to illustrate the place of sports in the Western culture.
Enumerates the several reasons for participating in individual and team sports activities.
Investigates how to prevent injuries when engaged in vigorous physical activities.
Explains the fundamental physiology involved in attaining a high level of physical condition.
Selects and explains the several factors contributing to an adequate night's sleep.

NUTRITION AND GROWTH

Grade 1

Relates why people eat (energy, growth, pleasure).
Explains the importance of a good breakfast and lunch.
Drinks fruit juices and milk.
Describes a pleasant, happy mealtime.
Distinguishes clean foods and utensils.
Identifies a wide variety of foods common to the community.

Grade 2

Recognizes a number of foods for various occasions.
Identifies individual differences in the rate of growth.
Chooses foods that help you grow (build tissue).
Chooses foods that help you "go" (energy).
Appraises sweets in the diet.

Grade 3

Demonstrates proper practices of eating: chewing, tasting, eating leisurely.
Discusses clearly how appetite may be improved.
Explains the importance of well-balanced meals to mental and physical efficiency.
Illustrates the many ways in which foods may be used: milk, fruit, etc.
Describes regularity in eating and the eating patterns in various cultures.

Grade 4

Investigates the essential function of carbohydrates, proteins, and fats in the human system.
Analyzes foods for vitamin and mineral sources.
Relates food products and eating practices to proper body weight — presently and in the future.
Describes the effect of cultural differences, customs and foods on eating practices.
Determines that physical growth and early mental capacity are influenced by a balanced diet.

Grade 5

Looks into the mechanics and elemental chemistry of digestion and elimination.
Acknowledges a variety of daily eating practices, most of which are within the acceptable range of eating behavior.

Illustrates how to promote good digestion by referring to before, during, and after mealtime activities.

Chooses foods of nutritional value because they contribute to physical fitness for games, sports, and work.

Relates food excesses and deprivation to animal and human growth, repair, energy, etc.

Grade 6

Analyzes animal and human nutrition requirements, noting differences and similarities.

Investigates the nature of malnutrition; its effect in dentition, bone growth, intellectual achievement, energy levels, etc.

Applies caloric measurements and food chart information to the building of selected menus.

Constructs menus for both young people (10–12 years of age) and old people that may be obtained in the home or in a restaurant.

Distinguishes fallacies, fads, and superstitions that distort the truth relative to foods and their use.

Cites elimination problems which relate to digestion and food choices.

DENTAL HEALTH

Grade 1

Brushes the teeth at the appropriate time and in the proper way.
Explains the loss of baby teeth and appearance of first 6-year molar.
Tells why people visit the dentist.

Grade 2

Demonstrates how to use powder or toothpaste.
Tells how the teeth contribute to appearance and help break foods down for swallowing.
Illustrates how raw foods help keep the teeth clean.
Shows what happens to the teeth when many sweets are a part of the diet.
Describes the need for regular dental inspections and care.

Grade 3

Shows how teeth may be cleaned without brushing.
Chooses foods that build strong teeth and bones.
Explains the value of clean, attractive teeth to relationships with others.
Describes the causes and prevention of toothache.

Grade 4

Draws the basic structure of the tooth and explains the parts.
Identifies the action of teeth in talking clearly and in the digestive process.
Describes the undesirable effects of tooth decay.
Portrays practices that may subject the teeth to injury.
Explains the several functions of the school dental hygienist.

Grade 5

Describes the function and importance of orthodontics.
Explains the meaning and consequences of properly handled cases of malocclusion.
Illustrates modern dental practice and the need for regular dental visits.
Cites the benefits of the way fluoride is applied to the teeth to help prevent tooth decay.

Grade 6

Tells how progress is being made at the sixth grade level toward the development of a full set of teeth.
Develops a logical argument in favor of water fluoridation and the reduction of tooth decay.
Illustrates the relationship of nutrition, aging, and other variables to bone and tooth decay.
Evaluates dentifrice advertisements in several ways.

BODY STRUCTURE AND OPERATION

Grade 1

Depicts how children grow tall and strong.
Tells the reasons for health examinations and tests of seeing and hearing.
Names the primary body organs and systems and tells what they do.

Grade 2

Demonstrates how the body moves using bones and muscles stimulated by nerves.
Illustrates how the body maintains various postures and positions: sitting, standing, walking, running.
Demonstrates various stunts, exercises and other movements to depict a wide range of human movements.

Grade 3

Explains how the eyes see and the ears hear using models, pictures, or diagrams.
Describes the cooperative action between the five senses.
Shows how eyeglasses help correct visual defects.
Shows how to protect the eyes and ears from injuries: in sports, while working, etc.
Demonstrates how the skeletal make-up functions to support the body and protect the organs.

Grade 4

Explains the body's need for fuel and how this works through the digestive system.
Cites the function of the skin, hair and nails in terms of health and appearance.
Depicts the various structural elements of the respiratory system.
Relates the speech function to the condition of the nose, tonsils, adenoids and teeth.
Illustrates how the larynx and epiglottis work.

Grade 5

Employs the means to cite the function of human cells, tissues, organs, and
systems.
Shows the mechanics of growth through cell division.
Relates enzymes to digestion.
Analyzes the circulatory system and the composition of the blood.
Seeks interrelationships of circulation, respiration, digestion and elimination.

Grade 6

Illustrates how the central nervous system, brain, and sense organs function and
how this relates to feelings.
Tells how muscles, bones, nerves and glands work together.
Explains elimination in relation to diet, constipation and frequency of bowel
movements.
Describes the reproductive structure and function of the body (referred to also
under Sex and Family Living Education).

PREVENTION AND CONTROL OF DISEASE

Grade 1

Maintains clean hands and keeps them away from mouth.
Explains the need for regular health examinations.
Describes the importance of vaccinations and immunizations.
Refuses to share "bites," whistles, straws, glasses, etc.
Demonstrates how to drink from a water fountain.

Grade 2

Cites ways to protect self and others from colds, sneezes, and sore throats.
Illustrates how to stay healthy through adequate amounts of food, water, sleep, and
exercise.
Tells what the hospital does for people who are ill.
Describes how disease organisms can travel from person to person.

Grade 3

Describes the germ theory and how people get sick.
Illustrates several ways in which various germs are spread.
Explains why some disease germs are contagious.
Avoids illness through practicing cleanliness, regular medical check-ups and
immunizations.
Tells how to prevent ear and eye infections.

Grade 4

Differentiates between harmful, harmless, and helpful germs.
Takes part in school activities designed to curtail disease.
Explains what can be done in the home to prevent the spread of disease.
Relates how several men and women of science have contributed to the conquering
of disease.

Grade 5

Analyzes the sources of infection: bacteria, viruses, fungi; people, animals, climate, insects, water, food.
Describes how immunizations are kept up to date.
Investigates how the spread of infections can be controlled.
Develops suggestions for the prevention of illnesses through the faulty storage of foods and medicines.

Grade 6

Describes the basic symptoms of common respiratory and childhood diseases. Explains controls.
Employs ways to care for sick in the home, and to tell others what can be done.
Cites ways in which the body builds its own immunity to disease.
Reorganizes several superstitions and evidences of quackery in relation to the control and cure of disease.

SAFETY AND FIRST AID

Grade 1

Demonstrates how to proceed to and from school safely.
Shows a number of general safety practices in the classroom.
Explains how to keep from accidents during and after school hours.
Gives accurate statement of personal identity when lost.
Tells where to seek help for injuries or illness.

Grade 2

Tells how policemen and firemen protect children.
Shows how to use playground equipment in a safe and fun fashion.
Treats strange animals and strange people in a proper way.
Demonstrates how to report accidents and illnesses.
Explains safety on the water, the school bus, and the family automobile.

Grade 3

Tells how to play safe in all seasons of the year.
Cites bicycle safety rules and how to maintain the bicycle in fine running condition.
Rides the bicycle skillfully and can demonstrate this at the school for others to see.
Describes eye, ear and face protection and shows personal responsibility for his own safety.
Explains fire prevention and fire safety in the home and school.

Grade 4

Shows how questionable water can be purified for drinking purposes.
Demonstrates elementary first aid practices.
Practices safety out-of-doors (insect bites, sunburn, poison ivy, etc.)
Is aware of accidents in the community and can tell how they might have been prevented.
Assists younger children in accident prevention.

Grade 5

Practices fire prevention at home and about the community.
Performs artificial respiration properly and explains water safety practices.
Exercises leadership in safety patrols and school safety councils.
Shows how to prevent eye, ear, and other injuries from accidents stemming from
    sports participation.

Grade 6

Performs first aid for minor injuries (cuts, burns, etc.)
Discriminates accurately between safe and unsafe medicines.
Describes personal safety at home (medicines, automobiles, rugs, stairways,
    electrical outlets, etc.)
Practices safety in recreational pursuits and in the choice of food products.
Investigates the several means of survival in a nuclear age.

MENTAL HEALTH

Grade 1

Knows a number of children and how to get along with them.
Develops new friends and new interests.
Shows feeling and consideration for others.
Enjoys caring for pets and discussing them.
Demonstrates ability to work by himself.
Seeks help when needed and knows why.
Controls emotions of fear and anger.

Grade 2

Has a sense of humor.
Shares experiences with others and willingly tries new things.
Accepts new responsibilities.
Demonstrates how to win and lose fairly, while having fun with others in a variety
    of situations.
Expresses feelings in an acceptable manner.
Overcomes difficulties and adjusts reasonably to disappointments.

Grade 3

Gains pleasure and satisfaction in helping others.
Works and plays to build self-control and self-reliance.
Develops new interests in hobbies, books, skills, etc.
Accepts others and makes new friendships in a wholesome way.
Expresses personal feelings through speech, play and dance.

Grade 4

Shows appropriate attitudes toward leadership and group participation.
Appraises personal capabilities and limitations.
Describes the variety of human emotions as they affect performance, personality
    and health in general.

Solves personal problems and shows how to live with handicaps.
Receptive to the suggestions of others and open-minded when dealing with others.

Grade 5

Contributes to group activity in school by exercising appropriate leadership and
fellowship.
Makes a number of plans and carries them out.
Registers pleasure in solving pertinent class and individual problems.
Describes both pleasant and unhappy attitudes and tells how to overcome worry.
Investigates the building of confidence and the reduction of tension through
successful accomplishments.
Is concerned for the feelings of others.
Obtains satisfaction from acceptable social behavior.

Grade 6

Portrays examples of the relationship of physical health to mental health.
Explains the meaning of recreation and how it along with rest contributes to mental
health.
Shares ideas and experiences with others and understands their inherent values.
Describes the nature of mental illness.
Exercises emotional control and self-confidence in difficult school and home
situations.
Identifies the relationship between the setting of personal goals and the attainment
of good mental health.

SEX AND FAMILY LIVING EDUCATION

Grade 1

Describes how a happy home life depends upon the contributions of each member
of the family.
Cooperates in the home, sharing work as well as fun.
Cares for the pets in the family or at school.
Accepts animals as part of family life.

Grade 2

Shows how several animals protect and feed their babies.
Recognizes that animals have babies like themselves.
Describes the many ways that happy families work and play together.
Names a variety of occasions when there are good times in a home and family.
Appreciates that boys and girls can play together, but that boys also play with boys,
and girls with girls.
Explains how the family prepares for, cares for, and loves the new baby.

Grade 3

Observes how parents make a home a pleasant place.
Describes elementary reproduction: all living things come from other living
things—illustrated by baby animals, plant life, and mothers and babies.
Shows how animals protect and feed babies in different ways.
Helps with family chores and the caring of younger family members.

Grade 4

Describes the unique contributions of men and women to society.
Explains how children inherit the way they look from mother and father.
Describes the growth of the human being in the body of the mother — where life
starts and develops.
Investigates the meaning of families as good neighbors.
Differentiates between the ovaries, testes, ovum, sperm, glands, hormones, etc.
Distinguishes inherited characteristics from characteristics not inherited.

Grade 5

Details the start of life and how body cells begin from a single cell, which divides
into two cells: terminology and structure.
Explains reproductive and growth process: egg cells, sperm cells, from egg to baby.
Describes elemental function of menstruation.
Investigates growth differences from ten to fourteen years of age: boy and girl
differences; more rapid maturation of girls.
Recognizes the contributions of both sexes to family life and society in general.

Grade 6

Describes the continuing process of physical growth and maturation toward
manhood and womanhood.
Explains how social, intellectual, and emotional growth are essential parts of the
maturation process.
Tells the several meanings of adolescence.
Describes puberty and is aware of the physical and mental occurrences which have a
bearing on peer group relationships.

ENVIRONMENTAL HEALTH

Grade 1

Contributes toward keeping the school, home, and neighborhood clean.
Explains the services performed by physicians, dentists, nurses and other selected
health personnel.
Describes how people are a part of the animal-plant world.

Grade 2

Relates how everyone is a member of the community.
Explains how items such as milk and water are kept clean, fresh and safe to drink.
Investigates how the community water supply is protected.
Tells how pets should be cared for to protect their health and the health of others.

Grade 3

Examines the problem of controlling insect pests and by what non-polluting means.
Shows how meat and other foods are handled in order to protect the purchaser.
Names public health functions and describes how many people help protect the
health of citizens: physician, dentist, hospital worker, automobile inspector,
barber, etc.

Grade 4

Indicates how health personnel work together to control the pollutants in the environment and the spread of disease: local government, professional personnel, and voluntary health workers.

Describes how water is made safe for swimming, for ice skating, and how it is purified for drinking.

Illustrates the duties of food inspectors.

Explains how playgrounds, parks and other recreational services help build health and maintain a healthful environment.

Grade 5

Explains the several roles of the voluntary health agency.

Describes how public health officials work with private citizens (even pupils) to control air, land, and water pollution.

Demonstrates how to purify water on a camping trip.

Cites the several important points associated with water fluoridation.

Investigates the problems associated with advancing technology while controlling thermal and nuclear pollution.

Grade 6

Relates school health service findings to the work of health care centers and other community agencies.

Interprets the hospital function as an essential service which is expensive, but worth the cost.

Explains rescue and ambulance services — a cooperative activity involving police, firemen, and hospitals.

Identifies local health leaders in the professions, business, public health, public works, planning, etc.

Evaluates land and water conservation practices in a community by relating this to environmental well-being.

Describes the several functions of the U.S. Environmental Protection Agency.

ALCOHOL, TOBACCO AND DRUGS

Grade 4

Describes beverages which contribute to growth.

Avoids coffee, tea and cola drinks and is aware of the reasons for this action.

Explains why smoking if started becomes habit-forming and is difficult to give up.

Describes inhalants and their effect on the body (glue sniffing, etc.)

Exercises precaution in taking any medicine without parental control and for prescription by a physician.

Investigates the life saving and beneficial uses of a number of drugs (aspirin, antibiotics, pain killers, etc.)

Grade 5

Describes in detail the several effects of tobacco smoking: minor effects: throat, appetite, tooth stain, bad breath, taste, smell, skin, etc.; major effects: heart, lungs, endurance, blood pressure, longevity, bronchitis, cancer, new births, etc.

Explains the relationship between smoking and athletic performance.

Investigates the wisdom of not starting to smoke, and how one lives with family and peers who smoke and yet remains a non-smoker.
Describes the negative effects of using barbiturates, amphetamines, hallucinogens and other mood modifying drugs.
Relates the several effects of alcoholic beverage to human problems: alcoholism, intoxication, etc.

Grade 6

Tells about the harmful effects of drinking alcohol — effects on digestion, circulation, nerves (thinking, acting, controlling), longevity, athletic performance, occupational performance.
Investigates alcoholism as a disease of the society and its culture.
Relates the use of alcohol in industry and medicine.
Investigates the difficulty of breaking the smoking habit.
Discusses the laws governing the sale of drugs.
Appreciates the need for discovering new drugs for the treatment of disease.

CONSUMER HEALTH

Grade 4

Relates how foods are purchased to provide well-balanced meals.
Describes the plight of the consumer and the need to understand the many health related products being sold.
Recognizes that everyone is a consumer of health products.
Reads newspaper and magazine articles relative to pure foods, proper labeling, food handling, and "truth in advertising."
Acknowledges that self-diagnosis and self-medication are poor practices, and that there is sometimes danger in using such items as dietary supplements, cosmetics and pep pills.

Grade 5

Cites scientific ways in which to purchase health items: consumer guides, medical-dental opinions, support from investigating agencies.
Relates the watchdog functions of agencies such as Food and Drug Administration, Federal Trade Commission, and the Post Office Department to fraudulent products.
Investigates how a careful consumer eventually helps to make a careful producer or manufacturer.
Discusses the special work of different kinds of doctors.
Relates misinformation and superstition to quackery and the resultant billion dollars a year loss to the unwise consumer.

Grade 6

Develops ways to evaluate advertised health products: sports equipment, pain-killers, dentifrices, cold tablets, "health" foods, vitamin pills, dietary substances.
Realizes that personal decision-making comes from adequate information and feelings.
Cites laws that exist to protect the consumer.
Examines media advertising, investigates FDA findings, and exercises caution in using new non-prescription items.

INDEX